The Essential Stratum Corneum

The Essential Stratum Corneum

Edited by

Ronald Marks FRCP FRCPath
Emeritus Professor of Dermatology, University of Wales College of Medicine, Skin Care Cardiff, Cardiff, UK

Jean-Luc Lévêque MD
L'Oréal Recherche, Clichy, France

Rainer Voegeli BSc
Pentapharm, Basel, Switzerland

MARTIN DUNITZ

First published in the United Kingdom in 2002
by Martin Dunitz Ltd, The Livery House, 7-9 Pratt Street, London NW1 0AE
Tel.: +44 (0) 20 74822202
Fax.: +44 (0) 20 72670159
E-mail: info@dunitz.co.uk
Website: http://www.dunitz.co.uk

A CIP record for this book is available from the British Library.

ISBN 1-84184-172-2

Distributed in the USA by
Fulfilment Center
Taylor & Francis
7625 Empire Drive
Florence, KY 41042, USA
Toll Free Tel.: +1 800 634 7064
E-mail: serve@routledge_ny.com

Distributed in Canada by
Taylor & Francis
74 Rolark Drive
Scarborough, Ontario M1R 4G2, Canada
Toll Free Tel.: +1 877 226 2237
E-mail: al_fran@istar.ca

Distributed in the rest of the world by
Thomson Publishing Services
Cheriton House
North Way
Andover, Hampshire SP10 5BE, UK
Tel.: +44 (0)1264 332424
E-mail: salesorder.tandf@thomsonpublishingservices.co.uk

Composition by Wearset Ltd, Boldon, Tyne and Wear
Printed and bound in Great Britain by Biddles Ltd, Guildford and King's Lynn.

Contents

Section II Pharmacology and percutaneous absorption

Section IV Clinical and cosmetic considerations

Contributors

SK Ahn
Department of Dermatology
Yonsei University Wonju College of Medicine
Wonju
Korea

K Alewaeters
Department of General and Biological Chemistry
Faculty for Physical Education and Physiotherapy
Vrije Universiteit Brussel
Brussels
Belgium

CE Allen
Department of Biomedical Sciences
CBD Porton Down
Salisbury
UK

M Andrian
L'Oréal Recherche
Aulnay-sous-Bois
France

Z Ashley
Department of Biomedical Sciences
CBD Porton Down
Salisbury
UK

C Baltenneck
L'Oréal Recherche
Aulnay-sous-Bois
France

AO Barel
Department of General and Biological Chemistry
Faculty for Physical Education and Physiotherapy
Vrije Universiteit Brussel
Brussels
Belgium

W Baschong
Ciba Specialty Chemicals
Basel
Switzerland

B Bautista
Unilever Research US
Edgewater NJ
USA

F Benech-Kieffer
L'Oréal Recherche
Aulnay-sous-Bois
France

D Bernard
L'Oréal Recherche
Clichy
France

D Black
CERPER
Hôtel Dieu St Jacques
Toulouse
France

U Bock
Head of Dermal Systems
Science Park Saar
Saarbrücken
Germany

ST Bradley
Department of Biomedical Sciences
CBD Porton Down
Salisbury
UK

I Brinkmann
Institut für Pharmazeutische Technologie
Technische Universität Braunschweig
Braunschweig
Germany

A Burgess
ICI Strategic Technology Group
Wilton
UK

A Casiraghi
Istituto di Chimica Farmaceutica e Tossicologica
Milan
Italy

C Caubet
L'Oréal Recherche
Clichy
France

GCh Charalambopoulou
National Center for Scientific Research 'Demokritos'
15310 Aghia Paraskevi Attikis
Greece

E Chatelain
Department of Biopharmacy
Spirig Pharma Ltd
Egerkingen
Switzerland

RP Chilcott
Department of Biomedical Sciences
CBD Porton Down
Salisbury
UK

EH Choi
Department of Dermatology
Yonsei University Wonju College of Medicine
Wonju
Korea

F Cilurzo
Istituto di Chimica Farmaceutica e Tossicologica
Milan
Italy

LI Ciortea
South Bank University
SEEIE
London
UK

P Clarys
Department of General and Biological Chemistry
Faculty for Physical Education and Physiotherapy
Vrije Universiteit Brussel
Brussels
Belgium

B Closs
SILAB
BP 213/19108
Brive Cedex
France

P Corcuff
L'Oréal Recherche
Aulnay-sous-Bois
France

CH Dalton
Department of Biomedical Sciences
CBD Porton Down
Salisbury
UK

G Daty
L'Oréal Recherche
Aulnay-sous-Bois
France

A Del Pozo
Dept Farmàcia I Tecnologia
Farmacèutica
Universitat de Barcelona
Barcelona
Spain

K De Paepe
Department of Toxicology
Vrije Universiteit Brussel
Brussels
Belgium

PJ Dooling
ICI Strategic Technology Group
Wilton
UK

F Dreher
L'Oréal Recherche
Aulnay-sous-Bois
France

PJ Dykes
Cutest Systems Ltd
Cardiff
UK

T Egelrud
Department of Dermatology
University Hospital Umeå
Sweden

AJ Emanuel
Department of Biomedical Sciences
CBD Porton Down
Salisbury
UK

KE Evans
ICI Strategic Technology Group
Wilton
UK

F Fiat
L'Oréal Recherche
Aulnay-sous-Bois
France

V Figueiredo
Institut für Spital-Pharmazie
Department of Dermatology
University Clinics
Kantonsspital Basel
Institute of Pharmaceutical Technology
University of Basel
Basel
Switzerland

D Födinger
Division of General Dermatology
University of Vienna
Vienna
Austria

E Fonseca
Universidad da Beira Interior
Covilha
Portugal

F Fouchard
L'Oréal Recherche
Aulnay-sous-Bois
France

HF Frasch
Health Effects Laboratory Division
National Institute for Occupational Safety and Health
Morgantown WV
USA

E Gabard
Iderma
Münchenstein/Basel
Switzerland

F Gafner
Pentipharm Ltd
Basel
Switzerland

Y Gall
CERPER
Hôtel Dieu St Jacques
Toulouse
France

J Gareiss
Nattermann Phospholipid GmbH
Cologne
Germany

P Garidel
Department of Physical Chemistry
Martin Luther University Halle-Wittenberg
Halle/Salle
Germany

M Ghyczy
Nattermann Phospholipid GmbH
Cologne
Germany

V Gillon
Laboratoires Sérobiologiques
Division de Cognis France
Pulnoy
France

F Girard
Laboratoire DERMASCAN
Villeurbanne
France

S Gottbrath
Institut für Pharmazeutische Technologie
Technische Universität Braunschweig
Braunschweig
Germany

M Guerrin
L'Oréal Recherche
Clichy
France

C Guinot
CERIES
Neuilly sur Seine
France

J Hadgraft
Skin and Membrane Transfer Research Centre
Medway Sciences
NRI University of Greenwich
Central Avenue
Chatham Maritime
UK

C Hadjur
L'Oréal Recherche
Aulnay-sous-Bois
France

M Haftek
Director of Research CNRS
Hospital E Herriot
Lyon
France

P Hallegot
L'Oréal Recherche
Aulnay-sous-Bois
France

E Haltner
Science Park Saar
Saarbrücken
Germany

CR Harding
Unilever Research
Colworth House
Bedford
UK

H Heise
Institute of Spectrochemistry and
Applied Spectroscopy
Dortmund
Germany

T Hirao
Shiseido Life Science Research center
2-12-1 Fukuura
Kanazawa-ku
Yokohama
Japan

SB Hoath
Skin Sciences Institute
Children's Hospital Research
Foundation
Cincinnati OH
USA

H Hönigsman
Division of Special and Environmental
Dermatology
University of Vienna
Vienna
Austria

JN Hughes
Department of Biomedical Sciences
CBD Porton Down
Salisbury
UK

D Hummel
Spirig Pharma Ltd
Egerkingen
Switzerland

SM Hwang
Department of Dermatology
Yonsei University Wonju College of
Medicine
Wonju
Korea

G Imanidis
Institute of Pharmaceutical Technology
University of Basel
Basel
Switzerland

RE Imhof
South Bank University
SEEIE
London
UK

E Jerschow
Chonnam National University
Medical School and Hospital
Kwangju
South Korea

C Jonak
University of Vienne
Vienna
Austria

H Jungmann
MBR Messtechnik GmbH
Gelsenkirchen
Germany

NK Kanellopoulos
National Center for Scientific Research
'Demokritos'
15310 Aghia Paraskevi Attikis
Greece

M Kietzmann
Institute for Pharmacology, Toxicology
and Pharmacy
Veterinary School of Hannover
Hannover
Germany

ES Kikkinides
Chemical Process Engineering
Research Institute
Center for Research and Technology
Hellas
Thermi-Thessaloniki
Greece

JY Kim
Chonnam National University
Medical School and Hospital
Kwangju
South Korea

MJ Kim
Department of Dermatology
Yonsei University Wonju College of
Medicine
Wonju
Korea

SJ Kim
Associate Professor
Department of Dermatology
Chonnam National University Medical
School & Hospital
Kwangju
South Korea

G Klosner
Division of Special and Environmental
Dermatology
University of Vienna
Vienna
Austria

C Kochhar
Institute of Pharmaceutical Technology
University of Basel
Basel
Switzerland

N Kuchina
Clinica Lenom
Rishon-Le-Zion
Israel

L Küpper
Institute of Spectrochemistry and
Applied Spectroscopy
Dortmund
Germany

C Kurdian
Laboratoire DERMASCAN
Villeurbanne
France

C Kuril
Institute of Pharmaceutical Technology
and Biopharmacetics
University of Vienna
Vienna
Austria

R Lambrecht
Department of General and Biological
Chemistry
Faculty for Physical Education and
Physiotherapy
Vrije Universiteit Brussel
Brussels
Belgium

P Lampen
Institute of Spectrochemistry
and Applied Spectroscopy
Dortmund
Germany

J Lasch
Department of Physical Chemistry
Medical Faculty
Martin Luther University Halle-
Wittenberg
Halle/Salle
Germany

J Latreille
CERIES
Neuilly sur Seine
France

DG Leahy
Skin Sciences Institute
Children's Hospital Research
Foundation
Cincinnati OH
USA

J Leclaire
L'Oréal Recherche
Aulnay-sous-Bois
France

C Leclerc
L'Oréal Recherche
Aulnay-sous-Bois
France

SH Lee
Department of Dermatology
Yonsei University College of Medicine
Seoul
Korea

I Le Fur
CERIES
Neuilly sur Seine
France

CY Lin
Institute of Clinical Pharmacy
College of Medicine
National Cheng Kung University
Tainan
Taiwan

YL Lo
Department of Pharmacy
Chia-Nam University of Pharmacy and
Science
Tainan
Taiwan

S Lopez
CERIES
Neuilly sur Seine
France

G Madry
L'Oréal Recherche
Aulnay-sous-Bois
France

S Maeder
Institute of Pharmaceutical Technology
University of Basel
Basel
Switzerland

PJ Matts
Procter & Gamble
Rusham Park Technical Centre
Egham
UK

F McGlone
Unilever Research
Port Sunlight
Bebington
UK

B Méhul
L'Oréal Recherche
Clichy
France

H Meldrum
Unilever Research
Colworth House
Bedford
UK

D Metze
Department of Dermatology
University of Münster
Münster
Germany

P Minghetti
Istituto di Chimica Farmaceutica e
Tossicologica
Milan
Italy

A-M Mirondo
L'Oréal Recherche
Aulnay-sous-Bois
France

W Mok
Unilever Research US
Edgewater NJ
USA

L Montanari
Istituto di Chimica Farmaceutica e
Tossicologica
Milan
Italy

A Moore
Unilever Research
Colworth House
Bedford
UK

F Morizot
CERIES
Neuilly sur Seine
France

CC Müller-Goymann
Institut für Pharmazeutische
Technologie
Technische Universität Braunschweig
Braunschweig
Germany

I Nicander
Department of Dermatology
Huddinge University Hospital
Huddinge
Sweden

L Norlén
Department of Physics
University of Geneva
GAP-Biomedical
Geneva
Switzerland

S Ollmar
Division of Medical Engineering
Karolinska Institutet Novum
Huddinge
Sweden

WS Park
Skin Research Institute
Pacific R&D Center
Yongin
Korea

JA Parkes
Department of Biomedical Sciences
CBD Porton Down
Salisbury
UK

A Patel
Department of Biomedical Sciences
CBD Porton Down
Salisbury
UK

C Patouillet
L'Oréal Recherche
Aulnay-sous-Bois
France

G Pauly
Laboratoires Sérobiologiques
Division de Cognis France
Pulnoy
France

D Pele
L'Oréal Recherche
Aulnay-sous-Bois
France

G Perie
Laboratoires Sérobiologiques
Division de Cognis France
Pulnoy
France

W Pittermann
Henkel KGaA
Düsseldorf
Germany

M Randeau
Laboratoire DERMASCAN
Villeurbanne
France

I Rantanen
Institute of Dentistry
University of Turku
Turku
Finland

X Ren
Exeter University
Exeter
UK

JS Rogers
Unilever Research
Colworth House
Bedford
UK

V Rogiers
Department of Toxicology
Vrije Universiteit Brussel
Brussels
Belgium

M Rohr
Director of Research
Institute Dr. Schrader
Holzminden
Germany

D Roseeuw
Department of Toxicology
Vrije Universiteit Brussel
Brussels
Belgium

J Sarramagnan
South Bank University
SEEIE
London
UK

G Schicksnus
Institut für Pharmazeutische
Technologie
Technische Universität Braunschweig
Braunschweig
Germany

R Schmidt
L'Oréal Recherche
Clichy
France

T Schmidt
Mepha Pharma
Aesch
Switzerland

S Schmitz
Science Park Saar
Saarbrücken
Germany

S Schnebert
LVMH
Branche Parfums & Cosmétiques
St Jean de Braye
France

A Schrader
Institute Dr. Schrader
Holzminden
Germany

A Scott
Unilever Research
Port Sunlight
Bebington
UK

G Serre
L'Oréal Recherche
Clichy
France

HM Sheu
Department of Dermatology
College of Medicine
National Cheng-Kung University
Hospital
Tainan
Taiwan

M Simon
Centre de Physiopathologie de
Toulouse-Purpan
Faculté de Médecine
Toulouse
France

JT Simonnet
L'Oréal Recherche
Chevilly-Larue
France

A Sirvent
Scientific Communication Manager
Laboratoire DERMASCAN
Villeurbanne
France

CW Smith
Exeter University
Exeter
UK

EW Smith
Ohio Northern University
College of Pharmacy
Ada, OH
USA

E Söderling
Institute of Dentistry
University of Turku
Turku
Finland

ED Son
Skin Research Institute
Pacific R&D Center
Yongin
Korea

KL Stefanopoulos
National Center for Scientific Research
'Demokritos'
15310 Aghia Paraskevi Attikis
Greece

ThA Steriotis
National Center for Scientific Research
'Demokritos'
15310 Aghia Paraskevi Attikis
Greece

AK Stubos
National Center for Scientific Research
'Demokritos'
15310 Aghia Paraskevi Attikis
Greece

K Subramanyan
Unilever Research US
Edgewater NJ
USA

C Surber
Institut für Spital-Pharmazie
Department of Dermatology
University Clinics
Kantonsspital Basel
Institute of Pharmaceutical Technology
University of Basel
Basel
Switzerland

H Tagami
Department of Dermatology
Tohoku University School of Medicine
1-1 Seiryo-machi
Aoba-ku
Sendai
Japan

M Takahashi
Shiseido Customer Satisfaction
Research Center
2-3-1 Hayabuchi
Tsuzuki-ku
Yokohama
Japan

T Tassopoulos
Institut für Spital-Pharmazie
Department of Dermatology
University Clinics
Kantonsspital Basel
Institute of Pharmaceutical Technology
University of Basel
Basel
Switzerland

JC Tsai
Institute of Clinical Pharmacy
College of Medicine
National Cheng Kung University
Tainan
Taiwan

E Tschachler
CERIES
Neuilly sur Seine
France
and Department of Dermatology
University of Vienna
Vienna
Austria

G Tolia
University of Cincinnati College of
Pharmacy
Cincinnati OH
USA

L Tosi
Istituto di Chimica Farmaceutica e
Tossicologica
Milan
Italy

H Traupe
Department of Dermatology
University of Münster
Münster
Germany

F Trautinger
Division of Special and Environmental Dermatology
University of Vienna
Vienna
Austria

C Valenta
Institute of Pharmaceutical Technology and Biopharmacetics
University of Vienna
Vienna
Austria

E Vanpee
Department of Toxicology
Vrije Universiteit Brussel
Brussels
Belgium

MP Verdier
L'Oréal Recherche
Aulnay-sous-Bois
France

A Vexler
Radiobiology and Biotechnology Laboratory
Hadassah University Hospital
Hadassah
Israel

M Visscher
Children's Hospital Medical Center
Cincinnati OH
USA

W Voss
Dermatest GmbH
Münster
Germany

RR Wickett
University of Cincinnati College of Pharmacy
Cincinnati OH
USA

N Widler
Pentapharm Ltd
Basel
Switzerland

JW Wiechers
Uniqema
Gouda
The Netherlands

A Winkler
Institut für Pharmazeutische Technologie
Technische Universität Braunschweig
Braunschweig
Germany

YH Won
Chonnam National University
Medical School and Hospital
Kwangju
South Korea

SJ Yun
Chonnam National University
Medical School and Hospital
Kwangju
South Korea

N Zahlan
ICI Strategic Technology Group
Wilton
UK

S Zellmer
Department of Physical Chemistry
Medical Faculty
Martin Luther University Halle-Wittenberg
Halle/Salle
Germany

Introduction

The stratum corneum appears thin and wispy and completely insignificant in routine formalin fixed and paraffin embedded histological sections. It was only when new techniques arrived on the scene allowing a glimpse into structure as it exists in life that some appreciation of its importance developed. The dissemination of knowledge about new techniques greatly assists the development of a discipline and is an important component of a symposium such as the one recorded here.

Currently stratum corneum research is undertaken by many disciplines including dermatologists, cosmetic scientists, physiologists, neonatologists, pharmaceutical scientists and bioengineers. The reason for the wide range of disciplines involved is compounded from the intrinsic interest of a complexly organised anucleate 15 μM thick structure that is vital to health and the practical problems associated with cosmesis and pharmacology of skin. The growing popularity of the subject is due to an increasing realization that the stratum corneum is the major barrier to all environmental insults whether these are climatic, toxic from xenobiotics or microbial. The health and well being of this structure also serves vital social and cultural functions as it is a major determinant of our appearance and of central interest to the cosmetic industry.

This publication stems from the third international symposium on the stratum corneum held in Basel in September 2001. The symposium consisted of 11 invited keynote lectures, 25 other oral presentations and 51 posters and was attended by a total of 260 participants. Any heterogeneity in the length of the contributions or in their format is due to the differing types of presentation, although these have now also been revised, in some cases extensively.

We are extremely grateful to the authors for responding so quickly to the request to submit manuscripts from their presentations and to the publishers for their forbearance and help at every turn. We are also very grateful to Pentapharm for all the practicalities in organising the symposium and their generous financial assistance as well as to L'Oréal for their generosity providing an educational grant for the publication of the proceedings.

Ronald Marks
Jean-Luc Lévêque
Rainer Voegeli

Section I
Stratum corneum anatomy and physiology

1
Ultrastructural aspects of the stratum corneum

M Haftek

Introduction

Stratum corneum (SC) is the final product of epidermal differentiation. In this perpetual process, keratinocytes divide in the deepest epidermal layers and their proliferation compensates, under normal conditions, for the loss of cornified cells at the skin surface. It is just before they desquame that keratinocytes, at the most advanced stage of their terminal differentiation, form a highly resistant, compact, and anucleated horny layer. The layer, which provides an essential attribute of cutaneous integument – a relative impermeability to water and water-compatible substances. This so-called 'occlusive barrier function' depends on the physical integrity of the SC and the adequate composition of its constituents.

As all the components of the SC, or at least their precursors, must be synthesized in the viable cell layers, the entire chain of subtle modifications occurring within the horny layer, and leading to the 'insensible' shedding of most superficial cells, appears to be pre-programmed. However, the epidermis is an interactive tissue, well adapted to the fluctuating environmental conditions, and a certain degree of feedback is also possible, in which the quality of the barrier influences keratinocyte proliferation and synthesis.[1] Nevertheless, what really happens in the horny layer is not easy to investigate. Besides biochemical analyses of shed or stripped cells vs entire isolated SC, most of the evidence could be provided by morphological studies, especially those combined with cytochemistry and performed in experimental settings allowing for targeted modifications of epidermal/SC homeostasis.[2–6]

Methods of investigation at the ultrastructural level

Among technical approaches allowing ultrastructural studies of the SC, schematically indicated in Figure 1.1, transmission electron microscopy (EM) is most frequently used.[7] This technique requires initial tissue

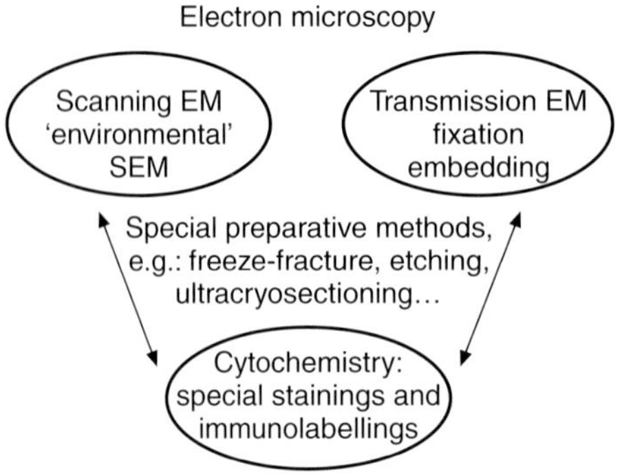

Figure 1.1
Main technical approaches in the ultrastructural studies.

fixation, typically aldehydic, and either embedding in polymerizable resins or cryovitrification allowing ultracryosectioning. Ultrathin tissue sections (60–90 nm thick), harvested on metal grids, may then be labelled and stained using various immuno- and cytochemical methods. In some instances, pre-embedding staining may be chosen, but this approach is usually disadvantaged by poor penetration of the reactants into the whole mount. The sections are counterstained with heavy metal salts and observed, in a microscope emitting an electron beam, as shades projected on to a fluorescent screen. Interpretation of the obtained images requires certain skills, since a three-dimensional situation should be deduced from a series of two-dimensional pictures. However, the host of information possible to retrieve using transmission EM is much larger than that obtainable with scanning EM, mainly because the latter approach visualizes only the surface of a studied sample and usually does not allow for very high resolutions.

Standard EM methods require complete dehydration of a studied tissue, because the observation takes place in the vacuum to avoid interactions of electron beam with gas particles. This may represent a handicap, since substitution of water with solvents may generate some artefacts. In standard techniques, the solution is a rapid and thorough fixation, which is most frequently incompatible with immunocytochemistry. However, there exist a couple of alternative methods allowing partial circumvention of the inconvenience. Samples may be quick-frozen, e.g. in liquid propane, and vitrified water (in an amorphous, non-crystalline state) can be sublimated and substituted with acrylic resins, under vacuum and at low temperature. For scanning EM, the use of a holder cooled with liquid nitrogen facilitates observation of frozen samples and so-called 'environmental' microscopes work with partial vacuum only, which allows for a brief visualization of low-hydrated samples, such as SC. In the latter cases, however, the ransom is a low energy of the electron beam being used and, therefore, the need to work at lower magnifications.

Supplementary information on cell structure and physical properties may be gained using such preparative techniques as freeze-fracture and etching. Frozen tissue, when broken at low temperature, would split mostly along specific interfaces, such as lipid bilayers of the cell membranes. In some instances, a controlled sublimation of water from the surface of the sample leads to exposure of the fractured cell's interior. A fine metallic cast of the exposed fracture plane is obtained by shadowing with platinum atoms projected at a sharp angle. When observed in transmission EM, such replicas give an impression of relief. In the SC, analysis of the actual path of splitting gives a valuable insight into the composition and structure of the extracellular spaces.[8]

An additional qualitative dimension is achieved by EM approaches such as spectral X-ray analysis, providing element composition of chosen structures, and X-ray diffraction studies, aimed at pinpointing the fine molecular arrangements, e.g. within crystalline-like spreads of the SC intercorneocyte lipids.

So far, however, the major sources of information on the SC structure and evolution, from its formation to desquamation, were special staining techniques combined with transmission EM. Cytochemistry and immunocytochemistry allow for detection and precise localization of such crucial components as enzymes and structural proteins. The use of modern acrylic resins, which are slightly hydrophilic and sufficiently fluid at low temperatures to allow freeze-substitution, is essential in post-embedding labellings. In such an approach, the targets of cytochemical reaction are readily accessible at the surface of ultrathin sections. This avoids the technical problems of pre-embedding labelling related to difficulties of a label penetration into whole tissue blocks. A range of electron-dense labels may be used, e.g. peroxidase or ferritin, with actual preference for corpuscular markers such as colloidal gold, which is available in a large variety of sizes compatible with multiple labellings. Tissue specimens may also be impregnated with ruthenium tetroxide, a highly oxidative reagent substituted for osmium tetroxide (RuO_4), used for tissue post-fixation in standard EM techniques. Ruthenium deposits, which are visible in EM, localize preferentially to water-compatible structural elements, such as proteins and polar parts of lipid molecules. This particularity has been used for the demonstration of lipid multilayers in the extracellular spaces of SC. Indeed, these intercorneocyte regions appear 'empty' on standard EM examination and only ruthenium staining reveals superimposed lipid layers, in which hydrophobic parts remain unaffected by RuO_4 and, thus, are electron-lucid.[9] Unfortunately, the use of both ruthenium staining and immunolabelling for simultaneous visualization of lipids and proteinic antigens proves impossible, because RuO_4 treatment suppresses immunoreactivity.[6]

Structural components of the SC and their function

In the early 1980s, Elias et al launched the 'brick and mortar' model of the SC.[10] According to his vision, the cellular 'bricks' are sealed and kept together by the lipidic 'mortar'. Although several aspects of SC morphology and function can be explained on the basis of the 'brick and mortar' theory, one major difference has been noted concerning SC cohesion and desquamation, namely that the principal factors responsible for maintaining attachment between corneocytes are not lipids but desmosomes.[11] Previously believed to be only rudimentary, non-functional elements persisting in the SC, these junctions appear to be crucial for the structural integrity of the SC barrier. Their progressive degradation leads to the liberation of cornified cells at the skin surface.[12]

Keratinocytes

The morphology of keratinocytes changes radically at the limit between the viable epidermis and the SC (Figure 1.2). All the intracytoplasmic

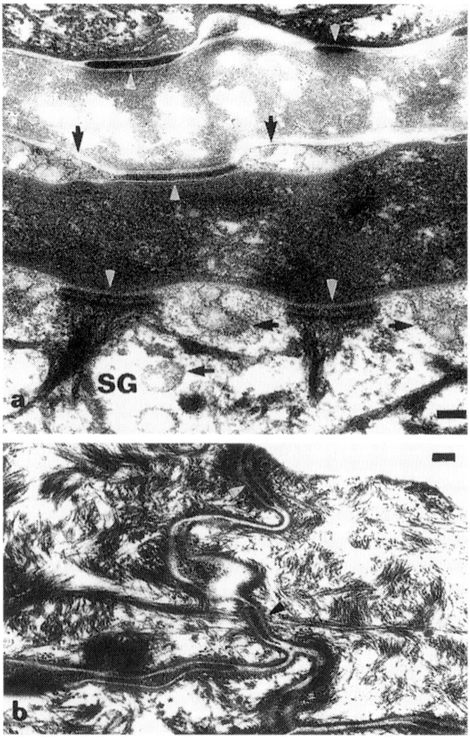

Figure 1.2

Standard transmission EM pictures of normal human SC. (a) At the limit with the underlying stratum granulosum (SG), lamellar bodies (arrows) are secreted into the interkeratinocyte spaces. Their contents may still be visualized in the lower SC, close to corneodesmosomes (arrowheads). Note that formation of corneocytes occurs very rapidly, most often without intermediate stages being observed, and it is associated with homogenization of the cell contents. (b) In the upper SC, biochemical processing of the amorphous material embedding keratin fibres makes cytoskeletal bundles reappear. The latter remain inserted into the junctional plaques (arrowhead) and are partially trapped at the corneocyte periphery in cornified envelopes. Bars = 100 nm.

organelles, including the nucleus, being rapidly degraded, the contents of the first corneocytes consist of keratin fibres embedded in an amorphous substance. The latter is issued largely from the transformation of profilaggrin, deposited in keratohyalin granules, to filaggrin.[13] The keratin cytoskeleton resists the proteolysis and intermediate filament bundles can be observed once again in the upper corneocytes, after further partial degradation of the amorphous matrix. The fact that some keratin bundles remain attached to the cell–cell junctions may testify to the mechanical functionality of such complexes, persisting in the SC and contributing to the tissue cohesion (Figure 1.2b).

The SC desmosomes differ morphologically from those present in the viable parts of the epidermis and are called corneodesmosomes. At least one new protein synthesized in the granular layer keratinocytes, corneodesmosin, becomes incorporated into the extracellular portion of these junctions (Figure 1.3).[14] Recent experimental evidence suggests an auxiliary cohesive function of corneodesmosin; however, its possible protective role against proteolysis of the principal transmembrane desmosomal cadherins cannot be excluded and remains an attractive idea.[15–17] Although corneodesmosomes look dense and homogeneous on standard EM, their striated nature, characteristic of regular desmosomes, can be revealed with a mild ruthenium staining (Figure 1.4). As RuO_4

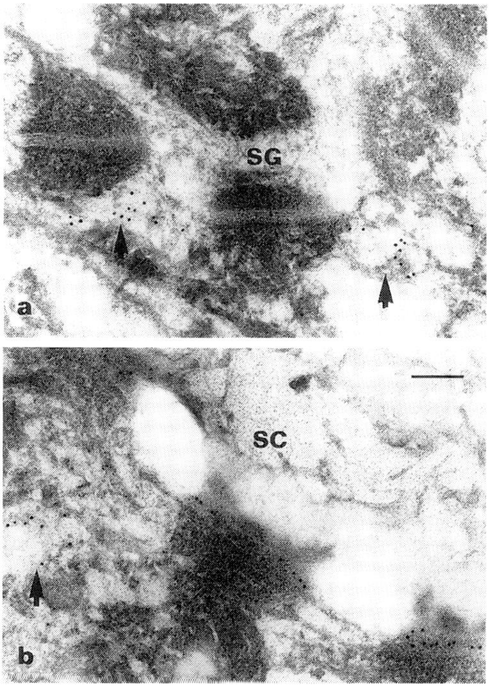

Figure 1.3

Immunogold labelling of ultrathin sections of normal human skin embedded in acrylic resin reveals the ultrastructural localization of corneodesmosin. The protein is secreted through keratinosomes (arrows) by the stratum granulosum (SG) keratinocytes (a). At the interface with the SC, the antigen becomes incorporated into the extracellular parts of desmosomes, during reorganization of these junctions into corneodesmosomes (b). Bar = 100 nm.

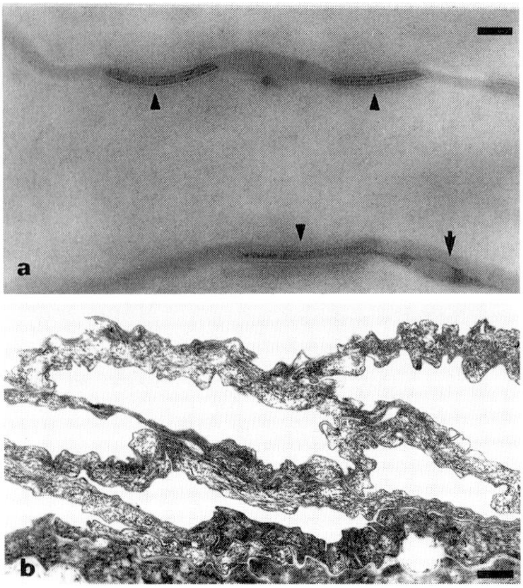

Figure 1.4

Corneodesmosomes represent hydrophilic spots in mostly hydrophobic SC interstices. (a) Ruthenium tetroxide, which poorly penetrates into the SC compactum, primarily stains the extracellular portions of corneodesmosomes (arrowheads) and the hydrophilic lacunae sometimes associated with the junctions (arrow). Bar = 100 nm. (b) 'Basket-weave' pattern of SC disjunctum induced by exposure to propylene glycol. Note the disappearance of the central, most accessible corneodesmosomes. Bar = 1 µm.

penetrates preferentially into corneodesmosomes, it reveals the hydrophilic nature of these junctions, surrounded by mostly hydrophobic extracellular substance.[6]

During their evolution towards corneocytes, the shape of keratinocytes changes dramatically. The cells flatten considerably and reduce in volume, whereas excess plasma membrane folds at the cell periphery creating indentations. Corneodesmosomes present in such indentations are less susceptible to degradation than ones spread over the relatively flat upper and lower sides of the corneocyte disk. In the lower SC, called stratum corneum compactum, corneocytes are tightly superimposed and attached by several corneodesmosomes. Further towards the SC surface, corneodesmosomes situated in the central parts of corneocyte disks start to disappear rapidly and the cells detach at these regions, forming a much looser SC structure – the SC disjunctum. A commonly observed 'basket-weave' pattern of the SC histology results from the artefactual expansion of the SC disjunctum (Figure 1.4b). Corneocyte desquamation follows the quasi-complete degradation of cell–cell junctions, including the lateral corneodesmosomes. Environmental conditions, and particularly hydration-related changes of the enzymatic activity and corneocyte volume, appear to be important regulators of desquamation.

Besides corneodesmosomes, incomplete strands of another type of cell–cell junction, the tight junction, could be observed with freeze-fracture in some cases of pathological SC. This type of linear junction, usually expressed in simple epithelia and responsible for sealing the extracellular compartments, could be important for the barrier function of the SC. Although proteins characteristic of tight junctions could be demonstrated in the normal epidermis, the structures themselves are only rudimentary and apparently not functional.[18]

Physical strength of the cellular 'bricks' and, thus, of the SC as a whole is considerably increased thanks to the deposition of the cross-linked cornified envelope. Several specific precursors of this highly resistant structure, e.g. involucrin, loricrin, small proline-rich proteins, are synthesized by keratinocytes and transformed by transglutaminase 1 at the cell periphery. In the process of cornified envelope formation, many other proteins present in this location get trapped and become definitively immobilized. Notably, this is the fate of keratins and desmosomal elements.[19] During corneocyte formation, the plasma membrane of viable cells is replaced by a ceramide monolayer, covalently bound to the underlying cornified envelope.[20] This lipid envelope functions as a template for accumulating extracellular lipid layers.

Extracellular substance

The extracellular compartment of the SC plays a key role both in the barrier function and desquamation. All the components of the extracellular substance present in the SC are produced by keratinocytes from the viable epidermal layers, essentially in the stratum granulosum. These products, rich in lipids but also containing various enzymes, are delivered by keratinosomes to the interface between the granular layer and the SC (Figures 2a and 3a). The vesicular structures that fuse with the apical membrane of granular keratinocytes often contain well-visualized, pre-formed lipid lamellae and, therefore, are also called lamellar bodies.

The barrier function of the SC and a relative water impermeability of this epidermal layer depend principally on the composition and the unique structural properties of the lipidic 'mortar'.[2,21] In contrast to the lower epidermis, where the production of phospholipids necessary for the constitution of cell membranes predominates, the lipids found in the SC are principally ceramides, free fatty acids, cholesterol, and cholesterol-3-sulphate. Lipid molecules belonging to these classes, each endowed with different physical properties, spontaneously constitute oriented layers, in which polar 'heads' and hydrophobic 'tails' segregate separately and alternate in a particular pattern.[22,23] Changes in spacing between the lipid sheets, visible with ruthenium staining as a succession of broad and narrow electron-lucent regions, testify to the evolution of the lipid sheet composition and suggest variations in functional properties.

Hydrolytic enzymes, which are also secreted at the base of SC, take an active part in remodelling the intercorneocyte spaces.[24] As they start to process their substrates, i.e. lipids, proteins and sugars, the molecular organization of the extracellular domains changes accordingly. Deglycosylation of sphingomyelin and of glucosylceramides is an important step in maturation of the SC lipids. The resulting ceramides, particularly of type 1, are essential for an efficient molecular riveting of the lipid bilayers and their occlusive barrier function.[23] In the upper layers of the SC, continuous modification of the lipid bilayers by a variety of lipases induces progressive loss of cohesion between the molecular strata. This, in turn, further favours the accessibility of substrates to specific hydrolases. The apparition of free fatty acids, the final product of lipid degradation, influences the SC pH and constitutes one of the regulatory factors of enzymatic activity.[25] Proteases, such as SC tryptic and chymotryptic enzymes or desquamin, are involved in the breakdown of the cell–cell junction proteins, leading to desquamation.[12,16,26–29]

Surface glycoproteins may be involved in the modulation of corneocyte interactions, as are the glycosylated extracellular portions of desmosomal cadherins involved in keratinocyte cohesion.[30] Indeed, pre-treatment with glycosidases appears to be prerequisite to desquamation, since it improves the corneodesmosome accessibility to proteases.[31]

The importance of various structural elements of the occlusive barrier and their modulating enzymes is highlighted by well-documented examples from human pathology and has often been confirmed experimentally (Table 1.1).[4,32–39]

Process of self-organization of components in the extracellular spaces of stratum corneum and desquamation of corneocytes

As mentioned previously, all the ingredients necessary for constitution of a properly functioning SC are prepared in the viable epidermal layers and delivered either to the cellular 'bricks' or to the extracellular 'mortar' at the moment of transition. What happens later on depends on this preprogramming and on the influence of environmental factors, because corneocytes themselves are no longer viable. Biochemical, cytochemical and X-ray diffraction analyses supply precise information on the exact composition of each SC compartment. It is, however, the privilege of morphological studies to put together the elements of the puzzle and to figure out, based on the structural and analytical data, how the SC components actually interact and cooperate to produce a constantly renewed occlusive barrier.

A closer look at the SC structure, following experimental modifications of the skin surface or in defined genodermatoses, reveals morphological evidence of progressive reorganization of the SC intercellular spaces.[4,6,38]

Using a short-term, ex vivo incubation system, we have followed the ultrastructural changes induced in the SC by simple occlusion or by con-

Table 1 Hydrolytic enzymes in the SC interstices.

Enzyme	Substrate: performed conversion	Functional modulation or pathology associated with insufficiency
Lipases		
acid lipase phospholipases A_2 (PLA_2) triacylgycerol lipase	triglycerides and phospholipids: => into free fatty acids	experimental inhibition of PLA_2 induces premature degradation of corneodesmosomes[25]
Sulphatases		
steroid sulphatase	cholesterol sulphate (ChS): => into cholesterol	X-linked ichthyosis: ChS inhibits SCCE, SCTE, TG1...[32,33]
Glycosidases	sugar groups on glycoproteins	
β-glucocerebrosidase	glucosylceramides:	Gaucher's disease, type 2:[35]
Ceramidases	=> into ceramides	impaired SC barrier
acid sphingomyelinase	sphingomyelin:	Niemann–Pick disease, subtype:[34]
Proteases		
SC chymotryptic enzyme (SCCE) SC tryptic enzyme (SCTE) desquamin	corneodesmosin, desmoglein 1 and other desmosomal cadherins: => into peptides	experimental inhibition of SCCE slows down desquamation;[27] accumulation of squames in case of mutation of a natural inhibitor – Netherton syndrome[36]

tact with a small-sized polar solvent, propylene glycol (Figure 1.5).[6] Our observations, using transmission EM and ruthenium or osmium tetroxide post-fixation, indicate that once the contents of keratinosomes are delivered to the intercellular space, spontaneous organization of the SC lipids in lamellar multilayers leads to partition of the extracellular compartment into larger hydrophobic and discrete hydrophilic domains. Such vesicular and composite non-hydrophobic domains were also noticed by other researchers using different experimental settings and visualization methods but were interpreted differently.[5,8,40] Formation of the lipid sheets and their progressive organization coincide with lateral displacements of hydrophilic lacunae towards corneodesmosomes, which represent the immobile hydrophilic elements in the extracellular spaces (see also Figure 1.4a). As hydrophilia is compatible with proteinic contents, such movements may be involved in the delivery of proteolytic enzymes to intercellular junctions. Interestingly, SCCE could be immunolocalized precisely in the vicinity of corneodesmosomes.[26] Fluidity of such a reorganization/displacement process is significantly enhanced by SC hydration, since, in the occluded skin, most of the hydrophilic domains were found to be in contact with the extracellular portions of corneodesmosomes.

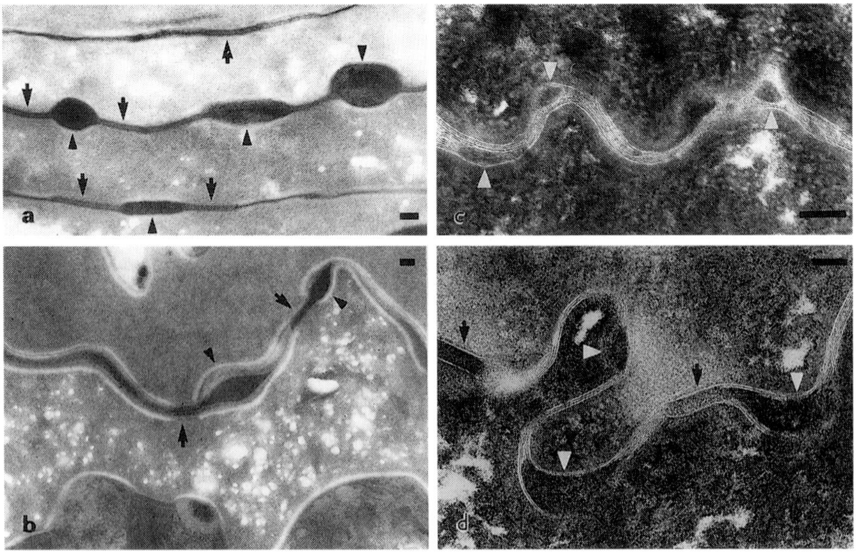

Figure 1.5

Lacunar domains in the intercorneocyte spaces of a normal human SC compactum stained with osmium (a,b) and ruthenium tetroxide (c,d). In non-occluded skin (a,c), the hydrophilic lacunae (arrowheads) remain fragmented and display composite contents. After occlusion (b,d), the hydrophilic elements are more apparent, homogenous, and are more frequently found in the immediate vicinity of corneodesmosomes (arrows). Bar = 100 nm.

This fits nicely with the fact that well-hydrated SC is characterized by an orderly desquamation.

The above-described ultrastructural observations are not contradictory with Norlén's model of the single gel phase of the intercellular barrier lipids.[41] The model predicts the most physically 'advantageous' organization of the lipid lamellae in a continuous spread, with no mosaic domains, and explains functional and morphological variations within the barrier lipids with changing molecular mobility and conformation of various lipid species. Although the seamless arrangement of carbohydrate chains according to the single-gel-phase model seems to be, indeed, optimal for the barrier lipid structure and function at the molecular level, the microscopic evidence of non-lipidic compartments in the SC interstices appears to be equally important for explanation of the 'programmed' evolution of this non-viable epidermal layer towards 'insensible' desquamation.

References

1. Proksch E, Holleran WM, Menon GK et al. Barrier function regulates epidermal lipid and DNA synthesis. Br J Dermatol 1993; 128:473–82.
2. Elias PM, Menon GK. Structural and lipid biochemical correlates of the epidermal permeability barrier. Adv Lipid Res 1991; 24:1–26.
3. Chapman SJ, Walsh A, Jackson SM et al. Lipids, proteins and corneocyte adhesion. Arch Dermatol Res 1991; 283:167–73.
4. Menon G, Ghadially R. Morphology of lipid alterations in the epidermis: a review. Microsc Res Tech 1997; 37:180–92.
5. Menon GK, Elias PM. Morphologic basis for a pore-pathway in mammalian stratum corneum. Skin Pharmacol 1997; 10:235–46.
6. Haftek M, Teillon MH, Schmitt D. Stratum corneum, corneodesmosomes, and ex vivo percutaneous penetration. Microsc Res Tech 1998; 43:1–8.
7. Haftek M. Immunoelectron microscopy. In: Kanitakis J, Vasilieva S, Woodley D, eds. *Diagnostic Immunohistochemistry of the Skin.* London: Chapman & Hall Medical 1998:19–28.
8. Van Hal DA, Jeremiasse E, Junginger HE et al. Structure of fully hydrated human stratum corneum: a freeze-fracture electron microscopy study. J Invest Dermatol 1996; 106:89–95.
9. Madison KC, Swartzendruber DC, Wertz PW et al. Presence of intact intercellular lamellae in the upper layers of the stratum corneum. J Invest Dermatol 1987; 88:714–18.
10. Elias PM, Grayson S, Lampe MA et al. The intercorneocyte space. In: Marks R, Plewig G, eds. *Stratum Corneum.* Berlin: Springer-Verlag 1983:53–67.
11. Chapman SJ, Walsh A. Desmosomes, corneosomes and desquamation. Arch Dermatol Res 1990; 282:304–10.
12. Egelrud T, Lundström A. The dependence of detergent-induced cell dissociation in non-palmoplantar stratum corneum on endogenous proteolysis. J Invest Dermatol 1990; 95:456–9.

13. Simon M, Sebbag M, Haftek M et al. Monoclonal antibodies to human epidermal filaggrin, some not recognizing profilaggrin. J Invest Dermatol 1995; 105:432–7.

14. Serre G, Mils V, Haftek M et al. Identification of late differentiation antigens of human cornified epithelia, expressed in re-organized desmosomes and bound to cross-linked envelope. J Invest Dermatol 1991; 97:1061–72.

15. Jonca N, Guerrin M, Hadjiolova K et al. Corneodesmosin, a component of epidermal corneocyte desmosomes, displays homophilic adhesive properties (paper in press). J Biol Chem 2002; 217:5024–9.

16. Lundström A, Serre G, Haftek M et al. Evidence for a role of G 36-19, a protein which may serve to modify desmosomes during cornification, in stratum corneum cell cohesion and desquamation. Arch Dermatol Res 1994; 286:369–75.

17. Haftek M, Simon M, Kanitakis J et al. Corneodesmosin is essential for keratinized epithelia and persists until desquamation occurs in both normal and pathological stratum corneum. Br J Dermatol 1997; 137:864–73.

18. Pummi K, Malminen M, Aho H et al. Epidermal tight junctions: ZO-1 and occludin are expressed in mature, developing, and affected skin and in vitro differentiating keratinocytes. J Invest Dermatol 2001; 117:1050–8.

19. Haftek M, Serre G, Mils V et al. Immunocytochemical evidence of the possible role of keratinocyte cross-linked envelopes in stratum corneum cohesion. J Histochem Cytochem 1991; 39:1531–8.

20. Swartzendruber DC, Wertz PW, Madison KC et al. Evidence that the corneocyte has a chemically bound lipid envelope. J Invest Dermatol 1987; 88:709–13.

21. Garson JC, Doucet J, Levèque JL et al. Oriented structure in human stratum corneum revealed by X-ray diffraction. J Invest Dermatol 1991; 96:43–9.

22. Schwartzendruber DC, Wertz PW, Kitko DJ et al. Molecular models of the intercellular lipid lamellae in mammalian stratum corneum. J Invest Dermatol 1989; 92:251–7.

23. Bouwstra JA, Gooris GS, Dubbelbelaar FER et al. Role of ceramide 1 in the molecular organisation of the stratum corneum lipids. J Lipid Res 1998; 39:186–96.

24. Menon GK, Ghadially R, Williams ML et al. Lamellar bodies as delivery systems of hydrolytic enzymes: implications for normal and abnormal desquamation. Br J Dermatol 1992; 126:337–45.

25. Fluhr JW, Kao J, Jain M et al. Generation of free fatty acids from phospholipids regulates stratum corneum acidification and integrity. J Invest Dermatol 2001; 117:44–51.

26. Sondell B, Thornell LE, Egelrud T. Evidence that stratum corneum chymotryptic enzyme is transported to the stratum corneum extracellular space via lamellar bodies. J Invest Dermatol 1995; 104:819–23.

27. Franzke CW, Baici A, Bartels J et al. Antileukoprotease inhibits stratum corneum chymotryptic enzyme. Evidence for a regulative function in desquamation. J Biol Chem 1996; 271: 21886–90.

28. Ekholm IE, Brattsand M, Egelrud T. Stratum corneum tryptic enzyme in normal epidermis: a missing link in the desquamation process? J Invest Dermatol 2000; 114:56–63.

29. Brysk MM, Bell T, Brysk H et al. Enzymatic activity of desquamin. Exp Cell Res 1994; 214:22–6.

30. Brysk MM, Rajaraman S, Penn P et al. Glycoproteins modulate

adhesion in terminally differentiated keratinocytes. Cell Tissue Res 1988; 253:657–63.

31. Walsh A, Chapman SJ. Sugars protect desmosome and corneosome glycoproteins from proteolysis. Arch Dermatol Res 1991; 283:174–9.
32. Nemes Z, Demeny M, Marekov LN et al. Cholesterol 3-sulfate interferes with cornified envelope assembly by diverting transglutaminase 1 activity from the formation of cross-links and esters to the hydrolysis of glutamine. J Biol Chem 2000; 275:2636–46.
33. Sato J, Denda M, Nakanishi J et al. Cholesterol sulfate inhibits proteases that are involved in desquamation of stratum corneum. J Invest Dermatol 1998; 111:189–93.
34. Schmuth M, Man MQ, Weber F et al. Permeability barrier disorder in Niemann-Pick disease: sphingomyelin-ceramide processing required for normal barrier homeostasis. J Invest Dermatol 2000; 115:459–66.
35. Holleran WM, Ginns EI, Menon GK et al. Consequences of beta-glucocerebrosidase deficiency in epidermis. Ultrastructure and permeability barrier alterations in Gaucher disease. J Clin Invest 1994; 93:1756–64.
36. Chavanas S, Bodemer C, Rochat A et al. Mutations in SPINK5, encoding a serine protease inhibitor, cause Netherton syndrome. Nat Genet 2000; 25:141–2.
37. Williams ML. Lipids in normal and pathological desquamation. Adv Lipid Res 1991; 24:211–62.
38. Fartasch M. Epidermal barrier in disorders of the skin. Microsc Res Tech 1997; 38:361–72.
39. Schmuth M, Yosipovitch G, Williams M et al. Pathogenesis of the permeability barrier abnormality in epidermolytic hyperkeratosis. J Invest Dermatol 2001; 117: 837–47.
40. Fartasch M, Bassukas ID, Diepgen TL. Structural relationship between epidermal lipid lamellae, lamellar bodies and desmosomes in human epidermis: an ultrastructural study. Br J Dermatol 1993; 128:1–9.
41. Norlén L. Skin barrier structure and function: the single gel phase model. J Invest Dermatol 2001; 117:830–6.

2

Update on desquamation and first evidence for the presence of the endoglycosidase heparanase 1 in the human stratum corneum

D Bernard, B Méhul and R Schmidt

Introduction

A balance between cell shedding at the surface of the epidermis and the proliferation in the basal layer of the epidermis is necessary for the formation of a normal stratum corneum (SC), to assure a physiochemical barrier against a hostile environment and to prevent water loss of our organism. The desquamation process is a precisely-controlled cascade of events, the molecular mechanisms of which are only known in part, actually representing a big puzzle which has to be put correctly in place. This article is divided into two parts: in the first part, a rather personal view of how the process of desquamation might occur is presented, and in the second part, a presentation of new data on the possible involvement of the endoglycosidase heparanase 1 in this process.

The substrates and enzymes implicated in the desquamation process

Twenty years ago, Elias et al[1] proposed the 'bricks and mortar model' to explain the mechanism of corneocyte adhesion (Figure 2.1). Extracellular lipids represent the mortar that sticks the bricks, corneocytes, together. This model was progressively revised by new hypotheses, e.g. that of Brysk et al,[2] where more adhesive mechanisms such as glycoprotein–lectin (G–L) interaction explained the cohesion of the SC. However, the strong cohesion attributed to G–L interactions could only be evidenced following lipid extraction, and no further confirmation by other research teams supported this theory. It is now generally accepted that SC cohesion is essentially mediated through inter-corneocyte structures, called corneosomes or corneodesmosomes,[3,4] which are desmosome-derived structures (Figure 2.1). Upon entry into the stratum disjunctum, corneocytes are characterized by a dramatic loss of non-peripheral corneodesmosomes, resulting in an inter-corneocyte binding which is reduced to the overlapping edges. The selective loss of non-peripheral corneodesmosomes and the retention of edge corneodesmosomes may reflect differential carbohydrate protection. The key event which eventually results in desquamation is the proteolysis of the corneodesmosomal proteins. Among these proteins, desmoglein I, a member of the cadherin family adhesion molecules, is believed to be one of the major desmosomal components, however barely detectable (degradation) in the uppermost layers of normal, healthy SC.[5] Other corneodesmosomal components, such as desmocollins,[6] desmoplakins (Bernard et al, unpublished results), or corneodesmosin,[4] are also progressively degraded during desquamation.[7]

Walsh and Chapman[3] described, as early as 1991, desquamation as a sequential action of glycosidases and proteases on corneodesmosomes. Using zymographic studies, several laboratories described the presence of proteases in the intercellular regions of the SC as (i) a chymotrypsin-like protease named Stratum Corneum Chymotryptic Enzyme (SCCE);[8] (ii) a trypsin-like protease named Stratum Corneum Tryptic Enzyme (SCTE);[9,10] (iii) a protease of the cystein protease family named Stratum Corneum Thiol Protease (SCTP);[11] and (iv) the aspartic protease Cathepsin D.[12] Some classical results obtained by zymography of stratum corneum extracts are presented in Figure 2.2. Table 2.1 summarizes some molecular information actually available for the above-described protease (note that the SCTP sequence has not been revealed until today). The cDNA-encoding SCCE and SCTE were isolated from a keratinocytes-derived library and these two proteases are tissue-specific.

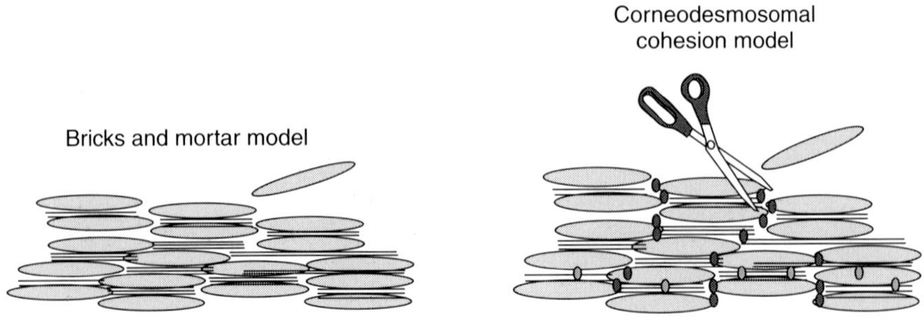

Figure 2.1
Corneocyte cohesion models.

Table 2.1 Some characteristics of the proteases potentially implied in the desquamation process.

Name	Protease class	Major MW (kDa)	Optimum pH	Differentiation related expression?	Genbank no
SCCE/KLK7	Serine protease	25	basic	yes	AF166330
SCTE/KLK5	Serine protease	30	basic	yes	AF135028
SCTP	Cysteine protease	34, 35	acid	yes	not determined
Cathepsin D	Aspartic protease	33, 48, 52	acid	yes	M11233

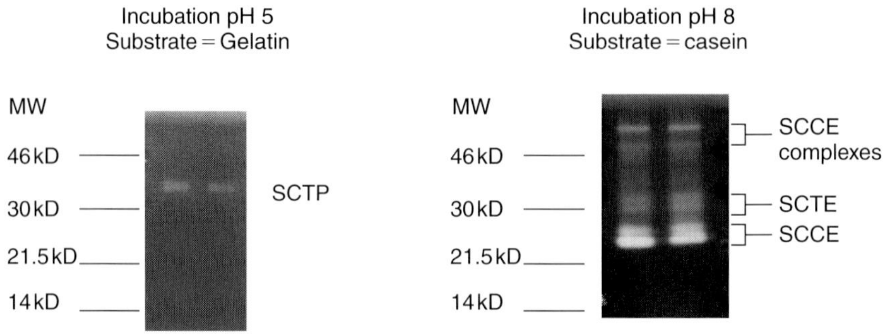

Figure 2.2

Zymography studies of proteases extracted from human SC. The zymography is useful to detect some of the major SC proteases. In this technique the substrate is directly incorporated in the electrophoresis gel prior to the migration of the SC sample. After the migration and a renaturing step the gel is incubated in a buffer adapted to the enzyme activity. At the end of the procedure, the gel is stained with coomassie blue, which stains the incorporated gelatin or casein. Non-stained band marks the proteolytic activities.

The in vitro desquamation models

Many of the above-described results were obtained with in vitro models. It is therefore important to be familiar with these models to judge the results and to eventually improve or create new models that will advance our understanding of desquamation.

In the first model, developed by Lundström and Egelrud (1988),[8] cell shedding from plantar stratum corneum was studied in vitro (Figure 2.3). Cell dissociation (desquamation) could be inhibited by chymotrypsin-like, trypsin-like, and cathepsin-D inhibitors, indicating the potential implication of certain proteases in the desquamation process.

In a second model (Figure 2.4), desquamation was assessed, based on the loss of immunoreactivity due to the degradation of a corneodesmosomal protein. Watkinson,[11] who developed this model, used an anti-desmoglein I antibody; however, desmocollin I, as well as corneodesmosin, degradation have also been studied in this model. The same model served to study the inhibition profile of specific protease inhibitors, revealing the potential roles of SCCE, SCTE, SCTP and Cathepsin D proteases in the desquamation process.

Regulation of the desquamation process

Few data are available concerning the regulation of the desquamation process. Undoubtedly, this process is much more complex, as is gener-

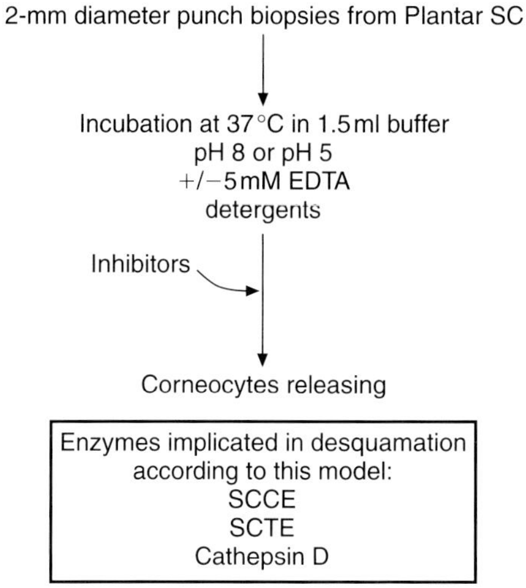

Figure 2.3

Desquamation models: the Lundström and Egelrud model.[8]
Flakes of plantar SC were cut parallel to the skin surface. After incubation, tubes containing the tissue were agitated in a vortex mixer. Released cells were then collected and quantified. The chelator EDTA increased the phenomenon. The cell release was optimal at pH 7–9 but was also significant at pH 6.

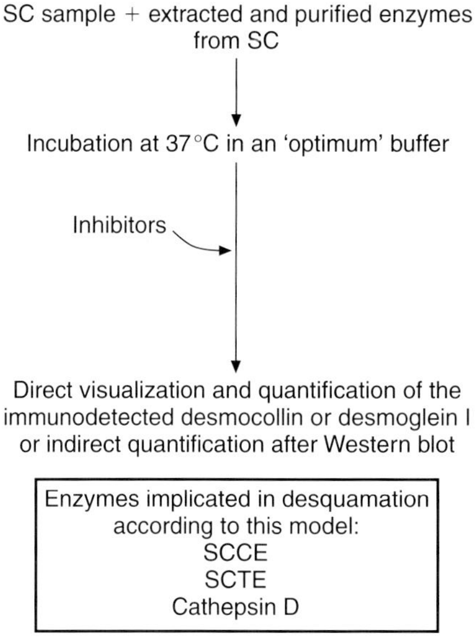

Figure 2.4

Desquamation models: the Watkinson model. After an incubation of an SC sample (obtained by stripping, surface biopsy or other methods), the residual desmosomal proteins are evaluated and quantified by fluorescence microscopy or by Western blot.

ally deduced from the in vitro experiments. Table 2.2 summarizes the main known factors affecting the enzyme activity and their occurrence during the epidermal differentiation process. It is not surprising that, in a recent paper,[13] humidity was identified to be a potent regulator of SCCE activity and, thus, corneocyte release. Another important regulating factor

Table 2.2 Potential factors regulating the enzymatic activities linked to the desquamation process.

Factors influencing the enzymatic activities in vitro	Occurrence of these factors during the epidermal differentiation
pH	pH gradient
Ionic strength	Ion gradient (Ca^{2+}...)
Temperature	Temperature gradient
Water content and state	Are modified
Substrate accessibility	Spatial arrangements of proteins
Coenzymes (ATP, NAD, FAD...)	At least ATP is present in the SC
Activators	Not known
Inhibitors	Numerous: Elafin, Cystatin A...
Allosteric regulators	Not known
Other enzymes	Numerous
Substrate modification	Oxidation, Ca^{2+} binding...

is the fact that proteases are frequently synthesized as inactive precursors requiring activation by other proteases. Figure 2.5 represents a schematic, hypothetical view of the proteolytic cascade during desquamation.

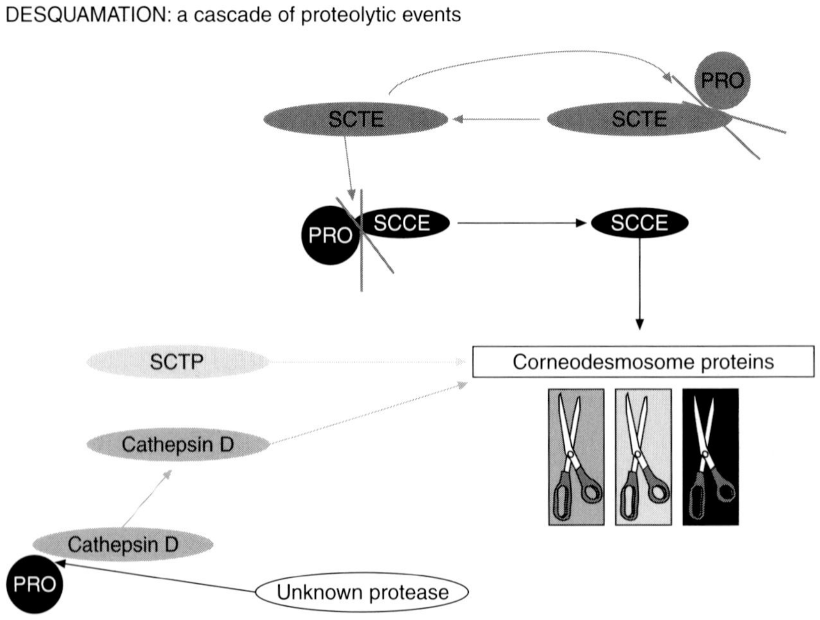

Figure 2.5

Schematic view of the cascade of proteolytic events leading to desquamation.

New data on the presence of (endo) glycosidases in the SC and their possible implication in the desquamation process

Walsh and Chapman[3] demonstrated: (i) that the addition of exogenous proteases induced no major changes in the corneodesmosomes' composition; (ii) the addition of exogenous glycosidases alone or added after protease treatment caused only mild fragmentation; and (iii) glycosidase treatment followed by the addition of exogenous proteases caused dramatic changes of the corneodesmosomal structures. These findings indicate that sugar moieties are present, protecting the corneodesmosomes from proteolysis by extracellular proteases. In their model, Walsh and Chapman demonstrated that endoglycosidases were more effective than exoglycosidases.

Until recently, no known endoglycosidase was described in stratum corneum. We demonstrated not long ago that at least one member of this enzyme family is expressed in human epidermis and is present in the stratum corneum.[14] By using FITC-labelled heparin sulfate as a substrate, a protein extracted from plantar human stratum corneum was clearly identified to exhibit heparanase activity. In a two-step, chromatographic procedure, the protein was purified to homogeneity. Sequence analysis revealed 100% homology with human heparanase 1 (Hpa1). In cultured human keratinocytes, reconstructed epidermis and normal human skin Hpa1 showed clearly a differentiation-related expression profile and that known inhibitors of keratinocyte differentiation, such as retinoids, block Hpa1 expression. From these results, we conclude that Hpa1, which is abundantly present in the human stratum corneum, might play an important role in the desquamation process, particularly in the pre-proteolytic processing of the protecting sugar moieties.

Conclusion

The process of desquamation resembles a cascade of events which are highly ordered in time and space, implicating the structural proteins of the corneodesmosomes, which are degraded by proteases to liberate the corneocytes. In recent years, our understanding of the structural proteins of the corneosomes, such as corneodesmosin, desmoglein I and desmocollin I, and the proteases possibly implicated in the degradation process has considerably advanced. We were able to demonstrate, for the first time, the presence of the endoglycosidase heparanase 1 in the stratum corneum, an enzyme which might trigger the first step in desquamation, the deglycosylation of corneodesmosomal proteins. A better understanding of the corneodesmosomal microenvironment, the spatial arrangement of corneodesmosomal proteins, and the identification of the biochemical modifications of these proteins at the molecular level will greatly contribute to a better understanding of the desquamation cascade.

References

1. Elias P, Grayson S, Lampe MA et al. The intercorneocyte space. In: Marks R, Plewig G, eds. *Stratum Corneum.* Berlin, Heidelberg: Springer-Verlag; 1983:53–67.
2. Brysk M, Rajaraman S, Penn P et al. Glycoproteins modulate adhesion in terminally differentiated keratinocytes. Cell Tissue Res 1988; 253:657–63.
3. Walsh A, Chapman SJ. Sugars protect desmosome and corneosome glycoproteins from proteolysis. Arch Dermatol Res 1991; 283:174–9.
4. Serre G, Mils V, Haftek M et al. Identification of late differentiation antigens of human cornified epithelia, expressed in re-organized desmosomes and bound to cross-linked envelope. J Invest Dermatol 1991; 97:1061–72.
5. Rawlings A, Harding C, Watkinson A et al. The effect of glycerol and humidity on desmosome degradation in stratum corneum. Arch Dermatol Res 1995; 287:457–64.
6. King IA, Tabiowo A, Purkis P et al. Expression of distinct desmocollin isoforms in human epidermis. J Invest Dermatol 1993; 100:373–9.
7. Lundström A, Serre G, Haftek M et al. Evidence for a role of corneodesmosine, a protein which may serve to modify desmosomes during cornification, in stratum corneum cell cohesion and desquamation. Arch Dermatol Res 1994; 286:369–75.
8. Egelrud T, Lundström A. A chymotrypsin-like proteinase that may be involved in desquamation in plantar stratum corneum. Arch Dermatol Res 1991; 283:108–12.
9. Egelrud T, Lundström A. The dependence of detergent-induced cell dissociation in non-palmoplantar stratum corneum on endogenous proteolysis. J Invest Dermatol 1990; 95:456–9.
10. Suzuki Y, Nomura J, Koyama J et al. The role of proteases in stratum corneum: involvement in stratum corneum desquamation. Arch Dermatol Res 1994; 286;249–53.
11. Watkinson WO 95/07686 patent 1995.
12. Horikoshi T, Arany I, Rajaraman S et al. Isoforms of cathepsin D and human epidermal differentiation. Biochim 1998; 80:605–12.
13. Watkinson A, Harding C, Moore A et al. Water modulation of stratum corneum chymotryptic activity and desquamation. Arch Dermatol Res 2001; 293:470–6.
14. Bernard D, Méhul B, Delattre C et al. Purification and characterization of the endoglycosidase heparanase 1 from human plantar stratum corneum: a key enzyme in epidermal physiology? J Invest Dermatol 2001; 117:1266–73.

3
One more look into the stratum corneum

R Marks

Even amongst both physicians and biologists, the stratum corneum (SC) has been a much undervalued structure and dermatologists have not, until quite recently, thought of this membrane as being of major importance. The reasons for this misperception are, first, that routine histological preparations deform and distort the stratum corneum so that it appears wispy and insignificant. Secondly, there has been a paucity of techniques that can afford an accurate view of this horny structure.

The skin surface biopsy (SSB) method was described in 1971,[1] and has been the subject of many publications since then (e.g. References 2–5). This technique provides an opportunity for inspecting the horny layer from most body sites in the state in which it exists in vivo. In addition, it enables the SC to be viewed in the horizontal dimension – the dimension in which it functions.

This short paper describes the technique and some of its less well-known and recently described applications.

Methods

The success of the technique relies on the use of rapidly bonding cyanoacrylate adhesives. Several different analogues have been used to take SSBs, including methyl, ethyl and octyl cyanoacrylate. They rapidly polymerize with minimal pressure in the presence of some moisture to form a very strong and optically transparent bond. In practice, a drop of the adhesive is placed on a clean glass microscope slide or a similarly sized flexible strip of transparent plastic material. The slide is then pressed against the skin site to be sampled. After some 20 seconds, the slide is gently 'rolled off' the skin, taking with it the SSB – an intact sheet of SC some two or three cells thick. The resulting SSB is undisturbed SC, which appears on the microscope slide precisely as it exists in vivo.

The polymerized cyanoacrylate of the SSB has very similar optical properties to glass, so that it is easy to examine the samples by ordinary light microscopy.

The taking of SSBs is quite painless – the worst discomfort arises from trapping hairs in the adhesive and then yanking these out inadvertently!

These adhesives appear non-toxic and, anyway, are completely removed with the taking of the specimen. In fact, several cyanoacrylates have been used for some years as tissue cements in wound repair. Recently, there has been a resurgence of interest in the use of octyl cyanoacrylate to repair small-incised wounds in what is sometimes termed 'needleless suture'.[6]

The fact that the adhesive bonds very rapidly can itself be a source of embarrassment if the operator is inexperienced and takes insufficient care, as fingers and other body parts can very easily become stuck together with only casual contact. Dowsing the affected area in acetone, which rapidly dissolves the adhesive, can readily solve this type of problem. Particular care must be taken when sampling facial skin to avoid injury to the eyes or lips. Only a very small amount of adhesive should be used and, to prevent the possibility of injury to the eyes, the procedure should only be performed with the subject sitting upright.

The use of skin surface biopsy to study percorneal penetration

The study of the absorption of drugs into the skin after topical application in vivo is beset by difficulties imposed by the complexities of the structure that the drug must cross. Measurement of blood levels after topical application of the preparation in question will provide some useful data but does not inform on the penetration of the drug into the skin. The SSB technique provides a simple way of tracking the movement of drugs through the SC and into the skin.

It is convenient to use radioactively tagged compounds for this purpose if these derivatives of the drug of interest are available. This enables the amount of penetrating drug in the SC strips of the SSB to be estimated easily, although it is also possible to trace the penetration of drugs using high performance liquid chromatography (HPLC) or enzyme-linked immunosorbent assay (ELISA) methods on the SSBs.

In practice, the ointment, cream or gel containing the drug agent is applied to the skin site being investigated and left undisturbed for 15 minutes, after which any excess is wiped off from an area of $2\,cm^2$. An SSB is then taken from this delineated site, followed by a second SSB from the same area, and then a third SSB followed by a fourth from the same site, i.e. samples are taken at increasing depth from the same site at a defined time. Similar SSB samples are taken at increasing depths from the SC at adjoining sites after wiping off the preparation remaining there for different defined periods. In this way, it is possible to build up a time and depth concentration profile. Should it be necessary to know the concentration of drug penetrating into the whole skin then full-thickness biopsies can be taken after taking the SSBs at the different sites.

We have used this technique to characterize the penetration of corticosteroids, imidazoles,[7] non-steroidal anti-inflammatory agents,[8] and antimicrobials.[9]

Detection of drugs in the stratum corneum

Hair has been used previously to determine the presence of drugs in the body and we have recently started a project to use the SSB sampling technique to characterize the presence and amounts of drug taken in the previous few days. This will be an important way of assessing patient compliance and an additional way of detecting administration of forbidden drugs.

Assessment of follicular obstruction and comedogenicity

When an SSB is taken from an obviously hairy site, inspection of the surface with a magnifying glass will reveal a hair and/or follicular debris projecting from many of the hair follicle openings. Much more follicular material is removed from an acne patient than from a control subject without acne. Comedolytic agents are used to try to 'loosen' the keratinous content of the follicular cavities so that they are more easily expelled. Use of the SSB technique to assess the amount of follicular debris that can be expelled is a simple test of comedolytic efficacy.

One important application of the ability to assess follicular content with the SSB technique is the human comedogenicity test. In former times, a 'rabbit ear test' was used to assess the propensity for topical applications to cause comedones to form. Human testing is now considered more suitable from all points of view, and we now routinely use the flank skin of human volunteers who have a mild grade of clinical acne (as that reassurance that they can produce comedones).[10]

The test preparations and a positive control (usually cocoa butter) are applied to the flank skin under occlusion over a 4-week period. At the end of the period of application, SSBs are taken from the treated sites and then examined by low power microscopy and scored on a short ordinal scale according to the amount of impacted horn in the follicular lumen.

Analysis of DNA content of skin surface biopsies

Clearly, it is possible to sample nuclear DNA from parakeratotic horn but it has always been thought that, in normal skin, epidermal nuclear DNA was completely destroyed during the process of keratinization. Recently, studies in our group have shown that this is not the case, as it has been possible to identify native DNA in SSBs from normal skin after using polymerase chain reaction (PCR) technique.[11] Quite understandably, SSBs from psoriatic lesions yielded very much more DNA.

The ability to study human DNA using a simple non-invasive technique opens the door to many opportunities for study of the human genome.

Assessment of mechanical function of the stratum corneum in vivo

Extensibility of the SC is a vital property of this structure, permitting movement and minor degrees of indentation without rupture. SSBs capture skin surface markings and allow the dimensions of the rectangles, rhomboids and diagonals to be measured. By extending the skin surface by a defined amount, using a flat metal frame or some other such device, and then taking a further SSB from the same site, the dimensions, when stretched, can be compared with those before stretching (Figure 3.1). This relationship portrays the ability of the surface horn to extend and is a potentially useful parameter.

Conclusion

The SC has been little investigated, despite its importance, because of inherent difficulties. The technique of SSB is simple, non-invasive and allows detailed study of the SC as it exists in vivo. It permits detailed

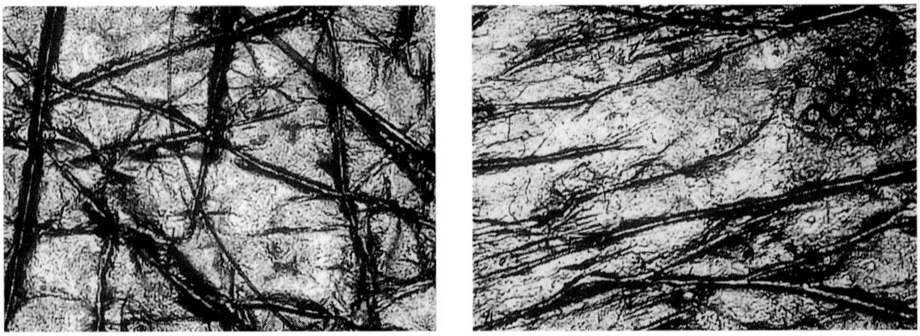

(a) (b)

Figure 3.1

(a) Photomicrograph of skin surface biopsy before stretching. (b) Photomicrograph of skin surface biopsy of a neighbouring area after stretching. Comparison of the geometry of the two patterns enables an assessment to be made of the extensibility of the skin surface.

microscopic inspection, analysis of its content and assessment of many aspects of its function.

Although the SSB technique was first described 30 years ago, new ways of using it to provide fresh information on the SC are continually coming to light.

References

1. Marks R, Dawber R. Skin surface biopsy: an improved technique for the examination of the horny layer. Br J Dermatol 1971; 84:117–23.
2. Marks R, Saylan T. The surface structure of the stratum corneum. Acta Derm (Stockholm), 1972; 52:119–25.
3. Marks R, Dawber RPR. In situ microbiology of the stratum corneum. Arch Derm 1972; 105: 216–21.
4. Marks R. Histochemical applications of skin surface biopsy. Br J Dermatol 1972; 86:20–6.
5. Griffiths WAD, Marks R. The significance of surface changes in parakeratotic horn. J Invest Dermatol 1973; 61:251–4.
6. Quinn J, Wells G, Sutcliffe T et al. A randomized trial comparing octylcyanoacrylate tissue adhesive and sutures in the management of lacerations. JAMA 1997; 277:1527–30.
7. Marks R, Dykes PJ, Williams DL et al. In vivo stratum corneum pharmacokinetics of econazole following once and twice daily application to human skin. J Dermatol Treat 1990; 1:195–7.
8. Marks R, Dykes PJ. Plasma and cutaneous drug levels after topical application of piroxicam gel: a study in health volunteers. Skin Pharmacol 1994; 7:340–4.
9. Dykes P, Hill S, Marks R. Pharmacokinetics of topically applied metronidazole in two different formulations. Skin Pharmacol 1997; 10:28–33.
10. Mills OH, Kligman AM. A human model for assessing comedogenic substances. Arch Derm 1982; 118:903–5.
11. Yahya H. Estimating the DNA content of stratum corneum by skin surface (MSc in Dermatology). UWCM, 1999.

4
Formation and function of the stratum corneum

SB Hoath and DG Leahy

Introduction

Eadem mutata resurgo – 'Though changed I arise again unchanged'.[1]

The concept of discrete structural and functional stratification constitutes a major organizing principle in epidermal biology.[2] The traditional segmentation of the epidermis into four distinct anatomical compartments is shown in Figure 4.1. The boundaries of the separate strata (basale, spinosum, granulosum, and corneum) are generally sharp and morphologically distinct. The first epidermal stratum, the stratum basale, rests upon the dermal–epidermal junction and is, by definition, a single cell layer thick. The fourth stratum, the stratum corneum begins with the process of programmed cell death and ends with desquamation at the surface of the body (environment). Only the junction between the stratum spinosum and stratum granulosum, based upon the inconstant morphological appearance of keratohyalin granules, is relatively ill defined.

The current study re-examines the traditional segmentation model of human epidermis (Figure 4.1). A rational model for epidermal stratification is proposed in which the stratum corneum optimally consists of 16 cell layers. In this model, the stratum corneum is the culmination of an ordered series of mutually-supportive segments containing 1, 4, 9, and 16 cells layers, respectively. The Langerhans cells, which migrate into the mid-epidermis, are considered a strategic cellular marker for the interface between the second and third epidermal segments. Evidence supporting this model is provided in terms of the number of cell layers within the stratum corneum and the immunolocalization of Langerhans cells in adult and newborn epidermis.

The mathematics of this model of epidermal stratification is related to the universal constant of gravitational acceleration and Φ proportionality.[3] The golden section ratio ($\Phi \sim 1.618034$) has long been connected with aesthetic considerations and typically occurs in nature where there is a need for structural stability under transformation.[4,5] The epidermis is note-

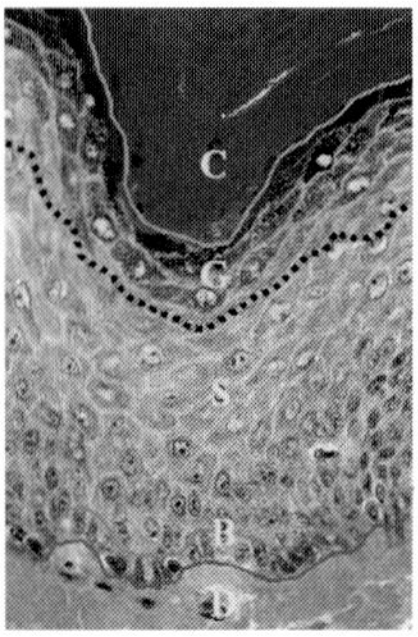

Figure 4.1

Microscopic cross-section of adult human epidermis. The usual nomenclature and position of the epidermal strata are shown; i.e. basale (B), spinosum (S), granulosum (G), and corneum (C). The thickening of the epidermis over the rete ridges at the edges of the micrograph is also indicated. (Figure adapted and modified from Wheater's *Functional Histology*, 4th ed. Churchill Livingstone: 2000.)

worthy as a biological structure closely linked to human perception and aesthetics. The epidermis is also characterized by structural stability in the face of continual transformation. The finding of a relationship between epidermal structure and Φ proportionality is, therefore, not entirely unexpected.

Methods and results

This study had two interrelated morphological objectives: 1) the determination of the number of cell layers in the stratum corneum in human newborn foreskin, and 2) the localization of epidermal Langerhans cells by immunocytochemistry in environmentally naive (newborn) and adult epidermis. Specifically, we tested the hypotheses that newborn stratum corneum comprises approximately 16 cell layers in thickness and that Langerhans cells migrate during development to a site within the suprabasal epidermis 4–5 cell layers from the basement membrane.

Experimentally, newborn foreskin and adult skin from the cheek or shoulder region were examined. Newborn skin samples were cryosectioned and underwent alkaline expansion for microphotography and counting of the cell layers in the stratum corneum, as previously described.[6] Newborn and adult samples were also paraffin-sectioned in a microtome. These sections were stained for Langerhans cells using an S100 antibody kit (DRACO) (Figure 4.2). The number of cell layers between the dermal–epidermal junction and the Langerhans cells was counted directly from stained sections. The following results were obtained: 1) The stratum corneum of human newborn skin measured 14.7 ± 0.3 layers thick – this result does not account for any cell layers shed during handling; 2) Langerhans cell localization in human newborn epidermis was difficult, with fewer cells noted than in the adult samples; 3) Langerhans cells in adult epidermis had a consistent suprabasal location measuring 4.15 ± 0.07 layers from the basement membrane

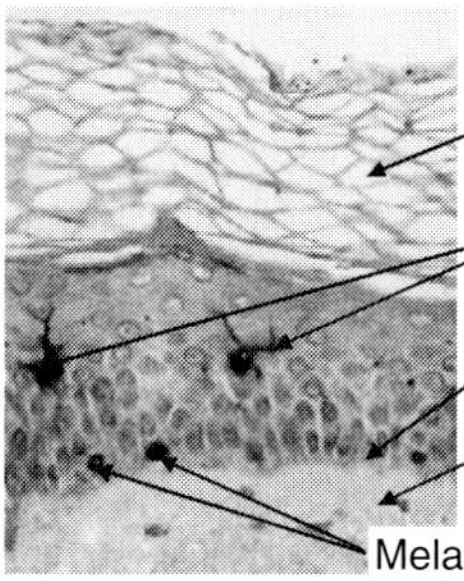

Figure 4.2
Immunolocalization of Langerhans cells by S100 antibody staining in adult human epidermis. The Langerhans cells have a dark-staining cell body and extensive branching dendrites. The cells shown are approximately four cell layers above the basal layer. The dendrites of the Langerhans cells extend upwards, presumably to subserve the role of LCs in antigen detection and immune function.

(N = 132); and 4) Langerhans cells in newborn epidermis were located significantly lower in the epidermis than adults, 2.0 ± 0.17 layers from the basement membrane (N = 34). These results are shown in Tables 4.1 and 4.2. Table 4.1, in addition, contains a review of the literature of the number of stratum corneum cell layers at different body sites.

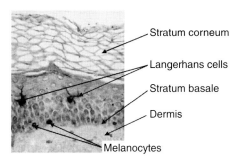

Taken as a whole, the results in Table 4.2, combined with the experimental algorithm, provide a logical rationale for the location of Langer-

Table 4.1 Numbers of cell layers in the stratum corneum

Region	No. of cell layers of SC	Reference
Abdomen	15–25	Brody[16]
	18	Smith et al[17]
	18 mean (15–21 range)	Holbrook and Odland[18]
	13 ± 4	Ya-Xian et al[19]
Flexor forearm	10.2–23.4 range	Blair[20]
	25	Odland[21]
	21.6 mean (16.7–30 range)	Holbrook and Odland[18]
	15 ± 4	Ya-Xian et al[19]
Thigh	19.3 (14.3–22.7 range)	Holbrook and Odland[18]
Back	9.6–20	Blair[20]
	19 (14–28 range)	Anderson and Cassidy[22]
	15.8 (14–21 range)	Holbrook and Odland[18]
Foreskin	14.7 ± 2.8	Hoath et al (present study)
Newborn rat (1 day old)	16.1 ($y = 0.13x + 13.07$) x = hours of age, y = SC layers	Hoath et al[6]

Table 4.2 Immunolocalization of Langerhans cells (No. of cells above basement membrane)

	Mean	SD	No. of samples
Adult skin	4.15	0.76	132
Newborn foreskin	2.00	1.02	34

hans cells in the suprabasal epidermis of adult humans. It is proposed that the migration of Langerhans cells within adult human epidermis places these important immunocompetent cells in a strategic position to mediate immunological interactions between the second and third epidermal segments. By hypothesis, Langerhans cells migrate to a tightly-organized, cellular 'ceiling', composed of nucleated keratinocytes in the third epidermal segment (cf. Figure 4.2). This third segment, together with the anucleated corneocytes in the fourth epidermal segment, the stratum corneum, constitutes the first line of defense against invasion by environmental toxins and microorganisms. When these two outer segments are breached, immunological host defenses involving Langerhans cells interactions are activated. This functional and structural demarcation, based on Langerhans cell location, calls into question the previously-used morphological criteria designating the two middle strata, respectively, as spinosum and granulosum.

Discussion

Recently, Bauer et al reported a 'strikingly constant ratio' of one Langerhans cell to 53 other epidermal cells in adult human breast skin.[7] This precise ratio of 1:53 supports the concept that the human epidermis is organized into morphologically-discrete, functional units. The definition of such Langerhans cell-containing units requires more information on the intraepidermal location of the Langerhans cells and their structural and functional relation to the various epidermal strata. The data presented in the current study supports the organization of the epidermis into a rational structure in which migratory Langerhans cells occupy a strategic location for immunosurveillence of 53 nucleated cells within the Malphigian epidermis. The number of supervised cells in an epidermal Langerhans unit, 53, is a function of Φ, where Φ is the golden section ratio (1.618034), 14 is the total number of layers of cells in the first three epidermal strata (the Malpighian epidermis), and 16 is the number of layers in the stratum corneum:

$$53 \sim \Phi^{14}/16.$$

The idea that Φ proportionality is integrally involved in the rational organization of the epidermis is evident elsewhere. Phi, the golden section ratio, underlies the Fibonacci series:

1, 1, 2, 3, 5, 8, 13, 21, ...infinity

Each number in this series is the sum of the two preceding numbers, and Φ is the ultimate ratio of two consecutive numbers as the series approaches infinity. An early segment of this series (3, 5, 8, 13) is encountered in the organization of epidermal barrier lipids in the intercorneocyte space of the stratum corneum (Figure 4.3).[8] This pattern is only observed in the interfollicular stratum corneum, and is not present in oral mucosa (Phil Wertz, personal communication, 2001). The working hypothesis underlying the (3, 5, 8, 13) arrangement is that the 13 nm repeat structure observed for stratum corneum lipid lamellae is necessary for optimal structural stability in a constantly changing environment. This structure provides a clue for linking lipid domains to other structures in the epidermis with Φ proportionality.

A provocative connection between Φ proportionality and stratum corneum development is evidenced in the relationship between surface area and body weight in newborn animals such as rodents. In the neonatal rat (age 0–3 days), Hoath et al reported that a log–log plot of the surface area of the stratum corneum versus body weight yielded a slope of 1.04 following linear regression analysis (Figure 4.4).[9] This finding contrasted with the expected slope of 0.67 based on simple surface area-to-volume relationships and differed from the empirical 0.75-power law observed in adult bioenergetics comparing adult animal species ranging in size from mice to elephants.[10] The finding that thc surface area of newborn animals plotted against body weight on a log–log plot has a slope greater than 1 is termed the 'neonatal violation' of the surface law of basal metabolism.[11]

In response to this experimental observation, the authors note that the conflicting powers of body mass reported in the allometric literature[3]

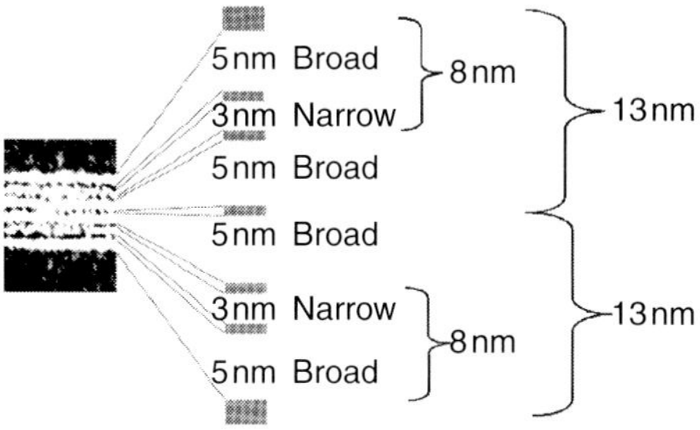

Figure 4.3

The organization of intercorneocyte lipid lamellae within the stratum corneum. The lamellar structure consists of a number of repeating layers of interdigitated lipids which appear as a series of regularly-arranged bands/lamellae on electron microscopy.[8] In normal human skin, the lamellar architecture of the lipid mortar consists of a series of repeating units of broad, narrow, and broad bands. This triplet sequence may range from only a few to several sets, but always there are triplet repeats. The 13 nm triplet repeats are composed of two units measuring 5 nm each, and one unit measuring 3 nm in thickness. The two differing units together measure 8 nm. The 3, 5, 8, 13 sequence is an early segment of the Fibonacci corioc.

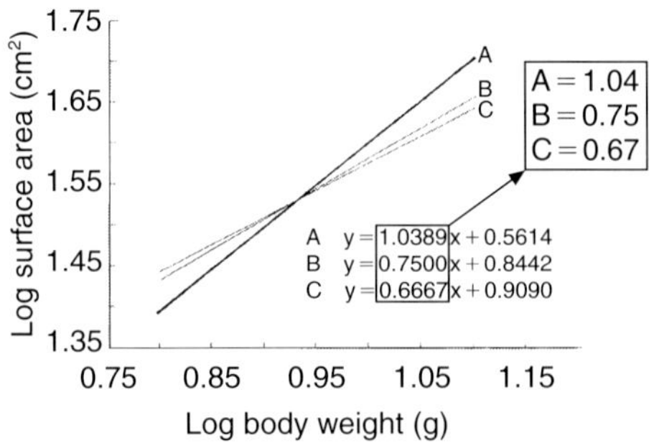

Figure 4.4

Relationship between total epidermal surface area and body weight in newborn rat pups. Data are plotted on a log–log plot with linear regression analysis. The empirically-derived slope of the regression line (line A) is approximately 1.04. Regression lines B and C were generated by fixing the mass exponent (slope of the log–log plot) at 0.75 and 0.67, respectively. Values are for postnatal animals aged 0–3 days. (Figure adapted and modified from Hoath et al.[9]

may, in fact, be reconciled by the reported neonatal violation of the body surface law. Assuming a fundamental mean Φ-proportionality for the structure of the human body, the divergence of the theoretically-expected adult body weight exponent (2/3) from the empirically-determined exponent (3/4) may be understood as directly proportionate to the exponent in the reported neonatal violation:

$$\Phi^{0.75}/\Phi^{0.666} = 1.0409.$$

It is further noteworthy that where 1.0397 ~ the neonatal exponent, 2.50290787509589 is the Feigenbaum alpha constant, and 4.66920160910299 the Feigenbaum delta constant:

$$(4.669/2.5029)\wedge 1/16 = 1.0397.$$

Thus, three widely different relationships all yield a solution of approximately 1.04. These relationships may be coincidental. On the other hand, the Feigenbaum constants are mathematical numbers governing the universal transition from ordered to chaotic behavior.[12] At the cellular and molecular levels, the process of stratum corneum desquamation similarly marks a transition from an ordered structure to an apparent chaotic state. The fact that the 1/16th root of the ratio of the Feigenbaum constants is equivalent to an empirically-derived ratio relating stratum corneum expansion to somatic growth of the newborn animal is worthy of further consideration. The further connection of these relationships to the Φ power law ratio, linking the allometric mass exponents of 2/3 and 3/4, begs a biological interpretation.

Allometry, in general, relates the relative growth rate of a part of an organism to another part or to the whole. In the proposed model, the epidermis is optimally constituted as a series of segments containing 1, 4, 9, and 16 layers each (Figure 4.5). These segments are not 'one after another', in the sense of distances traversed by a falling object, but rather 'one for another', in the sense of tissues or organs. In the case of a mass moving under the influence of gravity, the lengths traversed in equal intervals of time accord with the sequence 1, 4, 9, 16, etc. In the case of epidermal development, however, the boundary of the organism forms as a series of segments, *each of which forms the foundation for the subsequent segment.* Each part of the epidermis contributes to the functional and structural unity of the whole. This biological unity can be illustrated by considering the order of the segments as a series of ratios 1/4, 5/9, 14/16, 30/25 (Figure 4.6). The numerator of each element in this series is the sum of the preceding layers supported by the subsequent segment.

The ratio 30/25 is the first epidermal segmentation ratio greater than unity. 30/25 is the ratio in which the epidermis as a whole (1 + 4 + 9 + 16 = 30) is identified by the denominator, 25, first, as intrinsically related to the environment insofar as the denominator continues the sequence beyond the four epidermal strata (1, 4, 9, 16, 25), and, second, as a surface of closure or a 'bending back' that forms the epidermal barrier (9 + 16 = 25). This approach enables an understanding of the means whereby the epidermis can be simultaneously a molecular and cellular interface, which is open to the environment, and a psychological and perceptual interface, which is functionally closed. The ratio of 30/25 in this perspective brings to mind the close embryological relationship between the epidermis and the brain. Both the epidermis and the brain are ectodermal derivatives

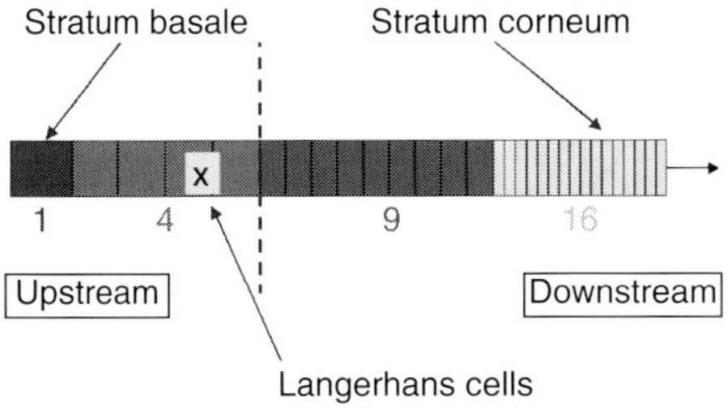

Figure 4.5

Proposed rational organization of adult human epidermis. The numbers of cell layers in the four epidermal segments are indicated. The stratum basale is the furthermost upstream segment and the stratum corneum the furthermost downstream. The approximate location of the Langerhans cells near the junction of the 2nd and 3rd epidermal segments is indicated.

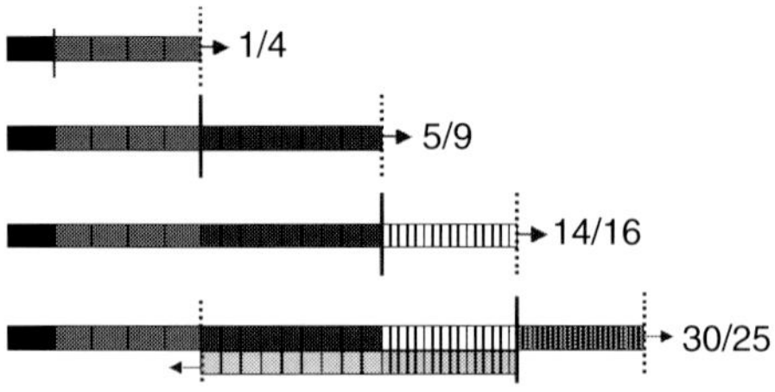

Figure 4.6

Epidermal segmentation ratios. In the proposed model, the interfollicular epidermis is considered to be optimally constituted as a series of segments containing 1, 4, 9, and 16 layers each (Figure 4.5). These segments can be considered as a series of ratios in which the numerator of each element in the series is the sum of the preceding layers supported by the subsequent segment. The segmentation ratios are less than unity until the entire epidermis constitutes the antecedent in the ratio 30/25. In the latter ratio, the denominator, 25, can be construed in two ways: first, as continuing the sequence of the squares of the natural numbers extending to the environment; i.e. 1, 4, 9, 16, 25; second, as constituting a surface of closure formed by union of the outer two strata (9 + 16 = 25) in which a 'bending back' or inflection occurs at the surface of the stratum corneum. It is this latter perspective which, hypothetically, gives rise to the concept of an epidermal barrier.

and both are primary evolutionary characteristics, distinguishing humans from all other primates.

This denominational identity of apparently differing orientations at the surface of the organism (Figure 4.6) resurrects, in a different context, the controversy between Pinkus and Ryan over 30 years ago as to the 'proper' direction of epidermal cell movement.[13,14] The traditional orientation, championed by Pinkus, views keratinocytes moving from the basement membrane to eventual sloughing at the environmental surface.[13] The opposite orientation, proposed by Ryan, presupposes an alternative view of the epidermis starting at the body surface.[14]

The latter orientation is conceptually consistent with the formation of the epidermal barrier as a combination of nucleated and anucleated cells in the third and fourth epidermal segments, respectively (Figure 4.6, left-facing arrow). Pinkus' orientation begs the question of the method by which the epidermal structure incorporates its relation to the environment (Figure 4.6, right-facing arrows). A mathematical hypothesis focusing on the development of the stratum corneum of the palms and soles has been formulated elsewhere.[15] According to this hypothesis, regional epidermal differentiation over the palms and soles incorporates the first environmental number; i.e. 25, in the mathematics of its thickening at those places where the epidermis most tangibly contacts its environment on a regular basis.

As reviewed above, the model proposed in this paper gives rise to similar, oppositely-oriented, mathematical expressions, which may have biological meaning in relation to the role of Φ proportionality in epidermal structure and function. Consider, for example, the ratios 1/4, 5/9, 14/16, and 30/25 derived from the proposed sequence of epidermal segments 1, 4, 9, 16. Viewing these ratios in order from the stratum basale to the stratum corneum, the following general numerical relations pertain where Φ = the golden section ratio ~ 1.618034:

$$(1/4)\ (5/9)\ (14/16)\ (30/25) \sim \Phi^{-4}$$

$$[(1/4)/(5/9)]/[(14/16)/(30/25)] \sim 1/\Phi.$$

Viewing these ratios in order from the stratum corneum to the stratum basale:

$$(25/30)\ (16/14)\ (9/5)\ (4/1) \sim \Phi^{4}$$

$$[(25/30)/(16/14)]/[(9/5)/(4/1)] \sim \Phi.$$

These Φ-based expressions support the hypothesis that commonly-perceived biological objects, such as the human epidermis, may, in fact, require a synthesis of divergent perspectives in order to quantitatively understand structure and function. These expressions hypothetically relate the sequential products and quotients of epidermal segmentation ratios under optimized conditions. Under such conditions, the vectorial addition of these opposite-facing expressions results in the following integral solutions:

$$\Phi^{-4} + \Phi^{4} = 7 \qquad \text{and} \qquad 1/\Phi + \Phi = 5^{1/2}.$$

Summary

Undoubtedly, the proposal of a single, rationally-organized, Φ-proportional model of optimal epidermal structure and function will meet resistance. Skepticism is welcome given the complexity and importance of the human skin interface. Two approaches to the mathematical model presented are foreseeable. First, a logico-mathematical structure of the epidermis and the stratum corneum may be discounted in the face of the extraordinary variability encountered in human epidermis. This variability is manifest within the same organism from time to time and region to region. Alternatively, the ability of a mathematical model to coherently describe the functional stratification of the human epidermis may lead to experimental considerations of the factors and conditions leading to the observed biological variability. The data presented in this paper and the biological examples in which Φ proportionality intersects epidermal barrier formation and function support the latter approach.

References

1. Bernoulli J. Epitaph on tombstone indicating the reproductive properties of the inscribed logarithmic spiral and its relation to phi proportionality. Basel, Switzerland; 1705.
2. Mancini A. Structure and function of newborn skin. In: Eichenfield L, Frieden I, Esterly N, eds. *Textbook of Neonatal Dermatology.* Philadelphia: W.B. Saunders Company; 2001: 18–32.
3. Leahy DG. The Langerhans-epidermal cell ratio and the structure of the epidermis (http://dgleahy.com/dgl/p24.html); 2002.
4. Herz-Fischler R. *A Mathematical History of the Golden Number.* Mineola, New York: Dover Publications; 1998.
5. Huntley H. *The Divine Proportion: A Study in Mathematical Beauty.* New York: Dover Publications; 1970.
6. Hoath S, Tanaka R, Boyce S. Rate of stratum corneum formation in the perinatal rat. J Invest Dermatol 1993; 100:400–6.
7. Bauer J, Bahmer FA, Worl J et al. A strikingly constant ratio exists between Langerhans cells and other epidermal cells in human skin. A stereologic study using the optical disector method and the confocal laser scanning microscope. J Invest Dermatol 2001; 116:313–18.
8. Wertz P, van den Bergh B. The physical, chemical and functional properties of lipids in the skin and other biological barriers. Chem Physics Lipids 1998; 91:85–96.
9. Hoath SB, Pickens WL, Tanaka R et al. Ontogeny of integumental calcium in relation to surface area and skin water content in the perinatal rat. J Appl Physiol 1992; 73:458–64.
10. Schmidt-Nielsen K. *Scaling: Why Is Animal Size So Important?* Cambridge, England: Cambridge University Press; 1984.
11. Sinclair J, Scopes J, Silverman W. Metabolic reference standards for neonates. Pediat 1967; 39:724–32.
12. Feigenbaum M. Universal Behaviour in Nonlinear Systems, Los Alamos Sci 1 (1980). In: Cvitanovic P, ed. *Universality in Chaos.* Bristol: Adam Hilger; 1984:49–84.
13. Pinkus H. The direction of growth of human epidermis. Br J Dermatol 1970; 83:556–64.
14. Ryan TJ. The direction of growth of epithelium. Br J Dermatol 1966; 78:403–15.
15. Leahy DG. The law of epidermal segmentation: The palms and soles hypothesis. (http://dgleahy.com/dgl/p24.html#footnote_13); 2002.
16. Brody I. An electron microscopic study of the fibrillar density in the normal human stratum corneum. J Ultrastruct Res 1970; 30:209–17.
17. Smith J, Fischer R, Blank H. The epidermal barrier: a comparison between scrotal and abdominal skin. J Invest Dermatol 1961; 36: 337–44.
18. Holbrook K, Odland G. Regional differences in the thickness (cell layers) of the human stratum corneum: an ultrastructural analysis. J Invest Dermatol 1974; 62:415–22.
19. Ya-Xian Z, Suetake T, Tagami H. Number of cell layers of the stratum corneum in normal skin – relationship to the anatomical location on the body, age, sex and physical parameters. Arch Dermatol Res 1999; 291:555–9.
20. Blair C. Morphology and thickness of the human stratum corneum. Br J Dermatol 1968; 80:430–6.
21. Odland G. Epidermis. In: Zelickson A, ed. *Ultrastructure of Normal and Abnormal Skin.* Philadelphia: Lea & Febiger; 1967:54–75.
22. Anderson R, Cassidy J. Variation in physical dimensions and chemical composition of human stratum corneum. J Invest Dermatol 1973; 61:30–2.

5
Morphological alterations in the stratum corneum of winter xerosis skin

A-M Minondo, P Hallégot, F Fiat and P Corcuff

As extensively described, the outermost layer of the human skin, the stratum corneum (SC), is generated by a stratified epithelium that is constantly renewing. A well-regulated desquamation is a prerequisite for an epidermal homeostasis. Moreover, SC moisturization is essential for the normal functioning of the skin. SC protects the organism against environmental stress and dehydration.[1] Strength and chemical resistance are provided by the anucleated flat cells, the corneocytes, with their characteristic rigid envelope linked to cytoplasmic keratin filaments. Corneodesmosomes, which join neighbouring corneocytes together, are the major cohesive structures within the inner SC. Retention of moisture and prevention of water loss depend on the filaggrin-derived hygroscopic components within the corneocytes and on the water-holding properties of the intercellular lipids.[2] These lipids consist of highly ordered lamellar unit structures. Actually, intracellular and extracellular components maintain tissue hydration and flexibility. The hydrolytic enzymes released by the lamellar bodies in the extracellular domains of the SC gradually modulate both lipid composition and desmosomal breakdown from the inner stratum compactum to the outer stratum disjunctum.[3,4] The enzyme-mediated degradation of corneodesmosomes requires the presence of condensed water.

Seasonal changes affect the condition of normal skin and may trigger various cutaneous disorders due to a decline in barrier function induced by decreased humidity.[5] Winter xerosis is a very common scaling disorder associated with hyperkeratinization: the shedding of dry flakes is observed whereas an imperceptible shedding of superficial corneocytes occurs in normal skin conditions. During the winter months, the skin is intrinsically more susceptible to dryness on the face, the arms, the hands and, more severely, on the legs. Dry skin with abnormal scaling of the SC is attributed to faulty desquamation and decreased water-retention properties of the SC. Xerosis is exacerbated when climatic conditions become cold and dry. The present aim of our ultrastructural studies is to illustrate the main structural entities involved in the dysfunction of xerotic SC. SC extracts, obtained by varnish-strippings from the legs of subjects with well-defined winter xerosis skin, were processed for transmission electron microscopy (TEM). Thin cross-sections, following osmium or ruthenium tetroxide postfixations, freeze-fracture replication procedure and fracture-label methods (developed by P Pinto da Silva), were performed.[6] Furthermore, one example of the improved skin xerosis condition induced by 15 days' treatment with a moisturizing product very rich in glycerol, can be shown on freeze-fracture replicas. Glycerol has been known as an effective moisturizer for decades and has consequently been widely incorporated into skincare products. However, its beneficial effects on skin xerosis have only quite recently been scientifically explained.[7,8]

Conventional TEM reveals the whole thick horny layer extracted from xerosis skin. It consists of thin, electron-dense corneocytes with indented contour (Figure 5.1a). Numerous corneodesmosomes are depicted in the upper SC layers (Figure 5.1b). Furthermore, the immunodetection of the specific corneodesmosomal protein, the corneodesmosin, on the fractured corneodesmosomes, demonstrates the presence of functional corneodesmosomes up to the upper SC layers in winter xerosis skin (Figures 5.2a and b). The abnormal retention of corneodesmosomes results in a failure to exfoliate continuously, and generates the accumulation of corneocytes at the skin surface.[9]

Following ruthenium tetroxide exposure, thin sections of xerotic SC clearly reveal the irregular distribution of lipid membranes with scarce intercellular bilayers in some areas, and numerous disorganized ones in saccular domains. These abnormally arranged lipid lamellae, interspersed within an amorphous material, are consistently located in inter-

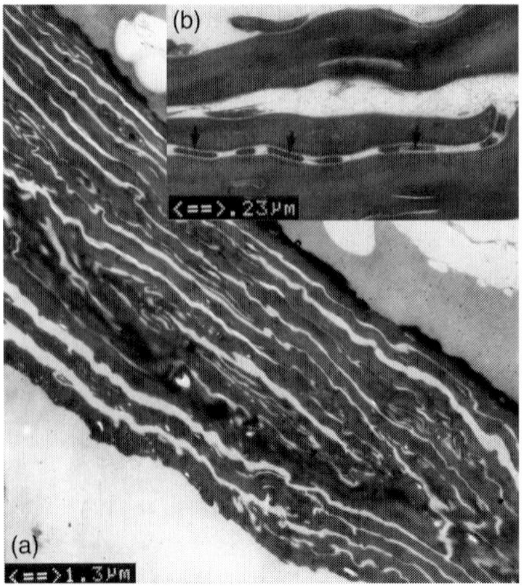

Figure 5.1

Conventional thin-section electron microscopy shows (a) the overview of the thick superficial xerotic SC extracted by varnish stripping, and (b) the presence of numerous corneodesmosomes in the upper SC layers (arrows).

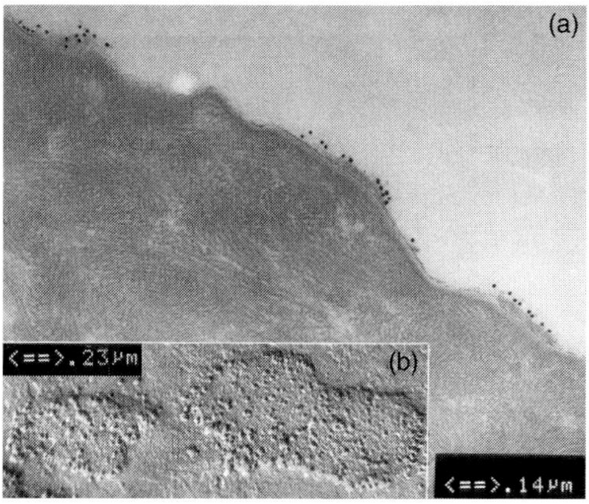

Figure 5.2

Freeze-fracture immunogold labelling was performed to reveal the fine localization of corneodesmosin within the fractured corneodesmosomes in the upper sheets of SC. (a) thin-section fracture-label method, and (b) Platinum/Carbon replica of fracture-labelled sample, displaying the two-dimensional distribution of the 10-nm gold particles on the fracture plane.

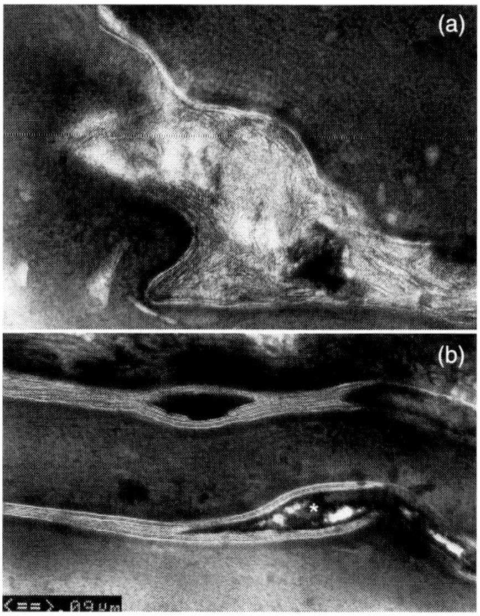

Figure 5.3

Thin sections of xerotic SC extracts reveal the complex intercellular material, following RuO_4 exposure. (a) Disorganized lipid lamellae are interspersed within amorphous material in a saccular domain, and (b) the lamellar bilayers insert into the lateral surfaces of degraded corneodesmosomal plugs. Some of them are squeezed against the corneocyte envelopes by an invasive flocculent material (*).

cellular dilatations, with pronounced indentation of the corneocytes (Figure 5.3a). A phase separation of the intercellular material can be deduced from this observation.

More or less advanced degradation of corneodesmosomal plugs is visualized within the extracellular spaces before the slow squame release. The lamellar bilayers insert into the lateral surfaces of the plug remnants. Invasive flocculent material swelling the SC interstice displaces the lamellar bilayers along the corneocyte envelopes (Figure 5.3b). Therefore, a separate non-lamellar phase is formed again. The freeze-fracture replica of the xerotic SC illustrates the intercorneocyte

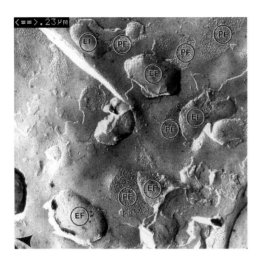

Figure 5.4

Platinum/Carbon replica from xerotic SC. The fracture planes, mainly parallel to the skin surface, display large areas of the corneocyte membranes and very sparse lamellar lipids within the SC interstice. Strikingly, a few prominent swellings are located at the level of corneodesmosomes, which are recognized as clusters of particles on the P face. EF, exoplasmic fracture face; PF, protoplasmic fracture face. Arrow in bottom left-hand corner indicates direction of platinum shadowing.

space fractured parallel to the scaly skin surface, showing a few prominent swellings located at the level of corneodesmosomes; sparse irregular laminae are also noted (Figure 5.4). This strikingly unusual image, never observed in healthy SC, suggests an altered structural lipid–desmosome interaction, which may generate disturbances in the desquamation process. Interestingly, the freeze-fracture replica of the moisturizing product-treated xerotic SC reveals broad laminae and very scarce residual corneodesmosomes within the most superficial SC interstices (data not shown). Moreover, deeper fracture planes display normal fractured corneodesmosomes surrounded by few regularly-distributed lamellar lipids (Figure 5.5). Actually, the moisturizing formulation restored xerotic skin condition to normal within 2 weeks.

Enhanced skin abnormalities during the winter season are clearly associated with dramatic perturbations to the ultrastructure of SC intercellular lipids.[10] The orderly bilayer architecture of these lipids is disrupted in the outer SC layers and their chemical composition is known to be modified.[11,12] Those changes result in a severely impaired barrier and contribute to increased transepidermal water loss.[13] The lamellar lipids no longer control the water flux within the SC efficiently. Thus, the reduced water content of xerotic SC exposed to a low relative humidity does not allow the optimal enzyme activity required for a controlled degradation of the extracellular cohesive portion of the corneodesmosomes. Moreover, as the enzymes mediate their action in the lipid matrix, the disrupted structural lipid–corneodesmosome interactions observed most likely prevent the enzymes reaching their substrates. Consequently, the disturbances in the desquamation process lead to the appearance of skin xerosis. Topical applications of glycerol-based products alleviate skin xerosis by correcting the morphological alterations. Glycerol has been

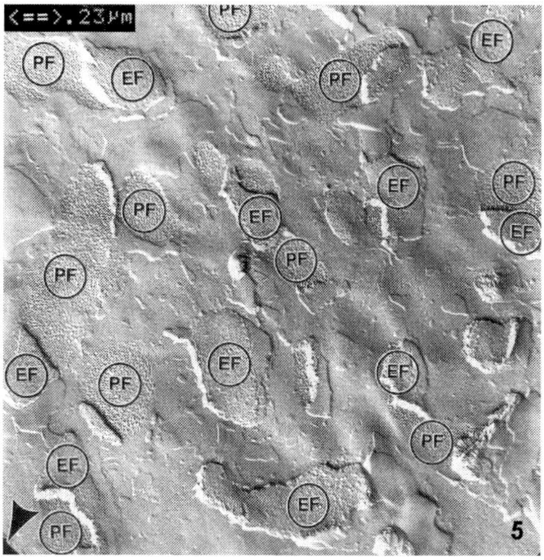

Figure 5.5

Replica from moisturizing product-treated xerotic SC illustrates normal freeze-fractured corneodesmosomal membranes surrounded by regular lamellar lipids. EF, exoplasmic fracture face; PF, protoplasmic fracture face. Arrow in bottom left-hand corner indicates direction of platinum shadowing.

shown to modulate the phase behavior of the SC lipids. It fluidizes these lipids and prevents their crystallization in low-humidity conditions. Glycerol allows recovery of the normal lipid organization mandatory for the restoration of an impermeable barrier. The resultant improved hydration allows normal corneodesmosomal degradation in the outer SC layers, which can, therefore, regularly exfoliate.[14,15]

Appendix

Freeze-fracture cleavage occurs at low temperature in the region of least resistance. Freeze-fracture of plasma membranes splits the hydrophobic core of the two opposite bilayers. The nomenclature used to label the freeze-fractured membranes distinguishes E and P faces exposed after fracturing. EF = Exoplasmic fracture face and PF = Protoplasmic fracture face. The arrowheads in the lower left corners of Figures 5.4 and 5.5 indicate the direction of the shadowing.

References

1. Elias PM. The stratum corneum revisited. J Dermatol 1996; 23: 756–68.
2. Laokawa G, Hattori M. A possible function of structural lipids in the water-holding properties of the stratum corneum. J Invest Dermatol 1985; 84:282–4.
3. Egelrud T. Desquamation in the stratum corneum. Acta Derm Venereol 2000; 208:44–5.
4. Piérard GE, Goffin V, Hermanns-Le T et al. Corneocyte desquamation (review). Int J Mol Med 2000; 6:217–21.
5. Denda M, Sato J, Tsuchiya T et al.

Low humidity stimulates epidermal DNA synthesis and amplifies the hyperproliferative response to barrier disruption: implication for seasonal exacerbations of inflammatory dermatoses. J Invest Dermatol 1998; 111:873–8.

6. Torrisi MR, Mancini P. Freeze-fracture immunogold labeling (review). Histochem Cell Biol 1996; 106: 19–30.
7. Rawlings A, Harding C, Watkinson A et al. The effect of glycerol and humidity on desmosome degradation in stratum corneum. Arch Dermatol Res 1995; 287:457–64.
8. Warner RR, Boissy YL. Effect of moisturizing products on the structure of lipids in the outer stratum corneum of humans. In: Lodén M, Maibach HI, eds. *Dry Skin and Moisturizers, Chemistry and Function*. CRC Press 2000: 349–69.
9. Simon M, Bernard D, Minondo A-M et al. Persistence of both peripheral and non-peripheral corneodesmosomes in the upper stratum corneum of winter xerosis skin versus only peripheral in normal skin. J Invest Dermatol 2001; 116: 23–30.
10. Fartasch M. Epidermal barrier in disorders of the skin. Microsc Res Tech 1997; 38:361–72.
11. Menon G, Ghadially R. Morphology of lipid alterations in the epidermis: a review. Microsc Res Tech 1997; 37:180–92.
12. Conti A, Rogers J, Verdejo P et al. Seasonal influences on stratum corneum ceramide 1 fatty acids and the influence of topical essential fatty acids. Int J Cosmet Sci 1996; 18:1–12.
13. Lévêque JL, Garson JC, De Rigal J. Transepidermal water loss from dry and normal skin. J Soc Cosmet Chem 1979; 30:333–43.
14. Summers RS, Summers B, Chandar P et al. The effect of lipids, with and without humectant, on skin xerosis. J Soc Cosmet Chem 1996; 47:27–39.
15. Fartasch M, Bassukas ID, Diepgen TL. Structural relationship between epidermal lipid lamellae, lamellar bodies and desmosomes in human epidermis: an ultrastructural study. Br J Dermatol 1993; 128:1–9.

6
The single gel-phase and the membrane-folding model for skin barrier structure, function and formation

L Norlén

Introduction

In contrast to the equilibrium situation in vitro, living systems are essentially open, non-linear, far from equilibrium, dissipative structures. A stop of the energy flow through the living system will eventually bring it to thermodynamic equilibrium, i.e. death. One striking feature of biological membranes is the apparent spontaneous self-organization. The basic question is whether this is the result of a local equilibrium, i.e. the intracell variations due to external fluxes are smaller than the local equilibrium fluctuations in the cell, or whether the exchange of energy with the surrounding, i.e. energy dissipation, is the source of internal order. Thus, in order to make predictions about the structure, function and dynamics of a system, like, e.g. the mammalian skin barrier, not only the composition and topology of, but also the gradients over, this system must be known in considerable detail.

Notwithstanding the spectacular progress made in the field of skin barrier research during the last 25 years, there still exist today rather few incontestable facts about the structure and dynamics of the lipid membranes constituting the skin barrier. This is certainly due to the compositional as well as functional complexity common to many biological systems, but also to the fact that epidermal cell-space is open (i.e. transversed by different gradients). It is consequently out of equilibrium, and, therefore, difficult to model in vitro.

The most serious problem, however, that skin-barrier research is confronted with is that we do not know what (irreversible) artefacts we introduce during standard sample storage and sample preparation procedures, e.g. electron microscopy and X-ray diffraction. Heat separation of epidermis, dehydration in a dessication chamber, storage in a freezer, solvent exposure, dehydration and fixation during preparation for electron microscopy, etc, are procedures that are likely to have profound effects on the structural organization of the lipid membranes constituting the skin barrier. This is especially so since, in their endogenous (i.e. in vivo) state, these membranes may not represent equilibrium structures, but may, instead, be stabilized by a feature of a secondary, or higher, minimum energy order (cf. above).

The most evident gradient over the skin barrier membrane system is in water chemical potential, with a water concentration of approximately 70–80% (w/w) of the living tissue inside the body and a variable water concentration of about 10–20% (w/w) of the outer stratum corneum in equilibrium with the often dry, environmental air.[1,2] Less is known about the remaining gradients and distributions over the skin, of importance for lipid phase-behaviour, such as gradients in ion concentrations, pH, gas concentrations (e.g. CO_2, O_2), lipid compositions and temperature. One important reason for this is the scarcity of topological data present today. In fact, the only incontestably known, structural features of the stratum corneum lipid matrix are that it is extracellular, continuous, multilamellar,[3,4] and at physiological conditions, largely 'crystalline' in character (i.e. has a low water content).[5–7] Virtually nothing is known about the actual lamellar organization, the distribution of water, ions and gases, the association of proteins, or the connectivity or genus (number of handles or holes) of the continuous membrane structure.

Despite the above-mentioned shortcomings, the data available today suffices for some far-reaching speculations to be made with respect not only to skin barrier structure and function, but also to the formation of this highly specialized membrane structure.

It was, thus, recently proposed that skin barrier formation may take place as a 'flattening' or an 'unfolding' of a three-dimensional, curved membrane structure into the flat, multilayered, two-dimensional lipid structure of the stratum corneum intercellular space, i.e. without fusion of so-called 'lamellar bodies'.[8] In fact, even the mere existence of 'lamellar bodies' was questioned. It was further postulated that the skin barrier, i.e. the intercellular lipid within the stratum corneum, exists as a *single and coherent* 'gel'-structure, or, equivalently, an extremely tightly packed liquid crystal which, under certain circumstances, may express true crystalline hydrocarbon chain organization in local cholesterol-deficient regions.[9] Below follows a short review of the newly-proposed *membrane folding model* and *single gel-phase model*, respectively.

Skin barrier formation

From a theoretical point of view, there are several serious difficulties that nature has to overcome if skin barrier formation is to take place via the massive membrane fusion/diffusion process proposed in the Landmann model.[10] More specifically, membrane budding, fusion and diffusion processes cost energy (due to large membrane curvature changes involved, cf. References 11 and 12), imply decreased control (due to the topology changes involved, i.e. the membrane disintegration and reintegration, respectively) over the barrier formation process (including water homeostasis and control thereof), and are time consuming (involves diffusion; fusiogenic processes do not macroscopically represent lipid phase transformations).

In fact, the whole process of skin barrier formation could, theoretically, be performed without energetically unfavourable processes such as membrane budding and membrane fusion, and without vesicular diffusion (i.e. slow transport, hours) of lipid components, through intersection-free* membrane folding/unfolding (cf. References 13 and 14).

It has, therefore, recently been proposed that skin barrier morphogenesis may take place via a continuous, highly dynamic process of 'intersection-free unfolding' (i.e. a continuous deformation of a single and coherent, curved three-dimensional† lipid structure (i.e. saddle-shaped) into a flat, two-dimensional‡ lipid structure) with a concomitant 'crystallization' of the developing stacked multilamellar lipid structure representing the skin barrier[8] (Figure 6.1). In fact, continuous, dynamic foldings/unfoldings between cubic (three-dimensionally hyperbolic, i.e. saddle-shaped) and lamellar (flat, two-dimensionally Euclidian) structures are present in numerous other biological systems, such as the endoplasmatic reticulum of metazoan cells,[14:94,15,16] and the thylacoid membrane of plant chloroplasts[13,14:140–1,17–19] (Figure 6.2).

The absence of geometric constraints during the proposed membrane 'flattening' or 'unfolding' would allow the skin barrier formation process to be extremely fast, i.e. momentary, since it basically represents a phase§ transformation from cubic-like to lamellar morphology. As the thermodynamics of this unfolding procedure are related to curvature energy, asymmetrical objects (e.g. proteins) that bind to both sides of the lipid bilayer could play a regulatory role.[20] It may, thus, be finely tuned by subtle stimuli. Skin-barrier formation taking place via an unfolding process consequently may be highly controlled and very fast (as compared to diffusion-dependent processes, cf. Reference 10).[8]

The profound difference between the Landmann model and the membrane folding model is that the Landmann model includes changes in

---

* i.e. ignore fusion.

† i.e. membrane constellation centred around a surface with *negative* average Gaussian curvature, or equivalently with genus higher than 1 (i.e. containing two or more handles or holes).

‡ i.e. membrane constellation centered around a surface with *zero* average Gaussian curvature, or equivalently with genus 1 (i.e. containing one handle or hole).

§ Note that the current use of the word 'phase' in a biological context is not necessarily reflecting thermodynamically stable phase-states.

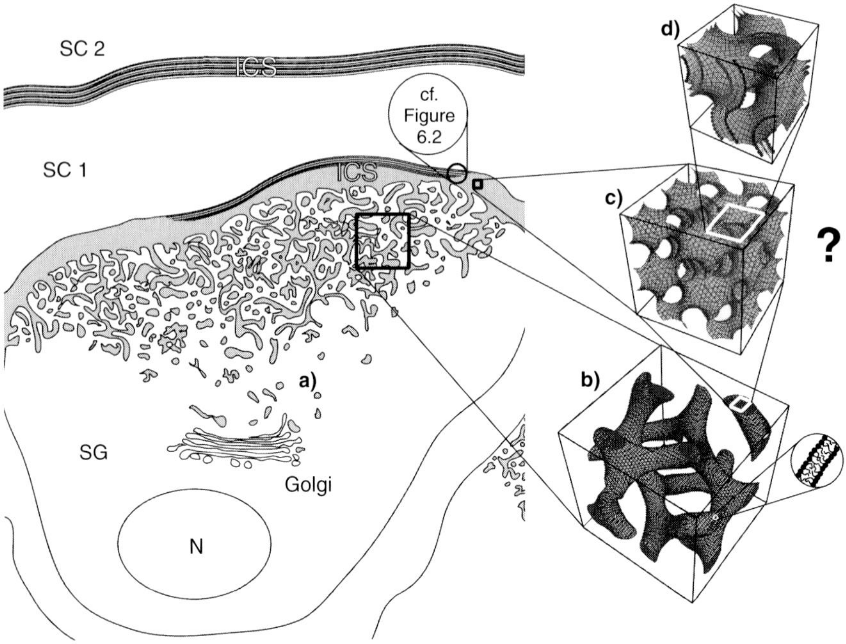

Figure 6.1

The membrane-folding model for skin barrier formation. Skin barrier formation taking place via a continuous, highly-dynamic process of 'intersection-free unfolding' of a single and coherent three-dimensional lipid structure with symmetry. Note that the trans-Golgi network and lamellar bodies of the uppermost stratum granulosum cells, as well as the multilamellar lipid matrix of the intercellular space at the border zone between stratum granulosum and stratum corneum, are visualized (light grey) as being parts of one and the same continuous membrane structure (a). Tentatively, the proposed single and coherent three-dimensional lipid structure with symmetry may consist of an *outer* folded membrane (e.g. cubic-like) with a large lattice parameter (> 500 nm) (b), and an *inner*, more highly-curved membrane with symmetry (c) expressing continuous foldings/unfoldings between cubic-like and lamellar morphologies (cf. Figure 6.2). Note that this detailed description of the proposed barrier-forming lipid structure is but one out of many possible, all of which share the basic idea of three-dimensional symmetry, continuity and dynamics. (d) Unit cell (schematic) of the proposed three-dimensional lipid structure (note the curved membrane) expressing intersection-free folding/unfolding. ICS: intercellular space; N: nucleus; SC 1: first stacked stratum corneum cell; SC 2: second stacked stratum corneum cell; SG: uppermost stratum granulosum cell. After Norlén,[8] with permission from Blackwell Science.

membrane topology, while topology is kept constant during barrier formation according to the membrane folding model.

The main advantages of the membrane folding model with respect to the Landmann model are the following:

(i) smaller energy cost (involves no budding or fusion);

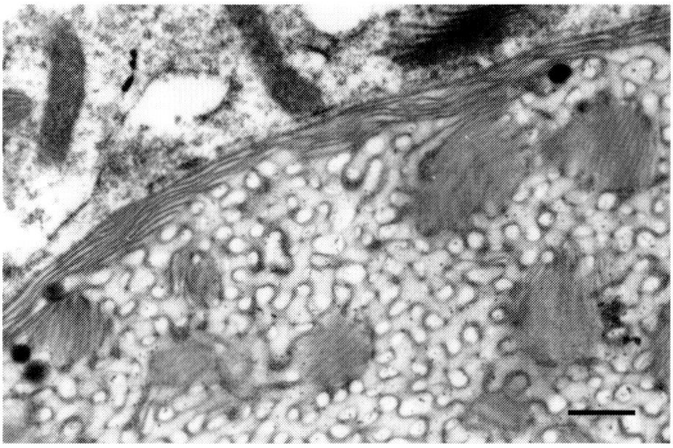

Figure 6.2

Continuous foldings/unfoldings between cubic and lamellar membrane structures in chloroplasts of the green alga Zygnema. Note the similarity of the rounded crystalline lamellar parts with 'lamellar bodies' of the stratum granulosum of mammalian skin. Transmission electron micrograph of the chloroplast Gyroid-based (G-type) cubic membrane morphology (cf. Reference 14). By the courtesy of Dr Yuru Deng. Scale bar = 0.5 μm.

(ii) conserves membrane continuity (preserves water compartmentalization and allows control thereof; membrane continuity essential for barrier function);
(iii) allows meticulous control (the thermodynamics of the unfolding procedure are related to curvature energy);
(iv) faster (milliseconds, since membrane unfolding basically represents a phase transition from cubic-like to lamellar morphology; involves no budding or fusion);
(v) membrane folding between lamellar and cubic-like morphologies is present in numerous biological systems (cf. References 14 and 21:257–338);
(vi) there is experimental evidence for an 'extensive intracellular tubulo-reticular cisternal membrane system within the apical cytosol of the outermost stratum granulosum' (Figure 6.3);[22]
(vii) it may explain the reported plethora of forms, numbers, sizes and general appearances of 'lamellar bodies' in TEM micrographs;[23,24]
(viii) it may partly explain the heterogeneous chain length distributions of epidermal lipids, through a stabilization of three-dimensional hyperbolic interfaces (showing variations in Gaussian curvature).*

* The molecules can then redistribute themselves over regions with variations in Gaussian curvature and therefore stabilize cubic-like interfaces. This is exemplified by the fact that a *reduction* in the monodispersity of self-assembled copolymer systems may significantly enhance the strength of these materials. Further, admixing polydisperse homopolymers to lamellar copolymer systems leads to the formation of bicontinuous hyperbolic mesophases.[25]

Skin barrier structure and function

Below, the general definition of a gel-phase is used, where 'gel-phase' signifies any highly 'condensed', or equivalently 'compressed' or 'crystallized', lamellar lipid phase with much reduced lateral diffusion of lipid molecules and low water content as compared to liquid crystalline phases, where the lipid hydrocarbon chains are 'melted' and lateral diffusion is practically unhindered. From a purely crystallographic point of view, this means that, in the absence of cholesterol, a 'gel-phase' has hexagonally-packed hydrocarbon chains (i.e. it is a loosely packed crystal) (cf. References 26:16–18,24–31;27:98–101;28:13–14,27) while in the presence of cholesterol, a 'gel-phase' is in fact an extremely tightly-packed liquid crystal (since no true crystalline X-ray wide-angle reflections can be obtained if cholesterol molecules are inserted between the lipid hydrocarbon chains). In summary, in cholesterol-deficient regions, a 'gel-phase' is, thus, a hexagonally packed crystal, while in cholesterol-enriched regions, a 'gel-phase' is an extremely tightly-packed liquid crystal. It should be noted, however, that density distributions of cholesterol can be present in membranes without any true thermodynamic lipid phase-separation. Further, given the high cholesterol content of the skin barrier lipid matrix (~45 mol% including cholesteryl esters[29,30]), a 'gel-phase' is here defined as an extremely tightly-packed liquid crystal,* which, under certain circumstances, may express true crystalline hydrocarbon chain packing in local cholesterol-deficient regions.

The most characteristic features of stratum corneum lipid composition[29–31] are (i) extensive compositional heterogeneity, (ii) almost complete dominance of saturated, very long hydrocarbon chains (20–36C), and (iii) large relative amounts of cholesterol (~35 mol%[29,30]). It is noteworthy that the stability of gel-phases increases with chain length, with compositional impurities (e.g. heterogeneity in chain length distributions) and with the presence of cholesterol.[28:27,43;32:412;33]

Accordingly, it was recently proposed that the skin barrier, i.e. the intercellular lipid within the stratum corneum, may exist as a single and coherent lamellar gel-phase.[9] Consequently, the lipid organization of the skin barrier may resemble that of non-ionic detergent-resistant membrane fragments (DRMs)† isolated from a variety of eukaryotic cells. These, like the skin barrier lipid matrix, are composed of a mixture of saturated long acyl-chain sphingolipids and cholesterol and, likewise, exist as a liquid-ordered structure.[34–38]

---

* i.e. a liquid ordered structure with low water content and limited or no lateral diffusion of lipid hydrocarbon chains.

† DRMs are thought to be derived from so-called membrane 'rafts'.

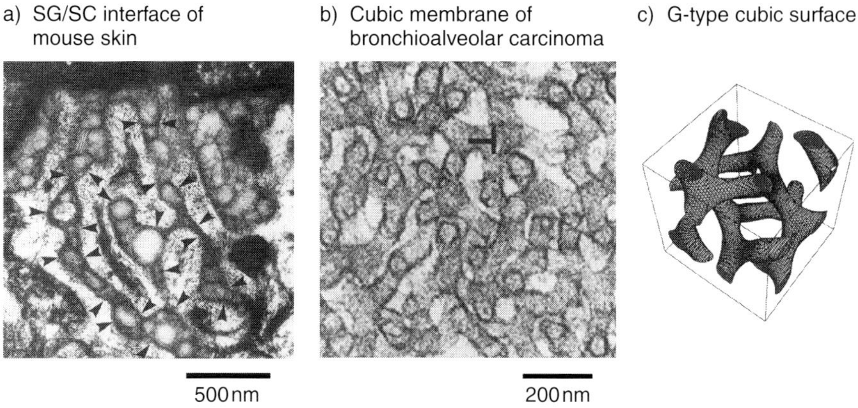

Figure 6.3

Cubic-like membrane or lamellar bodies? RuO_4 postfixated oblique section of the stratum granulosum/stratum corneum interface of mouse skin (a). Scale bar = 0.5 μm. After Elias et al,[22] with permission from Blackwell Science Publications. Note the similarity between the 'interconnected lattice' of 'lamellar bodies' in (a) and the swollen cubic membrane morphology of bronchioloalveolar carcinomas (b). Scale bar = 0.2 μm. After Ghadially[41] with permission from Edward Arnold Publishers. Mathematical 3D reconstruction of the G-type cubic morphology with a positive (>1) mean curvature level surface (c). After Norlén,[8] with permission from Blackwell Science Publications.

A single and coherent gel-phase may, in a biological context, be ideal as a barrier towards the environment. This is because it is a continuous lipid structure with pronounced compositional heterogeneity which may, irrespective of environmental (physiologically relevant) conditions, possess (a) low permeability (due to the close packing of the saturated, long hydrocarbon chains), at the same time as being (b) mechanically resistant (due to its 'plasticity' or 'pliability' rendered by the retained rotational disorder of the hydrocarbon chains in the hexagonal arrangement and/or cholesterol-enriched 'condensed' liquid crystal), and expressing (c) little or no tendency for phase transitions, phase separation or induction of 'pores' or non-lamellar structures.

The single gel-phase model differs in a most significant way from earlier models in that it clearly states that *no true thermodynamic (i.e. macroscopic) phase separation*, neither between liquid crystalline and crystalline phases (cf. the domain-mosaic model of Forslind[39]) nor between different crystalline phases with hexagonal and orthorhombic chain packing, respectively (cf. References 7 and 40), is present in the unperturbed barrier structure.[9]

References

1. Warner RR, Myers MC, Taylor DA. Electron probe analysis of human skin: determination of the water concentration profile. J Invest Dermatol 1988; 90:218–24.
2. von Zglinicki T, Lindberg M, Roomans GM et al. Water and ion-distribution profiles in human skin. Acta Derm Venereol (Stockh) 1993; 73:340–3.
3. Breathnach AS, Goodman T, Stolinski C et al. Freeze fracture replication of cells of stratum corneum of human epidermis. J Anat 1973; 114:65–81.
4. Elias PM, Friend DS. The permeability barrier in mammalian epidermis. J Cell Biol 1975; 65: 180–91.
5. Garson J-C, Doucet J, Lévêque J-L et al. Oriented structure in human stratum corneum revealed by x-ray diffraction. J Invest Dermatol 1991; 96:43–9.
6. Bouwstra JA, Gooris GS, Van der Spek JA et al. Structural investigations of human stratum corneum by small-angle X-ray scattering. J Invest Dermatol 1991; 97: 1005–12.
7. Bouwstra JA, Gooris GS, Salmon-de Vries MA et al. Structure of human stratum corneum as a function of temperature and hydration: a wide-angle X-ray diffraction study. Inter J Pharmaceut 1992; 84:205–16.
8. Norlén LPO. Skin barrier formation – the membrane folding model. J Invest Dermatol 2001; 17:823–9.
9. Norlén LPO. Skin barrier structure and function – the single gel-phase model. J Invest Dermatol 2001; 17:830–6.
10. Landmann L. Epidermal permeability barrier: transformation of lamellar granule-disks into intercellular sheets by a membrane-fusion process, a freeze-fracture study. J Invest Dermatol 1986; 87:202–9.
11. Helfrich W. Elastic properties of lipid bilayers: theory and possible experiments. Z Naturforsch 1973; 28c:693–703.
12. Fogden A, Hyde ST, Lundberg G. Bending energy of surfactant films. J Chem Soc Faraday Trans 1991; 87:949–55.
13. Landh T. From entangled membranes to eclectic morphologies: cubic membranes as subcellular space organizers. FEBS Lett 1995; 369:13–17.
14. Landh T. Cubic cell membrane architectures – taking another look at membrane bound cell spaces (thesis). Dept of Food Technology, Lund University, Lund, Sweden; 1996.
15. Oparka KJ, Johnson PC. Endoplasmatic reticulum and crystalline fibrils in the root protophloem of *Nymphoides peltata*. Planta 1978; 143:21–7.
16. Pathak RK, Luskey KL, Anderson RGW. Biogenesis of the crystalloid endoplasmic reticulum in UT-1 cells: evidence that the newly formed endoplasmatic reticulum emerges from the nuclear envelope. J Cell Biol 1986; 102: 2158–68.
17. von Wettstein D. The formation of plastid structures. Brookhaven Symp Biol 1959; 11:138–59.
18. Gunning BES. The greening process in plastids. 1. The structure of the prolamellar body. Protoplasma 1965; 60:111–30.
19. Deng Y, Landh T. The cubic gyroid-based membrane structure of the chloroplast in Zygnema (*Chlorophyceae zygnematales*). Zool Stud 1995; 34:175–7.
20. Fournier JB. Non-topological saddle-splay and curvature instabili-

ties from anisotropic membrane inclusions. Phys Rev Letters 1996; 76:4436–9.

21. Hyde S, Andersson S, Larsson K et al. *The Language of Shape. The Role of Curvature in Condensed Matter: Physics, Chemistry and Biology*. Amsterdam: Elsevier Science B.V.; 1997.
22. Elias PM, Cullander C, Mauro T et al. The secretory granular cell: the outermost granular cell as a specialized secretory cell. J Invest Dermatol Symp Proceedings 1998; 3:87–100.
23. Brody I. A light electron microscopy study of normal human stratum corneum with particular refernce to the intercellular space. Upsala J Med Sci 1989; 94:29–45.
24. Madison KC, Sando GN, Howard EJ et al. Lamellar granule biogenesis: a role for ceramide glycosyltransferase, lysosomal enzyme transport, and the Golgi. J Invest Dermatol Symp Proceedings 1998; 3:80–6.
25. Hasegawa H, Hashimoto T, Hyde ST. Microdomain structures with hyperbolic interfaces in block and graft polymers. Polymer 1996; 37:3825–33.
26. Hernquist L. Polymorphism of fats (thesis). Dept of Food Technology, Lund University, Lund, Sweden; 1984.
27. Small DM. *The Physical Chemistry of Lipids. Handbook of Lipid Research.* New York: Plenum Press; 1986.
28. Larsson K. *Lipids: Molecular Organisation, Physical Functions and Technical Applications.* Dundee, Scotland: The Oily Press; 1994.
29. Wertz PW, Swartzendruber DC, Kathi CM et al. Composition and morphology of epidermal cyst lipids. J Invest Dermatol 1987; 89: 419–24.
30. Norlén L, Nicander I, Lundh-Rozell B et al. Inter and intra individual differences in human stratum corneum lipid content related to physical parameters of skin barrier function in vivo. J Invest Dermatol 1999; 112:72–7.
31. Norlén L, Nicander I, Lundsjö A et al. A new HPLC-based method for the quantitative analysis of inner stratum corneum lipids with special reference to the free fatty acid fraction. Arch Derm Res 1998; 290:508–16.
32. Evans FD, Wennerström H. *The Colloidal Domain: Where Physics, Chemistry, Biology and Technology Meet.* New York: VCH Publishers; 1994.
33. Takahashi H, Sinoda K, Hatta I. Effects of cholesterol on the lamellar and the inverted hexagonal phases of dielaidoylphosphatidylethanolamine. Biochim Biophys Acta 1996; 1289:209–16.
34. Ahmed SN, Brown DA, London E. On the origin of sphingolipid/cholesterol-rich detergent-insoluble cell membranes: physiological concentrations of cholesterol and sphingolipid induce formation of a detergent-insoluble, liquid-ordered lipid phase in model membranes. Biochemistry 1997; 36:10944–53.
35. Brown DA, London E. Structure of detergent-resistant membrane domains: does phase separation occur in biological membranes? Biochem Biophys Res Commun 1997; 240:1–7.
36. Brown RE. Sphingolipid organization in biomembranes: what physical studies of model membranes reveal. J Cell Sci 1998; 111:1–9.
37. Ge M, Field KA, Aneja R et al. Electron spin resonance characterization of liquid ordered phase of detergent-resistant membranes from RBL-2H3 cells. Biophys J 1999; 77:925–33.

38. Xu X, London E. The effect of sterol structure on membrane lipid domains reveals how cholesterol can induce lipid domain formation. Biochemistry 2000; 39:843–9.
39. Forslind B. A domain mosaic model of the skin barrier. Acta Derm Venereol (Stockh) 1994; 74: 1–6.
40. Pilgram GSK, Engelsma-van Pelt AM, Bouwstra JA et al. Electron diffraction provides new information on human stratum corneum lipid organization studied in relation to depth and temperature. J Invest Dermatol 1999; 113:101–7.
41. Ghadially FN. Ultrastructural pathology of the cell and maxtrix. 3rd edn, vol 1. 1988, London: Butterworths.

7

Corneodesmosomal proteins are proteolysed in vitro by both SCTE and SCCE – two proteases which are thought to be involved in desquamation

M Simon, D Bernard, C Caubet, M Guerrin, T Egelrud, R Schmidt and G Serre

Introduction

Corneodesmosomes, the modified desmosomes of the stratum corneum (SC), are largely responsible for the strong corneocyte cohesion, and are crucial for a proper barrier function of the epidermis. Their degradation at the epidermal surface is of major importance for a normal desquamation process. In xeroses and various hyperkeratoses, as well as in palmoplantar skin, accumulation of scales is observed, and the number of corneodesmosomes persisting on the corneocyte surface in the upper SC is greatly increased. Two proteases present in the extracellular spaces of the cornified layer, the stratum corneum tryptic enzyme (SCTE) and the stratum corneum chymotryptic enzyme (SCCE), are thought to be involved in the degradation, but direct evidence of their role is still lacking.[1,2] SCCE and SCTE are serine proteases of the kallikrein family, synthesized as inactive pro-forms.

The major adhesive components of corneodesmosomes are two glycoproteins of the cadherin family, namely desmoglein 1 (Dsg1) and desmocollin 1 (Dsc1). Each desmosomal cadherin is known to exist as three different isoforms, encoded by three different genes, Dsg1 and Dsc1 being expressed in the uppermost layers of the epidermis.[3] Synthesized and secreted by granular keratinocytes, corneodesmosin (Cdsn) is also an adhesive glycoprotein, located in the extracellular part of corneodesmosomes. It is a 529-amino-acid long, glycine- and serine-rich protein. These amino acids form particular secondary structures, the so-called glycine loop-related domains, the function of which could be to interact with identical loops on the same or neighbouring proteins. During the maturation of the SC, Cdsn is progressively proteolysed.[4–6]

Until now, the enzymes involved in this proteolysis are not clearly identified.

To directly test the involvement of the two proteases in corneodesmosome degradation, we analysed in vitro the proteolytic activity of SCTE and SCCE towards these adhesive corneodesmosomal proteins.

Methods

Extracts of human epidermis were incubated with a fraction of human epidermis highly enriched in SCTE, with recombinant pro-SCCE, and with purified, either recombinant or epidermal, SCCE. Treatments were performed at a neutral pH of 7.4, and, also, after dialysis of the extracts, at a more acidic pH of 5.6, closer to the physiological pH of the SC. Proteins of the extracts were then separated by electrophoresis, stained with Protogold, and immunodetected with monoclonal antibodies directed to desmogleins (DG3.10) or Cdsn (F28–27), and with sera specific for either desmocollins or involucrin (a cornified cell envelope component).

Results

At pH 7.4, SCTE completely degraded Cdsn, and generated fragments of 48 and 35 kDa. Incubation in the absence of the enzyme was without effect on the protein. The enzyme also totally degraded desmocollins, whereas most of the other proteins in the extracts, as shown by Protogold staining, remained unaffected. In particular, desmogleins and involucrin were not cleaved (Figure 7.1). At pH 5.6, Cdsn was degraded by SCTE into fragments of identical molecular mass but with a somewhat lower efficiency. However, desmocollins were not proteolysed.

At pH 7.4, SCCE generated several Cdsn fragments, from 15 to 48 kDa. Incubation with recombinant inactive pro-SCCE or in the absence of enzymes was without effect on Cdsn. The active enzyme also induced degradation of desmocollins to immunoreactive fragments of 95 kDa. Most of the other proteins were not proteolysed (Figure 7.2). Identical results were obtained with both the epidermal and recombinant SCCE. At pH 5.6, proteolysis of Cdsn and desmocollins by SCCE was also observed, whereas the treatment was without effect on desmogleins and involucrin.

Conclusion

These results demonstrate that Cdsn and, to a lesser extent, desmocollins are in vitro substrates of both SCCE and SCTE. They suggest that

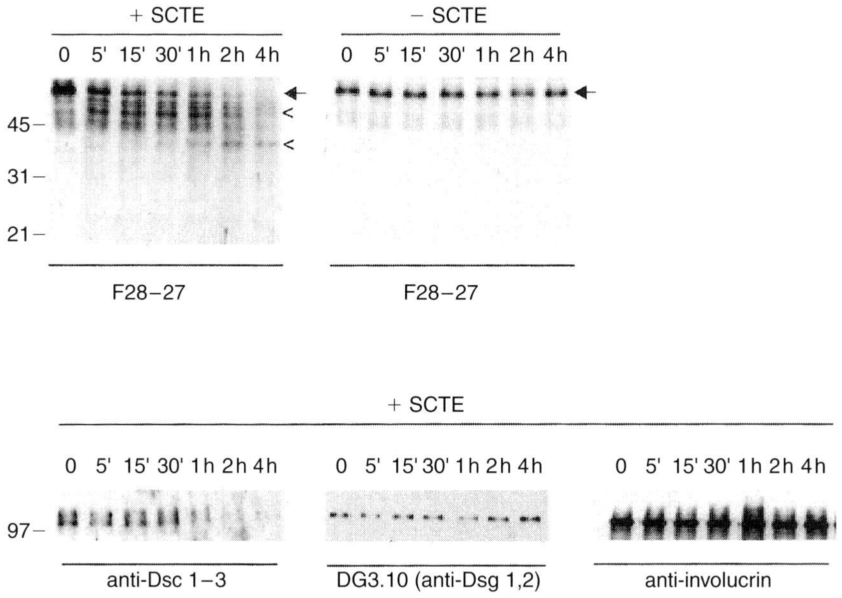

Figure 7.1

Effect of SCTE on epidermal proteins. Proteins extracted from human epidermis in the presence of a detergent were incubated with (+) or without (–) SCTE for increasing periods of time, as indicated on top of the plates. After stopping of the reaction, proteins were immunoblotted with F28–27 and DG3.10 monoclonal antibodies, and with sera directed against either desmocollins or involucrin, as indicated. Arrows indicate the 52–56 kDa Cdsn. Open arrowheads show the immunodetected Cdsn fragments. The position of molecular mass standards (kDa) is indicated on the left.

the proteases are involved in the proteolytic maturation of Cdsn in the SC and/or in the degradation of adhesive components of corneodesmosomes at the skin surface. They support previous studies that highlight the importance of both enzymes in desquamation. Therefore, a model of protease involvement in the degradation of corneodesmosome components and in desquamation can be proposed (Figure 7.3). Under an unknown signal, the inactive pro-SCTE is activated. In turn, the active SCTE is engaged in Cdsn processing, at the lower SC. It may also be the enzyme that activates SCCE. The active SCCE degrades Cdsn and Dsc1 in the upper SC. The protease that cleaves Dsg1 is not yet known, but may be one of the cysteine or aspartic proteases detected in the upper layer of the epidermis.

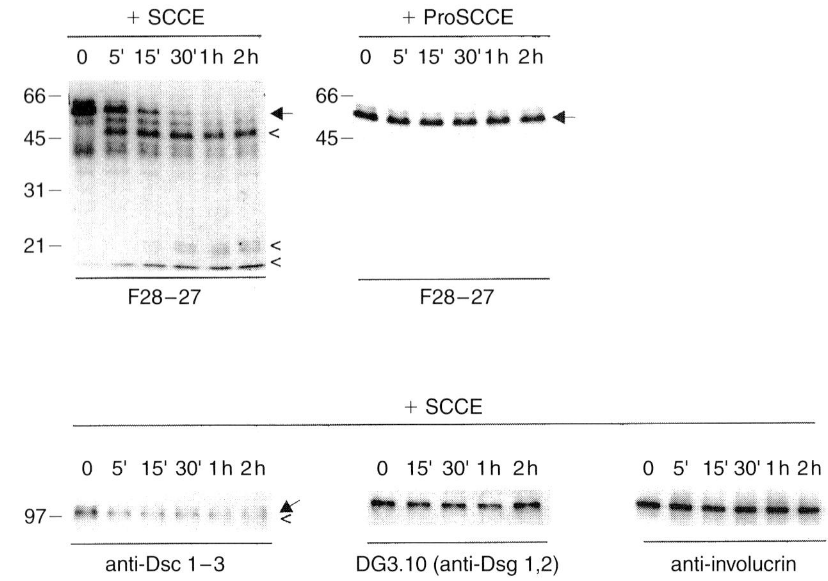

Figure 7.2

Effect of SCCE on epidermal proteins. Proteins extracted from human epidermis in the presence of a detergent were incubated with the active enzyme (+ SCCE) or with its inactive precursor (+ ProSCCE) for increasing periods of time. Proteins were then immunoblotted with F28–27 and DG3.10, and with sera directed against either desmocollins or involucrin. Arrows indicate either the 52–56 kDa Cdsn (top) or the 110 kDa desmocollins (bottom). Open arrowheads show the immunodetected protein fragments.

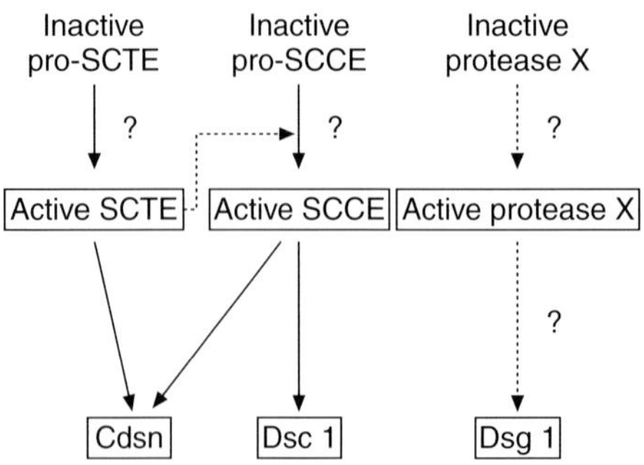

Figure 7.3

Involvement of proteases in desquamation: a model.

References

1. Hansson L, Strömqvist M, Bäckman A et al. Cloning, expression, and characterization of stratum corneum chymotryptic enzyme. J Biol Chem 1994; 269:19420–6.
2. Brattsand M, Egelrud T. Purification, molecular cloning, and expression of a human stratum corneum trypsin-like serine protease with possible function in desquamation. J Biol Chem 1999; 274:30033–40.
3. Arnemann J, Sullivan KH, Magee AI et al. Stratification-related expression of isoforms of the desmosomal cadherins in human epidermis. J Cell Science 1993; 104:741–50.
4. Guerrin M, Simon M, Montézin M et al. Expression cloning of human corneodesmosin proves its identity with the product of the S gene and allows improved characterization of its processing during keratinocyte differentiation. J Biol Chem 1998; 273:22640–7.
5. Simon M, Jonca N, Guerrin M et al. Refined characterization of corneodesmosin proteolysis during terminal differentiation of human epidermis and its relationship to desquamation. J Biol Chem 2001; 276:20292–9.
6. Jonca N, Guerrin M, Hadjiolova K et al. Corneodesmosin, a component of epidermal corneocyte desmosomes, displays homophilic adhesive properties. J Biol Chem 2002; 277:5024–9.

8
Calmodulin-like skin protein (CLSP): a new marker of keratinocyte differentiation

B Méhul, D Bernard and R Schmidt

After separating by two-dimensional gel electrophoresis, an extract of total proteins from human stratum corneum, two spots were extracted and analysed for their peptide sequence.[1] The resulting internal protein sequences provided evidence for the identification of a new calcium-binding protein. Cloning of the corresponding full-length cDNA was achieved by RT–PCR using keratinocyte libraries.[1] The cDNA had an open reading frame encoding for a calcium-binding protein of 146 amino acids, a new member of the calmodulin family.

Calmodulin is known to interact with several different target proteins.[2,3] Based on amino acid sequence analysis, our protein revealed only 52% homology with calmodulin.[1] RT-PCR studies of CLSP expression in 10 different human tissues indicated that our protein was particularly abundant in the epidermis, and directly related to keratinocyte differentiation. For these reasons, we named the protein CLSP.[4] A Western blot analysis, using a specific polyclonal antibody against CLSP, of extracts obtained from keratinocytes cultured either in low (0.1 mmol/1) or high (1.15 mmol/1) calcium,[5,6] showed that, in cultured keratinocytes, CLSP expression was strongly induced after stimulating cell differentiation by increasing the medium calcium concentration (Figure 8.1). The observation that non-differentiated keratinocytes do not express CLSP was confirmed by confocal microscopy analysis of a confluent keratinocyte culture.[4] Known modulators of epidermal differentiation, sodium butyrate[7] and a synthetic retinoid,[8] affected CLSP expression.[4] A more than 10-fold increase was observed in the presence of sodium butyrate (Figure 8.2), whereas the retinoid abolished CLSP expression almost completely (Figure 8.3); in contrast, calmodulin was not affected by these modulators (Figures 8.2 and 8.3), whereas CLSP expression correlates directly with the degree of keratinocyte differentiation in reconstructed human skin,[9] both at mRNA[1] and protein levels.[4] CLSP expression is restricted to the stratum granulosum and the lower layers of the stratum corneum in normal human epidermis (Figure 8.4).

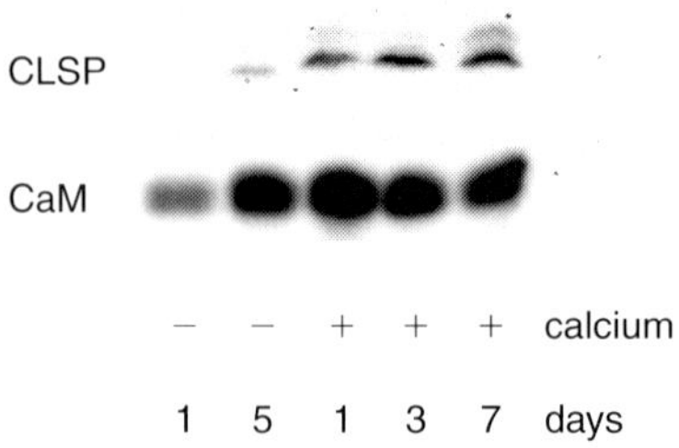

Figure 8.1

Western blot analysis of CLSP and calmodulin (CaM) expression in cultured human keratinocytes kept for several days in the presence of low (0.1 mmol/1)(–) and high (1.15 mmol/1)(+) calcium. Cell cultures were performed as described previously.[4]

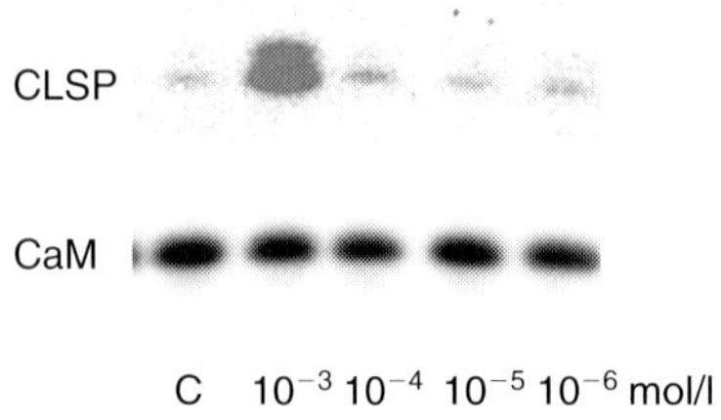

Figure 8.2

Western blot analysis of CLSP and CaM expression in the presence of increasing concentrations of sodium butyrate in a confluent, high-calcium keratinocyte culture as described previously.[4]

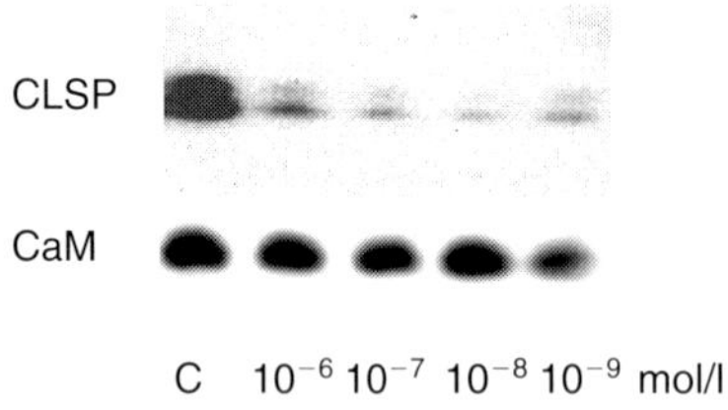

Figure 8.3

Western blot analysis of CLSP and CaM expression in the presence of increasing concentrations of CD 367, a synthetic retinoid in a confluent, high-calcium keratinocyte culture.[4]

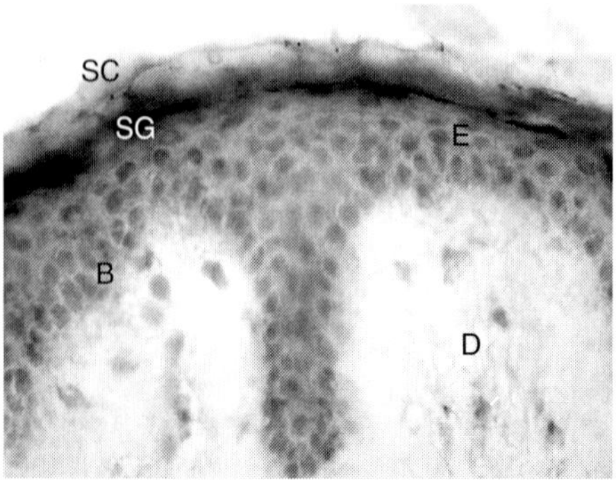

Figure 8.4

Immunohistological detection of CLSP in normal human skin using the polyclonal anti-CLSP antibody was performed as described previously.[14] Nuclei were counterstained with haematoxylin. E: epidermis; D: dermis; B: basal layer; SG: stratum granulosum; SC: stratum corneum.

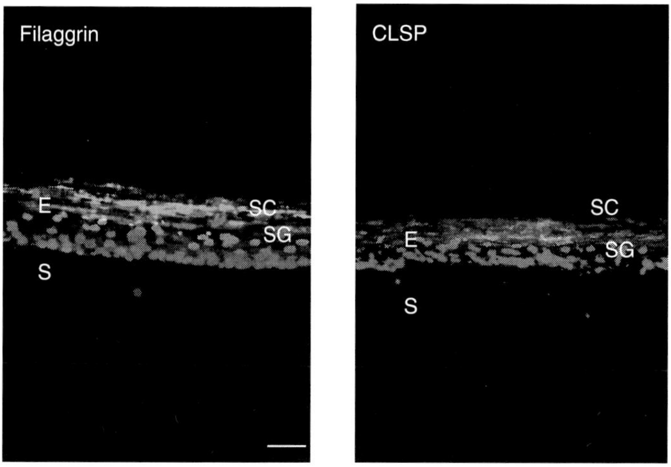

Figure 8.5

Immunofluorescence labelling of CLSP and filaggrin in reconstructed epidermis was performed as described previously.[4] Nuclei were stained with propidium iodine. S: substrate; E: epidermis; SG: stratum granulosum; SC: stratum corneum. Scale bar: 50 μm.

As for other markers of keratinocyte differentiation, including filaggrin, distribution is more diffuse in reconstructed epidermis, being present already in the deeper layers of the epidermis (Figure 8.5).[10,11] Expression of the cloned cDNA in *Escherichia coli* yielded a recombinant protein, which allowed further characterization of the new protein. rCLSP is able to bind calcium, and as calmodulin, exposes hydrophobic parts which most likely interact with target proteins.[1]

Epidermal proteins retained by the calmodulin affinity column are quantitatively and qualitatively distinct from those of the rCLSP column.[1] Sequencing of a potential target of CLSP (protein purified by affinity chromatography using rCLSP) revealed 100% identity with transglutaminase 3, a key enzyme in terminal keratinocyte differentiation.[12] The interaction in vitro between CLSP and transglutaminase 3 in the presence of calcium was confirmed using BIAcore technology with immobilized transglutaminase 3 on sensor chips (Figure 8.6). The interaction was abolished in the presence of EDTA. Transglutaminase 3 is a calcium-dependent enzyme, implicated in the cornified envelope formation,[13] indicating that CLSP might play a part in this process. Experiments to elucidate the exact role of CLSP in the physiology of normal human epidermis, particulary in the cornified envelope formation, are currently in progress.

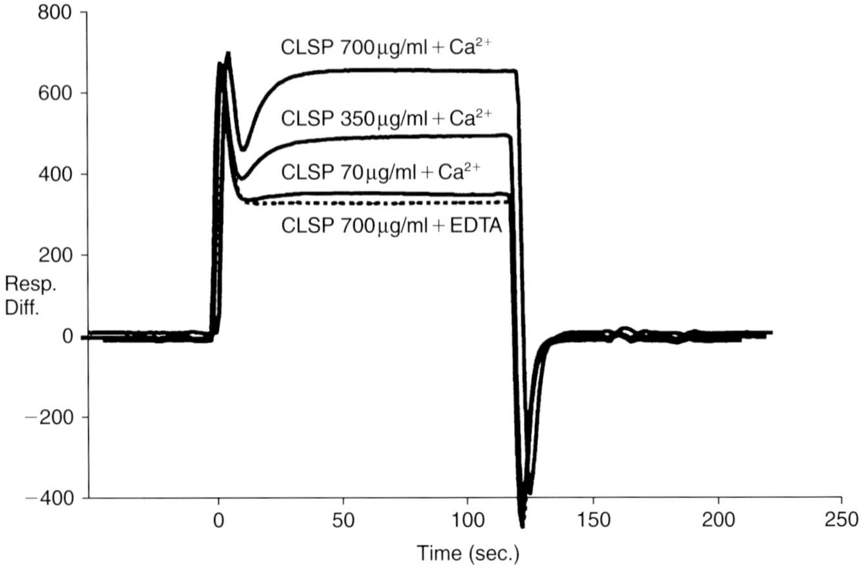

Figure 8.6

Calcium dependent interaction of rCLSP with immobilized transglutaminase 3 purified from plantar stratum corneum (BIACORE sensorgrams).

Acknowledgments

We are grateful to O Gournay-Zobiri, A Thomas-Collignon, C Collin and L Simonetti for their excellent technical assistance and appreciated very much the scientific discussions with Drs M Régnier and C Ferraris.

References

1. Méhul B, Bernard D, Simonetti L et al. Identification and cloning of a new calmodulin-like protein from human epidermis. J Biol Chem 2000; 275:12841–7.
2. Crivici A, Ikura M. Molecular and structural basis of target recognition by calmodulin. Annu Rev Biophys Biomol Struct 1995; 24: 85–116.
3. Tabernero L, Taylor DA, Chandross RJ et al. The structure of a calmodulin mutant with a deletion in the central helix: implications for molecular recognition and protein binder. Structure 1997; 5:613–22.
4. Méhul B, Bernard D, Schmidt R. Calmodulin-like skin protein: a new marker of keratinocyte differentiation. J Invest Dermatol 2001; 116:905–9.
5. Hennings H, Michael D, Cheng C et al. Calcium regulation of growth and differentiation of mouse epidermal cells in culture. Cell 1980; 19:245–54.
6. Watt FM. Keratinocyte cultures: an

experimental model for studying how proliferation and terminal differentiation are coordinated in the epidermis. J Cell Sci 1988; 90: 525–9.

7. Schmidt R, Cathelineau C, Cavey MT et al. Sodium butyrate selectively antagonizes the inhibitory effect of retinoids on cornified envelope formation in cultured human keratinocytes. J Cell Physiol 1989; 140:281–7.
8. Martin B, Bernadon JM, Cavey MT et al. Selective synthetic ligands for human nuclear retinoic acid receptors. Skin Pharmacol 1992; 5:57–65.
9. Tinois E, Tillier J, Gaucherand M et al. In vitro and post-transplantation differentiation of human keratinocytes growth on the human type IV collagen film of a bilayed dermal substitute. Exp Cell Res 1991; 193:310–19.
10. Schmidt R. Reconstructed human skin. Skin Pharmacol 1990; 3: 65–148.
11. Steven AC, Bisher ME, Roop DR et al. Biosynthetic pathway of filaggrin and loricrin: two major proteins expressed by terminally differentiating epidermal keratinocytes. J Struct Biol 1990; 104:150–62.
12. Lee SC, Jang SI, Yang JM et al. The proximal promoter of the human transglutaminase 3 gene. Stratified squamous epithelial-specific expression in cultured cells is mediated by binding of Sp1 and ets transcriptin factors to a proximal promoter element. J Biol Chem 1996; 271:4561–8.
13. Reichert U, Michel S, Schmidt R. The cornified envelope: a key structure of terminally differentiating keratinocytes. In Darmon M, Blumenberg M, eds. *Molecular Biology of the Skin*. London: Academic Press Inc; 1993:107–50.
14. Bernard D, Méhul B, Delattre C et al. Purification and characterization of the endoglycosidase heparanase 1 from human plantar stratum corneum: a key enzyme in epidermal physiology? J Invest Dermatol 2001; 117:1266–73.

9

Association of hsp27 with epidermal structural proteins and its expression in keratinization disorders

C Jonak, G Klosner, D Födinger, H Traupe, D Metze, H Hönigsmann and F Trautinger

Introduction

The synthesis of heat shock proteins (hsps) in all cells and tissues is stimulated by heat shock and other stressful conditions (e.g. heavy metals, infections, oxidation). These stress proteins enable the cell to resist further exposure to environmental or pathophysiological stresses.[1–6] Hsps can be found in all species so far investigated and have been highly conserved during evolution. The major function of hsp is to act as molecular chaperones – polypeptide chain-binding proteins.[7–11] Folding, transport, and interaction of bound proteins can be mediated by chaperones. Hsps enable renaturation or degradation of intracellular polypeptides that are damaged by hyperthermia or other forms of stresses.[12,13] Hsps also have a key role in physiological processes.[14–17] Hsps participate in transmembrane protein transport and mediate the three-dimensional folding of newly synthesized polypeptide chains. The heterogeneous group of hsps are divided into families, with respect to their molecular weight. According to this classification, hsp27 is a member of the 'small hsp', with a molecular weight of 27 kD. Its expression can be found in breast, uterus, cervix, placenta, platelets, epidermis and adnexal structures. The protein is situated in the cytoplasm, near the Golgi complex and, after stimulation, is predominantly translocated into the nucleus.[14,18]

Immunohistological studies demonstrated hsp27 expression in epidermal keratinocytes and hair follicles, and in the epithelium of the efferent duct of sweat glands.[19–21] The pattern of hsp27 expression in epidermis correlates with keratinocyte differentiation and, therefore, hsp27 can be regarded as a differentiation marker in these cells. On the other hand, hsp27 is absent in undifferentiated keratinocyte-derived malignancies. Tumour development was delayed in animals inoculated with hsp27-overexpressing squamous cell carcinomas.[15,22,23]

In the subcorneal epidermal layers, specific differentiation-associated proteins are highly expressed and are crosslinked to form the cornified cell envelope (CCE), a process that is catalysed by the action of transglutaminase 1. The CCE is a highly insoluble structure beneath the plasma membrane of terminally differentiated keratinocytes. The CCE is a 15-μm thick layer of proteins, crosslinked by isodipeptide and disulfide bonds. Major proteins of the CCE are loricrin, filaggrin, involucrin, cystatin A, a cysteine-rich protein (CRP), and the 'small proline-rich' proteins (SPRRs).[21,24–28] Formation of this complex protein polymer without chaperone action is probably not possible, and would result in improper structures. In search of a chaperone of the CCE, we thought that, owing to its epidermal expression, hsp27 could fit the bill.

To investigate whether there is a physical association between hsp27 and proteins of the CCE or other structural proteins of epidermal keratinocytes, we perfomed double-staining immunofluorescence and immunoelectron microscopy on normal human skin and immunohistochemistry on a panel of different ichthyoses.

Materials and methods

Immunofluorescence

Samples of normal human skin (n = 15) were obtained from surgical specimens and immediately snap frozen. Cryosections (17 μm) were stained with a biotinylated monoclonal antibody (moAb) against hsp27 (Stress Gen) and rhodamin-avidin (Molecular Probes). Subsequently, one of the following reagents was used for double staining: FITC-phalloidin (Molecular Probes); moAb to pan-keratin (NeoMarkers) and transglutaminase (Bio Trend); polyclonal antibody (poAb) to filaggrin (Babco) and loricrin (Babco).

Samples were analysed by confocal laser scan microscopy (Zeiss).

Immunohistochemistry

Detection of hsp27 was performed on 25 formalin-fixed, paraffin-embedded skin tissue samples of different ichthyoses (Table 1). Specimens were stained with a sensitive, three-step immunoperoxidase technique.

Immunoelectron microscopy

Cryostat sections (15 μm) of unfixed tissue were prepared and processed for preembedding immunogold labelling. After incubation with anti-hsp27 moAb (StressGen), sections were further reacted with streptavidin gold conjugate (BritishBioCell). For double labelling, sections were incubated with biotinylated anti-hsp27 moAb and rabbit anti-filaggrin poAb (Babco), or with biotinylated anti-hsp27 moAb and rabbit anti-loricrin poAb (Babco).

Results

Coexpression of hsp27 with epidermal structural proteins in normal human epidermis

Subcorneal colocalization of hsp27 with keratin, filaggrin, loricrin and transglutaminase 1 was detected in over 60% of the samples. No colocalization of hsp27 with actin was observed.

Subcorneal colocalization of hsp27 and keratin confined to a narrow subcorneal layer was found in 11 out of 14 samples (Figure 9.1A).

Coexpression of hsp27 and filaggrin was found in 50% of the investigated samples (7 out of 14). The colocalization pattern in four samples was formed to cytoplasmatic granules within the upper epidermal layers. One sample showed colocalization in a broad subcorneal layer (Figure 9.1B). Few isolated clusters of subcorneal keratinocytes with hsp27–filaggrin colocalization were detected in two samples. With electron

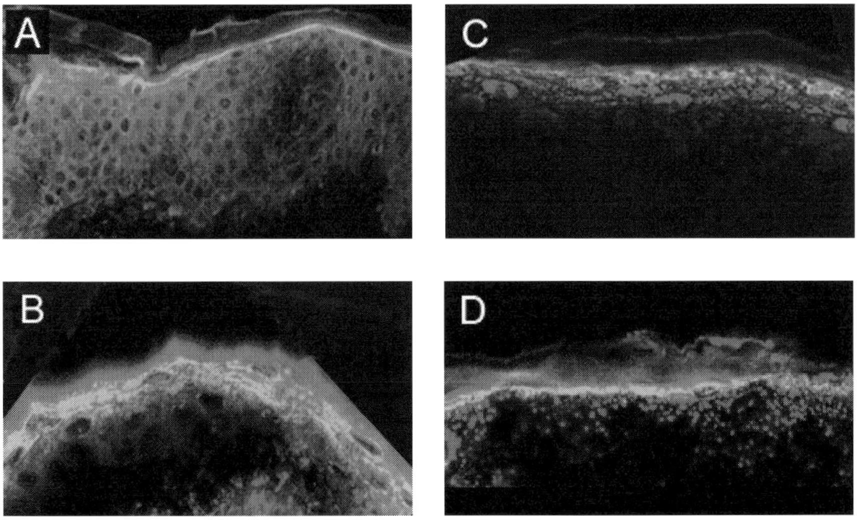

Figure 9.1

Immunofluorescence and confocal laserscan microscopy of normal human skin.
(A Colocalization of hsp27 and keratin is confined to a narrow subcorneal layer. For filaggrin (B), loricrin (C), and transglutaminase 1 (D), similar patterns of colocalization were observed.

microscopy, both antigens were found to be in association with intermediate filaments in suprabasal keratinocytes (Figures 9.2A and B).

Seven out of thirteen samples showed subcorneal colocalization of loricrin and hsp27. In five of these, colocalization was confined to isolated single cells. In two samples, these cells formed a continuous band of colocalization (Figure 9.1C). With electron microscopy, both antigens were found in association with intermediate filaments in suprabasal keratinocytes (Figures 9.2C and D).

Colocalization of hsp27 with transglutaminase 1 was found in 6 out of 13 samples, and was confined to a continuous subcorneal band, similar to the coexpression pattern that had been demonstrated for loricrin (Figure 9.1D).

Expression of hsp27 in different ichthyoses

Twelve different hereditary and acquired skin diseases associated with an ichthyotic phenotype were investigated. With the exception of X-linked dominant chondrodysplasia punctata and bullous congenital ichthyotic erythroderma, the pattern of expression of hsp27 was identical to normal human skin. Results are summarized in Table 9.1.

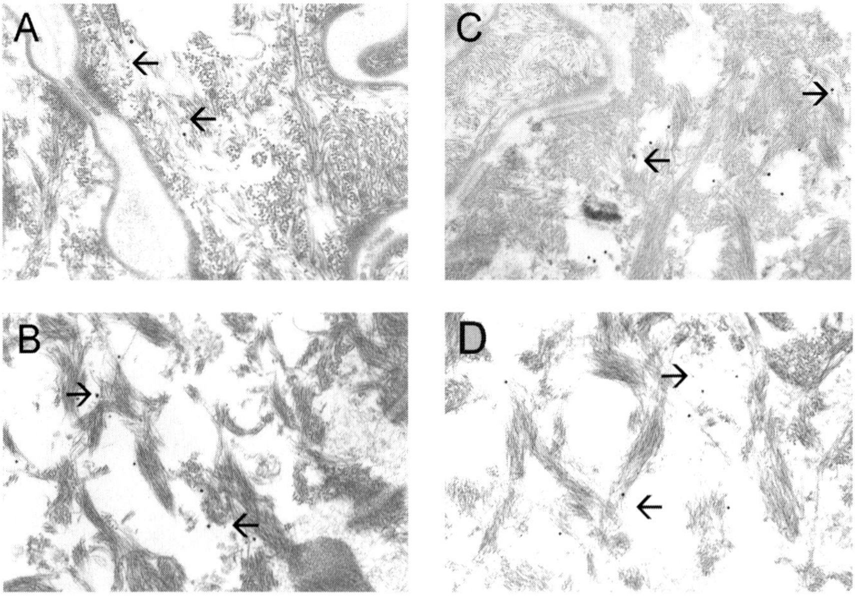

Figure 9.2

Preembedding double-label immunogold electron microscopy reveals association of hsp27, loricrin, and filaggrin with tonofilaments. (A) Upper epidermis; hsp27 (5 nm gold), indicated by arrows; filaggrin (10 nm gold). (B) Lower epidermis; hsp27 and filaggrin. (C) Upper epidermis; hsp27 and loricrin (10 nm gold). (D) Lower epidermis; hsp27 and loricrin.

Table 9.1 Expression of hsp27 in a panel of different ichthyoses. N indicates the number of cases investigated, and the expression of hsp27 within the epidermis is indicated by (+) or (–).

Diagnosis	N	Hsp27
Acquired ichthyosis	1	+
Autosomal-dominant lamellar ichthyosis	2	+
Anhydrotic epidermolytic ichthyosis	1	+
Autosomal-recessive lamellar ichthyosis (TG1–)	2	+
Autosomal-recessive lamellar ichthyosis (TG1+)	2	+
Bullous congenital ichthyosiform erythroderma (Brocq)	2	+/–
X-linked dominant chondrodysplasia punctata (Conradi–Hünerman–Happle)	5	–
Ichthyosis vulgaris	2	+
Netherton syndrome	3	+
Sjögren–Larsson syndrome	1	+
Child syndrome	1	+

Discussion

Colocalization of hsp27 with keratins, transglutaminase, loricrin, and filaggrin was found in 60% of the samples. Their colocalization with hsp27 was always confined to a narrow subcorneal layer, close to the CCE. This might imply that hsp27 is involved in CCE formation, a complex process that might need the help of a molecular chaperone for the correct assembly of the CCE proteins. Hsps and other chaperones have been described as cooperating in protein folding and assembly in the form of so-called chaperone machines.[5] Our results, together with earlier studies, suggest the existence of chaperone machines in the epidermis, since the major chaperones, hsp72, 73, and 90, are expressed in normal human epidermis without prior stress exposure.[29,30] In some cases, colocalizations were confined to single keratinocytes instead of cohesive bands. This might be explained by the fact that, in normal human skin, keratinization is not synchronized and individual keratinocytes differ in their state of differentiation at a given time point. As immunohistological stainings are snapshots, only these cells will stain positively when, at the time of investigation, hsp27 is associated with the specific substrate under investigation.

Although all antigens tested were expressed in every tissue sample, colocalization with hsp27 was absent in 20–40% of biopsies. Colocalization of hsp27 with one cornified envelope protein did not predict for colocalization with others. Thus, no consistent pattern of colocalization could be revealed. This interindividual variation can be explained by factors such as biopsy site and age. Further studies will be necessary to define the correlation between hsp27 expression, colocalization with structural proteins of the epidermis, and individual factors.

The specific expression and colocalization pattern of hsp27 in normal human epidermis points to a function of hsp27 in epidermal differentiation and keratinization. Lack of hsp27 might thus be associated with dyskeratinization. This hypothesis led us to the investigation of hereditary keratinization disorders. Whether the absence of hsp27 in chondrodysplasia punctata and its reduced expression in epidermolytic hyperkeratosis is associated with the clinical phenotype remains a matter of speculation; this will have to be addressed in further studies at the molecular level.

References

1. Carper SW, Duffy JJ, Gerner EW. Heat shock proteins in thermotolerance and other cellular processes. Cancer Res 1987; 47:5249–55.
2. Leppä S, Sistonen L. Heat shock response – pathophysiological implications. Ann Med 1997; 29:73–8.
3. Lindquist S. The heat-shock response. Ann Rev Biochem 1986; 55:1151–91.
4. Lindquist S, Craig EA. The heat-shock proteins. Annu Rev Genet 1988; 22:631–77.
5. Morimoto RI, Santoro MG. Stress-inducible responses and heat shock proteins: new pharmacologic targets for cytoprotection. Nat Biotechnol 1998; 16:833–8.
6. Schlesinger MJ. Heat shock proteins. Biol Chem 1990; 265: 12111–14.
7. Ellis RJ. The molecular chaperone concept. Semin Cell Biol 1990; 1: 1–9.
8. Gething MJ, Sambrook J. Protein folding in the cell. Nature 1992; 355:33–45.
9. Hartl FU, Hlodan R, Langer T. Molecular chaperones in protein folding: the art of avoiding sticky situations. TIBS 1994; 19:20–5.
10. Jakob U, Gaestel M, Engel K, Buchner J. Small heat shock proteins are molecular chaperones. J Biol Chem 1993; 268:1517–20.
11. Rothman JE. Polypeptide chain binding proteins: catalysts of protein folding and related processes in cells. Cell 1989; 59: 591–601.
12. Hightower LE. Heat shock, stress proteins, chaperones, and proteotoxicity. Cell 1991; 66:191–7.
13. Pinto M, Moranges M, Bensaude O. Denaturation of proteins during heat shock. In vivo recovery of solubility and activity of reporter enzymes. J Biol Chem 1991; 266: 13941–6.
14. Ciocca DR, Oesterreich S, Chamnes GC et al. Biological and clinical implications of heat shock protein 27,000 (Hsp27): a review. J Natl Cancer Institute 1993; 85:1558–70.
15. Kindås-Mügge I, Trautinger F. Increased expression of the M(r) 27,000 heat shock protein (hsp27) in in vitro differentiated normal human keratinocytes. Cell Growth Differ 1994; 5:777–81.
16. Morimoto RI. Heat shock: the role of transient inducible responses in cell damage, transformation, and differentiation. Cancer Cells 1991; 3:295–301.
17. Samali A, Orrenius S. Heat shock proteins: regulators of stress response and apoptosis. Cell Stress Chaperones 1998; 3: 228–36.
18. McClaren M, Isseroff RR. Dyn-

namic changes in intracellular localization and isoforms of the 27-kD stress protein in human keratinocytes. Invest Dermatol 1994; 102:375–81.

19. Welsh MJ, Gaestel M. Small heat-shock protein family: function in health and disease. Ann N Y Acad Sci 1998; 851:28–35.
20. Trautinger F, Kindas-Mügge I, Dekrout B et al. Expression of the 27-kDa heat shock protein in human epidermis and in epidermal neoplasms: an immunohistological study. Br J Dermatol 1995; 133:194–202.
21. Gandour-Edwards R, McClaren M, Isserroff RR. Immunolocalization of low-molecular-weight stress protein HSP 27 in normal skin and common cutaneous lesions. Am J Dermatopathol 1994; 16:504–9.
22. Kindås-Mügge I, Herbacek I, Jantschitsch C et al. Modification of growth and tumorigenicity in epidermal cell lines by DNA-mediated gene transfer of M(r) 27,000 heat shock protein (hsp27). Cell Growth Differ 1996; 7:1167–74.
23. Kindås-Mügge I, Micksche M, Trautinger F. Modification of growth in small heat shock (hsp27) gene transfected breast carcinoma. Anticancer Res 1998; 18: 413–17.
24. Hohl D. Cornified cell envelope. Dermatologica 1990; 180: 201–11.
25. Ishida Yamamoto A, Eady RA, Watt FM et al. Immunoelectron microscopic analysis of cornified cell envelope formation in normal and psoriatic epidermis. J Histochem Cytochem 1996; 44: 167–75.
26. Ishida Yamamoto A, Iizuka H. Structural organization of cornified cell envolopes and alterations in inherited skin disorders. Exp Dermatol 1998; 7:1–10.
27. Jarnik M, Simon MN, Steven AC. Cornified cell envelope assembly: a model based on electron microscopic determinations of thickness and projected density. J Cell Sci 1998; 111:1051–60.
28. Steinert PM, Candi E, Kartasova T et al. Small proline-rich proteins are cross-bridging proteins in the cornified cell envelopes of stratified squamous epithelia. J Struct Biol 1998; 122:76–85.
29. Boehncke WH, Dahlke A, Zollner TM et al. Differential expression of heat shock protein 70 (HSP70) and heat shock cognate protein 70 (HSC70) in human epidermis. Dermatol Res 1994; 287:68–71.
30. Trautinger F, Trautinger I, Kindås-Mügge I et al. Human keratinocytes in vivo and in vitro constitutively express the 72-kD heat shock protein. J Invest Dermatol 1993; 101:334–8.

10

The effect of change in epidermal calcium gradient on stratum corneum lipid and epidermal differentiation

EH Choi, W-S Park, E-D Son, SM Hwang, MJ Kim, SK Ahn and SH Lee

Introduction

Lamellar bodies (LBs) are the source of lipid composition of the stratum corneum (SC). SC intercellular lipid bilayers formed from secreted LBs are the most important structure of the permeability barrier. The cornified cell envelope (CE), formed during the terminal differentiation of keratinocytes, is a specialized structure covalently bound with SC intercellular lipids. This forms a structurally and functionally complete permeability barrier. Also, during epidermal differentiation, specific keratins are synthesized.[1] After barrier perturbation with acetone or tape stripping, transepidermal water loss (TEWL), LB secretion, epidermal lipid synthesis and keratins K10, K6, K16 and involucrin expression increase as a homeostatic response. The loss of calcium from the upper epidermis, following barrier disruption, signals the increased synthesis and secretion of LB.[2] Sonophoresis of calcium-free solutions, which decreases calcium concentrations in the upper epidermis without disrupting the barrier, also induces LB synthesis and secretion.[3] We previously reported that iontophoresis induced an increase in LB secretion without an increase in TEWL. This came from changes in the epidermal calcium gradient, which were observed by electron microscope.[4]

We performed this study to elucidate whether changes in the epidermal calcium gradient by iontophoresis can increase SC lipids and enhance terminal differentiation in vivo.

Materials and methods

Eight- to twelve-week-old, hairless mice were used. Following anaesthesia with an intraperitoneal injection of 4% chloralhydrate, patches (3.46 cm²)

containing only three drops of distilled water, which is needed for electric current on skin, were attached to the flanks of the hairless mice. A direct current (6 V, 0.6 mA) with a duty ratio (2:1) by an iontophoresis device was used to pass a current through the skin for 2 hours. TEWL, checked by Tewameter TM210 (Courage+Khazaka, Germany) was measured before and immediately after the current. A skin biopsy was taken from a negative site at 2 hours after the current for lipid analysis, and at 2 hours, 12 hours, and 36 hours after the current for immunohistochemical stains for CE proteins.

Lipid analysis

Epidermal sheets were obtained by first removing whole skin samples from hairless mice. Extractable lipids from the dried epidermal sheets were obtained using the method of Bligh and Dyer.[5] Chromatography was performed on silica gel HPTLC plate (60F254, 20 × 10 cm, Merck). An automated TLC sampler III ATS3 (Camag, Basel, Switzerland) was used to apply standards. Plates were developed using a Camag AMD instrument with the solvent system in (1) methanol/chloroform/water (19:79:2), (2) methanol/chloroform/ethyl ether/hexane (20:25:40:15), (3) chloroform/ethyl ether/hexane (25:50:25), (4) ethyl ether/hexane (52:48), and (5) ethyl ether/hexane (5:95). After charring, the lipids on the HPTLC plates were quantified with a TLC2 scanner II and Camag TLC evaluation software (ver. 3.15) (Camag, Basel, Switzerland). Lipid amounts were quantitated by cochromatography against known standards.

Immunohistochemical stains

Frozen specimens were used for immunohistochemical stains. All anti-K5, anti-K10, anti-K6, anti-involucrin and anti-loricrin antibodies were purchased from BabCO (Richmond, CA, USA).

Results

TEWL was not changed after iontophoresis, as in our previous report. Total lipid content showed a higher increase in the 2-hour-iontophoresis skin than in the untreated control. Sphingolipids containing mainly ceramides, and neutral lipids, containing cholesterol, free fatty acid and triglycerides, increased after the current. But phospholipid, a representative polar lipid, decreased after the current (Figure 10.1).

Expression of K10 showed an increase in suprabasal portions at 12 hours, K6 focally in stratum granulosum and stratum spinosum at 36 hours, and involucrin at 12 hours, but loricrin did not change (Table 10.1).

Fraction (μg/mg SC)	Untreated control ( ) : % of lipids (n = 4)	Iontophoresis (negative) for 2 h ( ) : % of lipids (n = 4)
Sphingolipids	5.05 (17.67)	6.67 (10.85)
Neutral lipids	18.05 (63.16)	46.4 (75.47)
Cholesterol	8.94 (31.27)	16.10 (26.19)
Free fatty acid	4.15 (14.51)	5.59 (9.09)
Triglycerides	3.45 (12.08)	19.55 (31.80)
Cholesterol ester	1.51 (5.29)	5.16 (8.39)
Phospholipid	2.45 (8.57)	1.89 (3.07)
Other lipids Galactocerebroside Squalene, etc	3.03 (10.60)	6.52 (10.61)
Total lipids	28.58 (100.00)	61.48 (100.00)

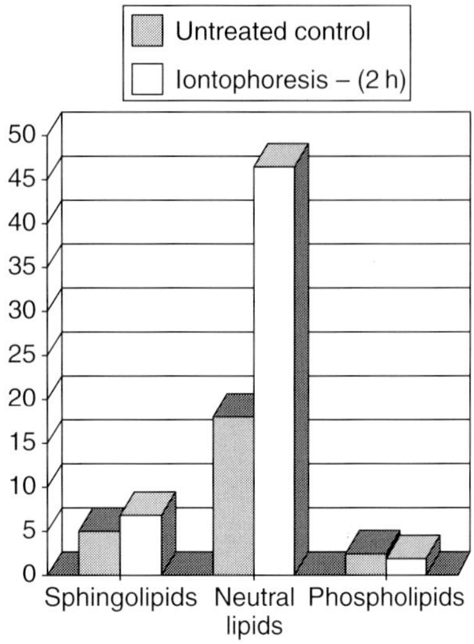

Figure 10.1

Effect of iontophoresis on stratum corneum lipid content

Table 10.1 Summary of immunostaining of keratin K6 and involucrin after tape-stripping and negative iontophoresis.
Expression of K6 appeared in the basal layer and stratum basale (SB) at 12 hours after tape-stripping and iontophoresis and then extended to whole epidermis at 36 hours. Expression of involucrin was increased at 12 hours after tape-stripping and iontophoresis.

	Keratin K6				Involucrin			
	SC	SG	SS	SB	SC	SG	SS	SB
Normal	–	–	–	–	+/–	++	–	–
2 h after Tape-stripping	–	–	–	–	+/–	++	–	–
12 h after Tape-stripping	–	+/–	+	+	+	++	+/–	–
36 h after Tape-stripping	–	+++	+++	+++	+	++	+	–
2 h after Iontophoresis	–	–	–	–	+/–	++	–	–
12 h after Iontophoresis	–	–	+/–	+/–	+	++	+	–
36 h after Iontophoresis	–	+/–	+	+	+	+++	+	–

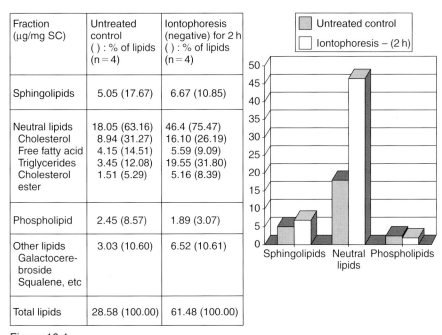

SC, Stratum corneum; SG, stratum granulosum; SS, stratum spinosum; SB, suprabasal layer

Discussion

It was known that polar lipids, like phospholipids, change to non-polar lipids, like sphingolipids and neutral lipids, along with terminal differentiation.[6] Therefore, an increase of non-polar lipids in the SC means an increase of terminal differentiation of the keratinocytes.

The change in the epidermal calcium gradient by iontophoresis in vivo can induce an increase in sphingolipids and neutral lipids in the SC, which means there is an acceleration of terminal differentiation, and change in the expression of CE proteins, a marker of keratinocyte terminal differentiation.

Acknowledgement

This study was supported by a grant from the Korea Science and Engineering Foundation, Republic of Korea (KOSEF 98-0403-18-01-3).

References

1. Ekanayake-Mudiyanselage S, Aschauer H, Schmook FP et al. Expression of epidermal keratins and the cornified envelope protein involucrin is influenced by permeability barrier disruption. J Invest Dermatol 1998; 111:517–23.
2. Lee SH, Elias PM, Proksch E et al. Calcium and potassium are important regulators of barrier homeostasis in murine epidermis. J Clin Invest 1992; 89:530–8.
3. Menon GK, Price LF, Bommannan B et al. Selective obliteration of the epidermal calcium gradient leads to enhanced lamellar body secretion. J Invest Dermatol 1994; 102:789–95.
4. Lee SH, Choi EH, Feingold KR et al. Iontophoresis itself on hairless mouse skin induces the loss of the epidermal calcium gradient without skin barrier impairment. J Invest Dermatol 1998; 111:39–43.
5. Bligh EG, Dyer WJ. A rapid method of total lipid extraction and purification. Can J Biochem Physiol 1959; 37:911–17.
6. Wertz PW, Michniak BB. Epidermal lipid metabolism and barrier function of stratum corneum. In: Kydonieus AF, Wille JJ, eds. *Biochemical Modulation of Skin Reactions: Transdermal, Topicals, Cosmetics*. Boca Raton: CRC Press LLC, 2000:35–44.

11

Expression analysis of stratum corneum chymotryptic enzyme and its precursor at the surface of human epidermis, using affinity-purified anti-peptide antibodies

M Simon, D Bernard, M Guerrin, T Egelrud, R Schmidt and G Serre

Introduction

Several proteases that belong to the kallikrein family, a subfamily of serine-proteases whose genes are located in a single locus at 19q13.3–13.4, are expressed in the late stages of human epidermal differentiation. Among them, the stratum corneum chymotryptic enzyme (SCCE) is synthesized by granular keratinocytes as an inactive precursor (pro-SCCE) that is activated by proteolytic cleavage of a short amino-terminal domain. SCCE is thought to be involved in corneodesmosome proteolysis and desquamation.[1] To characterize SCCE metabolism, and to analyse the expression of SCCE and pro-SCCE in the uppermost stratum corneum (SC), antibodies either specific for pro-SCCE or directed against both proteins were produced.

Methods

Rabbit sera were developed against synthetic peptides corresponding to various parts of pro-SCCE: serum A against peptide A_{23-31}, corresponding to the region specific for the precursor, and serum B against a mixture of three peptides, distributed along the sequence of the active enzyme (B_{71-84}, C_{87-99} and $D_{169-183}$). Specificity of the affinity-purified antibodies was tested on recombinant pro-SCCE (produced in C127 cells) and on the derived active SCCE. To precisely characterize the molecular forms of SCCE present near the epidermis surface, total proteins of superficial SC were obtained from six different individuals by varnish-stripping and analysed by immunoblotting. The same extracts were also immunodetected with G36-19, a monoclonal antibody to corneodesmosin, an adhesive component of corneodesmosomes.[2]

Results

The affinity-purified antibodies directed to the peptide A_{23-31} only detected pro-SCCE, whereas the antibodies directed to the three other peptides recognized both pro-SCCE and SCCE (Figure 11.1). The reactivity of these antibodies was suppressed by incubation in the presence of the peptide(s) used for their production. When the antibodies were used to investigate pro-SCCE in the varnish-stripping extracts, the precursor was, surprisingly, always detected. SCCE was also detected in all the extracts. The amounts of both pro-SCCE and SCCE were shown to differ from one individual to another. Moreover, the amount of SCCE was shown to be inversely related to that of the pro-enzyme. Interestingly

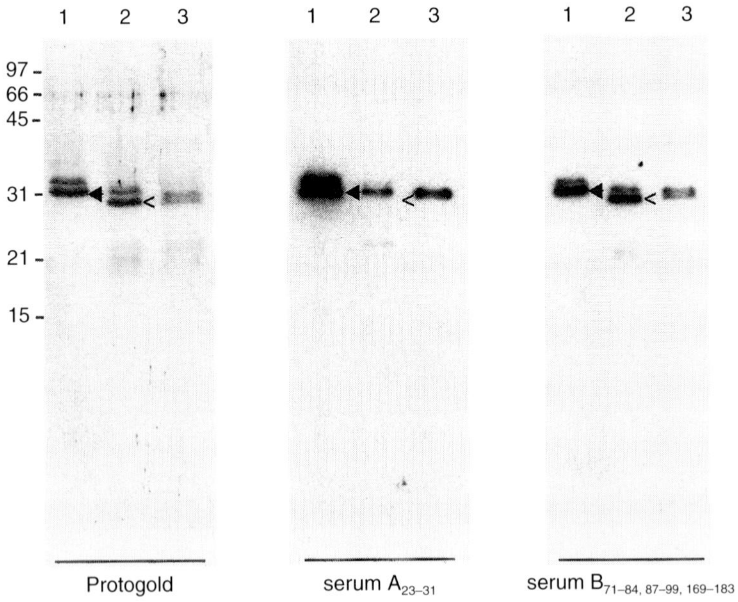

Figure 11.1

Specificity of the sera directed to pro-SCCE and SCCE. Purified recombinant pro-SCCE (lane 1) and SCCE (lane 2), and a fraction of plantar stratum corneum extracts highly enriched in pro-SCCE and SCCE (lane 3) were separated by SDS-PAGE, transferred to membranes and either stained with Protogold or immunodetected with the sera, as indicated. The black and empty arrowheads show the non-glycosylated recombinant pro-SCCE and SCCE, respectively.

enough, the amount of immunodetected corneodesmosin was low in the extracts that were characterized by a high SCCE content. This suggests that, at the epidermis surface, SCCE is the (or one of the) enzyme(s) that degrades corneodesmosin, and that desquamation may be regulated by the activation of pro-SCCE.

References

1. Hansson L, Strömqvist M, Bäckman A et al. Cloning, expression, and characterization of stratum corneum chymotryptic enzyme. J Biol Chem 1994; 269:19420–6.
2. Jonca N, Guerrin M, Hadjiolova K et al. Corneodesmosin, a component of epidermal corneocyte desmosomes, displays homophilic adhesive properties. J Biol Chem 2002; 277:5024–9.

12

Non-invasive evaluation of cornified envelope maturation in the stratum corneum

T Hirao, M Takahashi and H Tagami

Aims

Cornified envelopes (CEs) provide a basis for barrier function of the stratum corneum (SC). We have recently established a non-invasive method to evaluate CE maturation.[1] This method is based on the fact that involucrin antigenicity in immature CEs was stronger than that in mature CEs, whereas immature CEs were less hydrophobic than mature CEs. The purpose of this study was to demonstrate the significance of CE maturation in the SC, using this evaluation method.

Methods

The outermost SC samples were collected by non-invasive tape stripping. CEs were prepared by extensive boiling and washing of the SC in a buffer containing sodium dodecyl sulphate (SDS) and dithiothreitol, and stained with anti-involucrin followed by fluorescein-isothiocyanate (FITC)-labelled secondary antibody, to evaluate loss of antigenicity during maturation, and with Nile red to assess their hydrophobicity. Fluorescence images were obtained by observation using a fluorescence microscope.

To compare the appearance of immature CEs with parakeratosis, corneocytes were dissociated by incubation of the tape-stripped SC in 20 mmol/l SDS-80 mmol/l N,N'-dimethyldodecylamine oxide. They were stained with anti-involucrin followed by FITC-labelled secondary antibody, and with propidium iodide to detect retention of nuclei.

To examine the potential ability of immature CEs in the SC to mature, the face SC was incubated ex vivo in the air with controlled humidity at 37°C, followed by evaluation of CE maturation by the method mentioned above. To elucidate the effect of moisturization on CE maturation in vivo, the faces of healthy volunteers were treated with a moisturizing cream daily for 6 weeks.

Results

Appearance of immature CEs in the SC with impaired barrier function

Immature CEs, which were stained with involucrin, but not with Nile red, were detected in the SC with impaired barrier function, such as those of the face (Figure 12.1), and involved areas of psoriasis and atopic dermatitis, and experimentally-induced dermatitis.

Involucrin-positive immature CEs were not always associated with parakeratosis, which is often used as a marker for hyperkeratosis, since there were four types of corneocytes: involucrin (+) nuclei (+), involucrin (+) nuclei (–), involucrin (–) nuclei (+), and involucrin (–) nuclei (–).

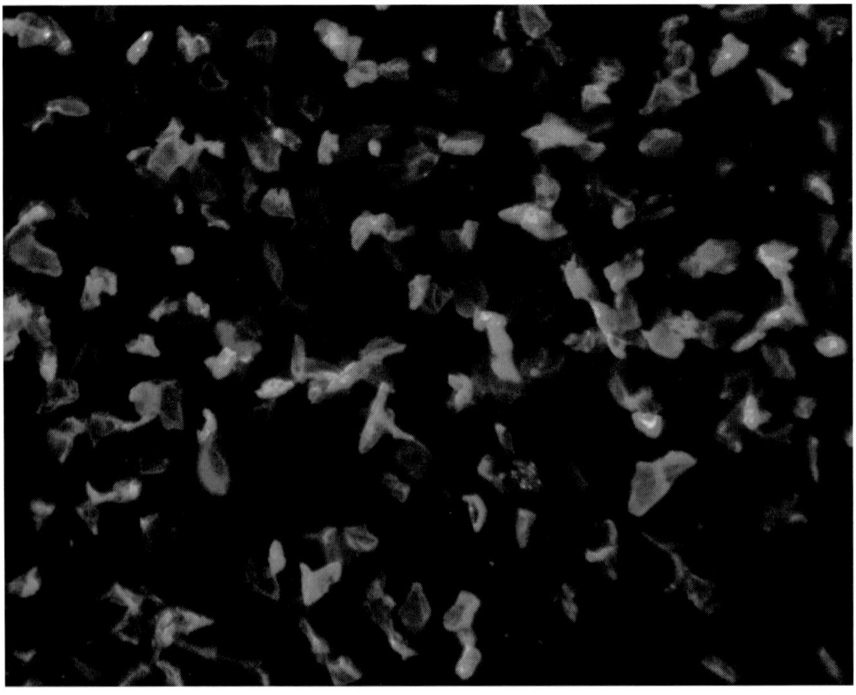

Figure 12.1

Immature CEs detected in the face SC. Involucrin-positive immature CEs (brighter ones) and Nile positive mature CEs (darker ones) were observed.

Maturation of CEs ex vivo and in vivo

Ex vivo incubation of the outermost SC of the face under humidified conditions resulted in conversion of immature CEs to mature CEs. Biochemical analyses revealed that the maturation was mediated by transglutaminase, suggesting that immature CEs have the potential ability to mature. This maturation was inhibited under low humidity conditions, and replenished by application of moisturizers to SC samples prior to the incubation. The appearance of immature CEs in the face was significantly reduced by daily application of moisturizing cream, suggesting that appropriate skin care can promote CE maturation, together with promotion of barrier function of the skin.

Conclusion

CE maturation is one of the crucial events for the barrier function of the skin, and moisturization is effective to promote CE maturation. Our staining method is useful for the evaluation of CE maturation without any serious invasive procedure.

Reference

1. Hirao T, Denda M, Takahashi M. Identification of immature cornified envelopes in the barrier-impaired epidermis by characterization of their hydrophobicity and antigenicities of the components. Exp Dermatol 2001; 10:35–44.

13
Organization of the intercellular spaces of human palmo–plantar stratum corneum

H-M Sheu and J-C Tsai

Introduction

Stratum corneum (SC) is the final product of the epidermal terminal differentiation. It consists of corneocytes embedded in a lipid-rich environment. Besides the extracellular lipids, the intercorneocyte spaces also contain corneodesmosomes or desmosomal remnants and lacunae of unknown origins. It has been found that transepidermal water loss is highest in palms and soles,[1] and lipid content is lowest in palmo–plantar SC.[2] However, little is actually known about the organization of the intercellular lipid lamellae of human palmo–plantar SC[3] and its interaction with corneodesmosomes and lacunaes within intercorneocyte spaces. The aim of the present work was to observe the intercorneocyte spaces and to understand if there is qualitative or quantitative structural difference between the palmo–plantar and non-palmo–plantar SC.

Materials and methods

Specimens

Skin biopsies were performed from the normal palm (eight), sole (six) and non-palmo–plantar skin (eight).

Ruthenium tetroxide staining for SC intercellular lipid bilayers

Skin samples were minced into approximately 1-mm^3 pieces, and fixed overnight (more than 16 hours) at 4°C in 2% glutaraldehyde, 2% paraformaldehyde with 0.06% calcium chloride in 0.1 mol/l sodium cacodylate buffer, pH 7.3. The samples were washed three times with washing buffer and then post-fixed in 0.2% ruthenium tetoxide (RuO_4) (Polysciences, Warrington, PA, USA) with 0.25% potassium ferricyanide in 0.1 mol/l cacodylate buffer, pH 7.2, at 4°C for 1 hour. After rinsing in buffer, they were dehydrated in a graded ethanol series, propylene oxide, and then embedded in Epoxy resin (Merck, Darmstadt, Germany). Thin sections were post-stained with uranyl acetate and lead citrate and examined under a JOEL JEM-2000 EXII electron microscope.

Results and discussion

Electron micrograph of palmo–plantar SC by RuO_4 staining revealed that the intercellular spaces between corneocytes were composed of abundant corneodesmosomes, various numbers of lipid lamellae and the putative pore structure, lacunae[4] (Figure 13.1). In the palmo–plantar SC, more than 50% of the intercellular spaces were occupied by corneodesmosomes, in contrast to less than 20% in the non-palmo–plantar area. In general, the multilamellar lipid sheets are less extensive in palmo-plantar than in non-palmo–plantar areas. Typical six-lucent-band arrangements with broad-narrow-broad-broad-narrow-broad pattern were observed both in palmo–plantar (Figure 13.2a) and non-palmo–plantar areas. However, in palmo–plantar areas, foci with uniformly spaced lucent bands are frequently observed (Figure 13.2b). Recent in vitro studies with isolated pig skin demonstrated that the barrier function in the broad-narrow-broad three-layers pattern is superior to only one uniform lipid bilayer.[5] Similar lucent bands of uniform width were also observed in porcine palatal SC, which has been known to have a poor permeability barrier.[6] Finally, large swirls of many disorganized lipid lamellae with uniformly spaced lucent bands are sometimes seen in the dilated intercellular spaces of palmo–plantar SC. This disorganized

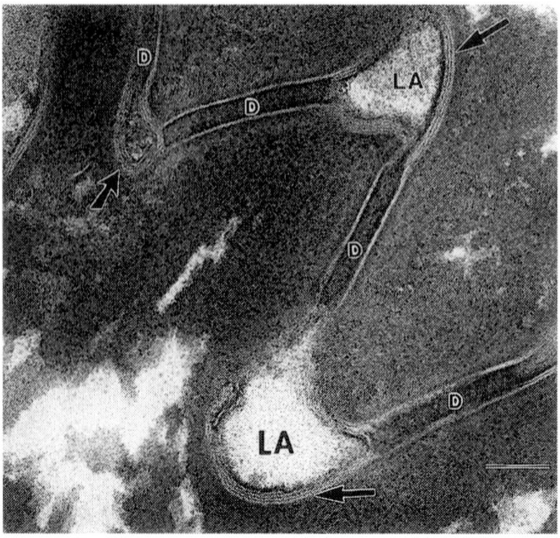

Figure 13.1

Electron micrograph of stratum corneum from the palm. RuO_4 staining revealed that the intercellular spaces between corneodesmosomes (D) are composed of lipid lamellae (arrows) and a putative pore structure, lacunae (LA). In general, relatively few lipid lamellae are observed as compared with the non-palmo–plantar skin. Bar = 100 nm.

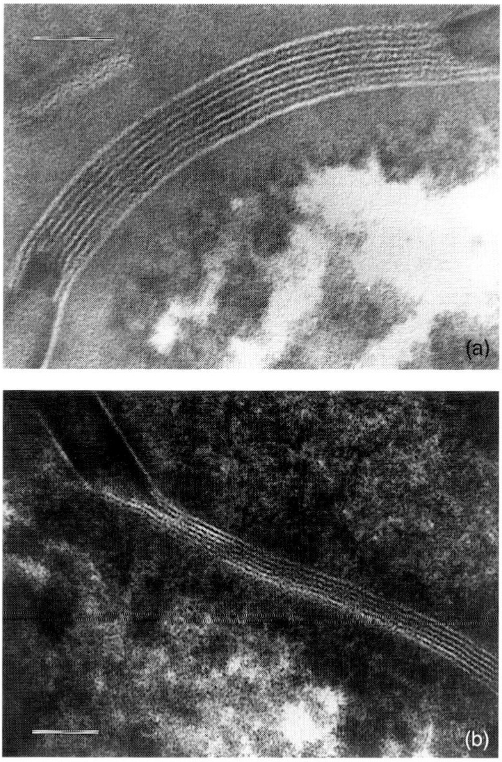

Figure 13.2

Electron micrograph of SC from the sole. Besides the typical pattern of broad-narrow-broad lucent lamellae (a), uniform broad lucent bands are frequently observed in the palmo–plantar SC (b). Bar = 50 nm.

lamellar material seems to imply poorer barrier function. A similar structure has also been described recently in palatal SC.[6]

Conclusion

The present results suggest that the multilamellar lipid sheets are less extensive in palmo–plantar than in non-palmo–plantar SC. Meanwhile, the palmo-plantar SC also shows considerable variation and poorer organization of their lipid lamellae. These structural differences may partially explain the high water permeability of the palms and soles.

Acknowledgments

This work was supported by a grant from the National Science Council of the Republic of China (NSC 89-2314-B-006-093).

References

1. Scheuplein RJ, Blank JH. Permeability of the skin. Physiol Rev 1971; 51:702–47.
2. Lampe MA, Burlingame AL, Whitney J et al. Human stratum corneum lipids: characterization and regional variations. J Lipid Res 1983; 24:120–30.
3. Egelrud T, Lundström A. Intercellular lamellar lipids in plantar stratum corneum. Acta Derm Venereol (Stockh) 1991; 71:369–72.
4. Menon GK, Elias PM. Morphological basis for a pore-pathway in mammalian stratum corneum. Skin Pharmacol 1997; 10:235–46.
5. Bouwstra JA, Gooris GS, Dubbelaar et al. Role of ceramide 1 in the molecular organization of the stratum corneum lipids. J Lipid Res 1998; 39:186–96.
6. Swartzendruber DC, Manganaro A, Madison KC et al. Organization of the intercellular spaces of porcine epidermal and palatal stratum corneum: a quantitative study employing ruthenium tetroxide. Cell Tissue Res 1995; 279:271–6.

14
Rapid infrared spectrometric quantitation of stratum corneum lipid content

J-C Tsai, C-Y Lin, H-M Sheu and Y-L Lo

Introduction

Stratum corneum (SC), the outermost layer of the skin, serves as a barrier to both water loss and to penetration of exogenous substances. Such barrier properties are mediated by a series of lipid multilayers, enriched with ceramides, cholesterol and free fatty acids, segregated within the SC interstices. Various studies[1,2] have indicated that SC lipid content is defective in pathologic states that are accompanied by compromised barrier function. SC lipid content of these physiologic and pathologic states is usually determined by gravimetric measurement following organic solvent extractions.[3] These procedures are time-consuming, rather tedious to carry out, and involve hazardous solvents. Fourier transform infrared (FTIR) spectroscopy, which is used to measure the vibrational modes of the functional groups of molecules, is sensitive to molecular structure, conformation and environment of the biomolecules. The objectives of the study were to establish quantitative relationships between IR spectral characteristics of C–H stretching region and SC lipid content, and to develop a method of measuring SC lipids by FTIR, which is fast and requires no solvents.

Materials and methods

Isolation of porcine stratum corneum

Sheets of SC were prepared by treating porcine skin, dermatomed to 500 µm, with 0.5% trypsin, in phosphate-buffered saline, pH 7.4, for 18 hours at 4°C. The isolated SC sheets were dried overnight and stored in a desiccator.

FTIR spectroscopy

The IR spectra of isolated porcine SC sheets were recorded using a Nicolet Magna 560 FTIR spectrometer, equipped with an MCT detector and OMNIC software for data acquisition. Resolution was set at 4 cm^{-1}. Each spectrum represented the average of 64 scans. Spectral analysis by curve-fitting was performed using GRAMS/32 software between 2800–3000 cm^{-1}.

Gravimetric measurement of stratum corneum lipids

The lipid extractions of the ground porcine SC were performed at 2-hour intervals, with each of a series of chloroform/methanol mixtures. The lipid extracts were filtered, concentrated under nitrogen, and dried in a vacuum. The residue was then dissolved in a chloroform/methanol (2:1) mixture. Total SC lipid weight was determined by weighing the lipid residue after evaporating an aliquot in an aluminum pan on a Mettler balance (sensitivity = 2 μg).

Results and discussion

The peak area of both the CH_2 symmetric (2850 cm^{-1}) and asymmetric (2920 cm^{-1}) stretching bands in the IR spectra of progressively solvent-extracted porcine SC sheets was decreased with increasing amount of SC lipids removed. As shown in Figure 14.1, peak area ratios of CH_2 to CH_3 asymmetric stretching bands in the IR spectra of 46 isolated porcine SC samples were correlated to SC lipid content ($y = 0.036x + 0.648$, $r^2 = 0.90$), with the standard error of measurement of 1.91%. The FTIR method provides a fast and accurate measurement of SC lipid content,

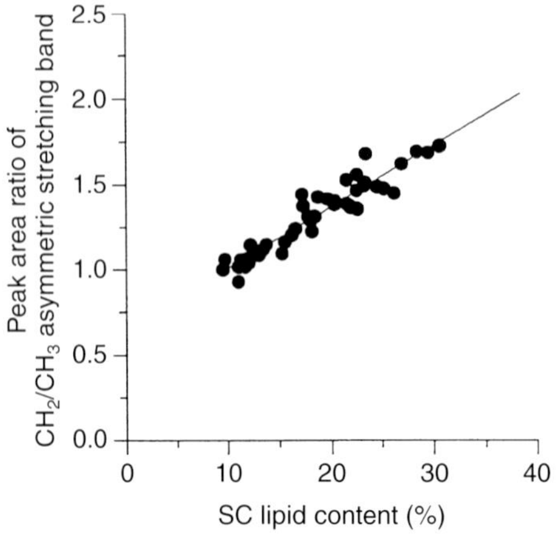

Figure 14.1

Peak area ratio of CH_2/CH_3 asymmetric stretching bands as a function of SC lipid content (N = 46).

and potentially can be developed as a non-invasive technique for human SC lipid quantitation in vivo with the assistance of fiber-optic accessories.

Acknowledgments

This work was supported by a grant from the National Science Council of Taiwan (NSC 89-2320-B006-145).

References

1. Elias PM, Williams ML, Maloney ME et al. Stratum corneum lipids in disorders of cornification. Steroid sulfatase and cholesterol sulfate in normal desquamation and the pathogenesis of recessive X-linked ichthyosis. J Clin Invest 1984; 74:1414–21.
2. Yamamoto A, Serizawa S, Ito M et al. Stratum corneum lipid abnormalities in atopic dermatitis. Arch Dermatol Res 1991; 283:219–23.
3. Wertz PW, Downing DT et al. Free sphingosine in human epidermis. J Invest Dermatol 1990; 94: 159–61.

15

The combination of neutron scattering techniques for the study of hydration of porcine stratum corneum

GCh Charalambopoulou, ThA Steriotis,
KL Stefanopoulos, ES Kikkinides and AK Stubos

Aims

A wide range of methods with the aim of efficiently studying the structure of either human or animal stratum corneum (SC) has so far been employed. Emphasis has been put on the investigation of SC's lipid phase ultrastructure by using scattering techniques, such as small- and wide-angle X-ray scattering.[1–3] In contrast, attempts at investigating SC using neutron scattering have been few, and not always successful.[4] Nevertheless, neutron scattering is a non-destructive structural analysis tool, appropriate for providing information about inhomogeneties as large as 1 μm, and can often prove more useful than X-rays, especially in the context of pharmaceutical sciences. In the present work, different versions of neutron scattering were, for the first time, successfully used for the investigation of the effect of hydration on the biphasic structure of porcine SC. The primary goal was to obtain data concerning microscopic details of SC, as well as to investigate structural changes induced by interaction with various molecules. This information can further feed the efforts of understanding, modeling and, finally, predicting SC transport processes.

Methods

Three different scattering techniques, relevant to scales of SC structure of different lengths, were used. Ultra-Small Angle and Small Angle Neutron Scattering (USANS and SANS), as well as Neutron Diffraction (ND) experiments were performed on the Double Crystal Diffractometer (V12a), SANS Instrument (V4) and Membrane Diffractometer (V1), in the facilities of Hahn–Meitner Institut, Berlin. The SC samples, originating from the epidermis of porcine skin, were hydrated in situ to relative humidities, ranging from 0% to 100%, with a home-made, portable absorption apparatus.

Results and conclusions

USANS was used for the study of the bulk properties of the lipid phase of SC during hydration.[5] The qualitative examination of the scattering curves, recorded for samples with different water content, revealed swelling mechanisms for both lipid and protein regions (Figure 15.1).

At the same time, the dry samples' spectra were mathematically processed in order to obtain information about the dimensions of the SC biphasic geometry, in terms of the correlation function.[6] By adopting the

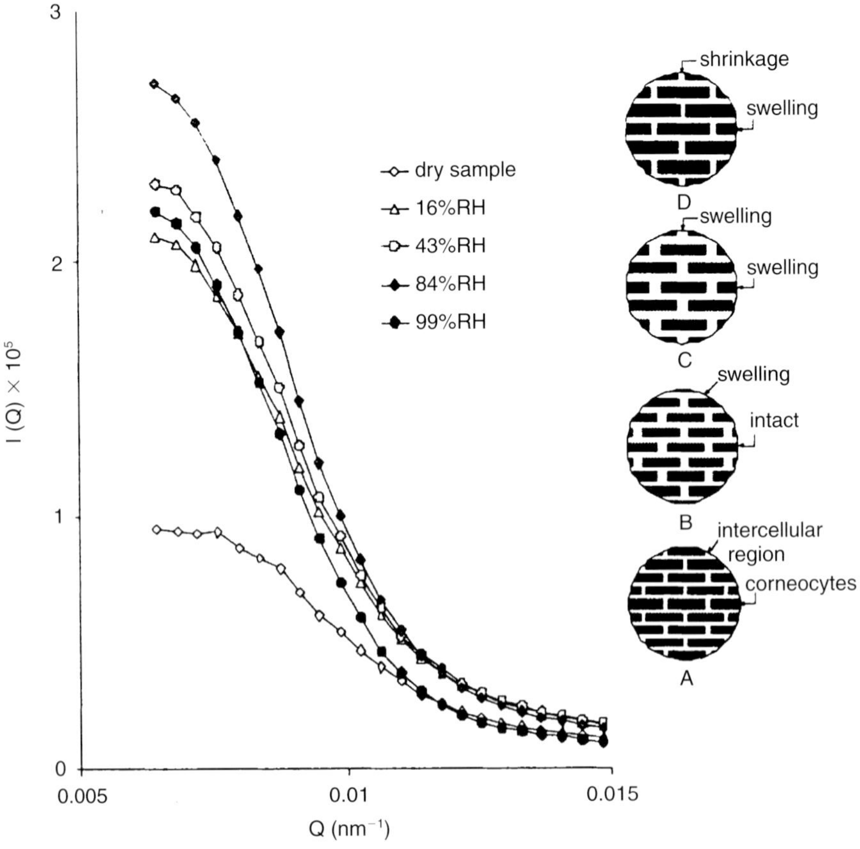

Figure 15.1
Ultra-Small Angle Scattering curves of porcine SC at various RH.

two-dimensional 'brick-and-mortar' model, an attempt was made to numerically produce SC model structures that matched the experimentally determined correlation function. The most appropriate values for the corneocyte thickness and the surrounding lipid gap were found in the range 0.6–1 μm and 0.05–0.1 μm, respectively. The effect of the variation of corneocyte length could not, however, be detected, as length scales of such magnitude are clearly outside the USANS resolution.

Moving towards smaller-length scales, SANS was used for the investigation of the hydration effect on the organization of the lipid bilayers. The obtained spectra (Figure 15.2) showed a shoulder at $Q = 1\,nm^{-1}$[7] in good agreement with previous SANS measurements.[3] This result indicates an ~6 nm periodicity in the lipid phase, reflecting the size of one bilayer. Towards lower scattering angles, a shoulder appears at $Q = 0.195\,nm^{-1}$, which corresponds to a periodicity of 32.2 nm.

Finally, the ND method was employed, ultimately aiming to enable the localization of water molecules in the two phases of SC. The resulting scattering pattern of fully hydrated SC (Figure 15.3) was characterized by a strong diffraction peak at $Q = 1\,nm^{-1}$, which corresponds to a periodicity of 6.28 nm. The second order peak was also clearly observed at $Q = 2\,nm^{-1}$. It should be noted that the lamellar structure of the SC lipid phase is clearly revealed by a neutron technique, for the first time. This preliminary, but significant, result is considered to be only the starting point, encouraging future experimentation. The continuation of this work is already under way.

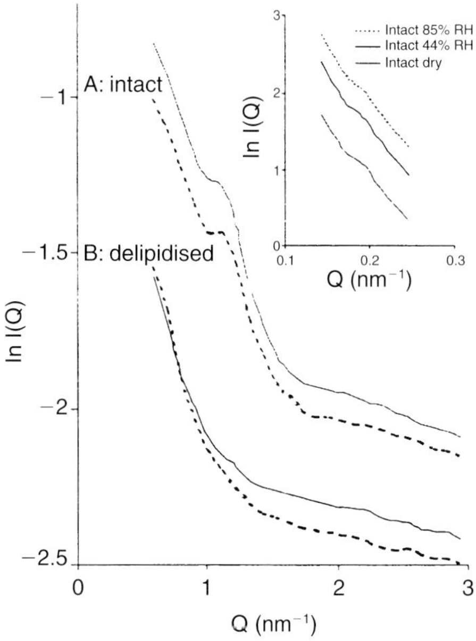

Figure 15.2

Small Angle Scattering curves of intact and delipidized porcine SC.

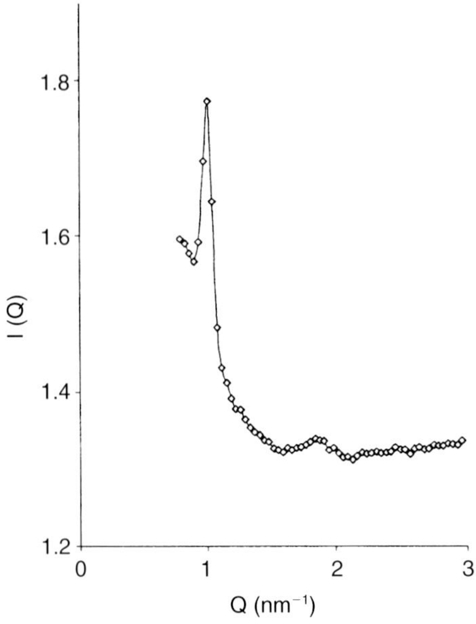

Figure 15.3
Diffraction pattern of fully hydrated porcine SC.

References

1. Friberg SE, Osborne DW. Small-angle X-ray diffraction patterns of stratum corneum and a model structure for its lipids. J Dispersion Sci Tech 1985; 6:485–95.
2. Bouwstra JA, Gooris GS, Van der Spek JA et al. Structural investigations of human stratum corneum by small-angle X-ray scattering. J Invest Dermatol 1991; 97: 1005–12.
3. Bouwstra JA, Gooris GS, Bras W et al. Lipid organisation in pig stratum corneum. J Lipid Res 1995; 36:685–95.
4. Watkinson AC, Hadgraft J, Street PR et al. Neutrons, surfaces, and skin. In: Potts RO, Guy RH, eds. *Mechanisms of Transdermal Drug Delivery*. First edn. New York: Marcel Dekker 1997:231–65.
5. Charalambopoulou GC, Steriotis TA, Mitropoulos AC et al. Investigation of water sorption on porcine stratum corneum by very small angle neutron scattering. J Invest Dermatol 1998; 110: 988–90.
6. Charalambopoulou GC, Karamertzanis P, Kikkinides ES et al. A study on structural and diffusion properties of porcine stratum corneum based on very small angle neutron scattering data. Pharm Res 2000; 17:1085–91.
7. Charalambopoulou GC, Steriotis TA, Stefanopoulos KL et al. Investigation of lipid organization on stratum corneum by water absorption in conjunction with neutron scattering. Physica B 2000; 276–8:530–1.

Section II
Pharmacology and percutaneous absorption

16
Crossing the barrier

J Hadgraft

Introduction

It has been estimated that some 60% of the population suffers from a dermatological disorder, and that 25% of this number requires medical intervention. However, skin disorders are very difficult to treat. This, in part, is due to the superb barrier properties of the stratum corneum, which results in very low topical bioavailability. The unique barrier properties of the stratum corneum are a direct consequence of the mechanism by which xenobiotics permeate. The route appears to be a tortuous one around the dead, dense corneocytes. The permeant, therefore, diffuses in the intercellular channels, which contain structured lipid bilayers. The molecule, therefore, not only has a tortuous path, but also has to cross, sequentially, lipophilic and hydrophilic domains. In addition, the polar head groups of the lipids hold the alkyl chains in close proximity. This means that the methylene groups close to these head groups are relatively rigid in nature and the diffusing molecule experiences a microenvironment that is rather viscous in nature.[1]

There are a number of possible means of improving transport through the channels. The drug should be applied to the skin at as high an activity state as possible. The driving force for diffusion is the chemical potential gradient, which, under normal circumstances, will be a maximum when the formulation is saturated with the drug.[2] For identical formulations, a 1% suspension of an active will give the same flux as a 5% one. It is not always the concentration that is present that determines the bioactivity.[3]

Even if the drug is applied at as high an activity as possible, the amount that is absorbed is usually very small, and other approaches have to be used to enhance permeation. These can be either chemical or physical means. In general, the major approaches used for local delivery use chemical enhancement strategies. These will be discussed later. An additional problem in dermal delivery is that the drugs that are used have often been developed for other routes of administration and, therefore, they do not possess optimum physicochemical properties for partition and diffusion into and across the skin. As the mechanisms of skin permeation are better understood at a molecular level, it is possible to make general statements about the properties that an ideal permeant should have. It should:

1. be small,
2. have a low melting point,
3. possess a log(octanol–water partition coefficient) ~ 2,
4. have good solubility in both water and oils, and
5. have a minimum number of pendant functional groups capable of hydrogen bonding.

When drugs are specifically designed for topical use, these criteria should be considered, but, of course, remembering that the therapeutic activity of the drug also needs to be taken into account. It is sometimes better to select a compound that is less bioactive but permeates the skin to its site of action.[4] Where there is no opportunity to design the drug ab initio and a compound is selected that does not permeate particularly well, there are various enhancer approaches. The different ways this can be achieved is best understood by considering Fick's first law of diffusion. Steady state fluxes (J) are given by:

$$J = KDA\Delta c/h \qquad (16.1)$$

where K is the partition coefficient between the stratum corneum and the applied vehicle, D is the 'average' diffusion coefficient, A is the diffusional area with pathlength (h), and Δc is the concentration difference between the donor and receptor phase. The variables which can be influenced are therefore D, K, or both. As mentioned above, under normal circumstances, it is only possible to vary c up to the solubility limit. Supersaturated states can be prepared and, if they can be stabilized, they can be used to give enhanced fluxes.[5] This is seen in Figure 16.1.

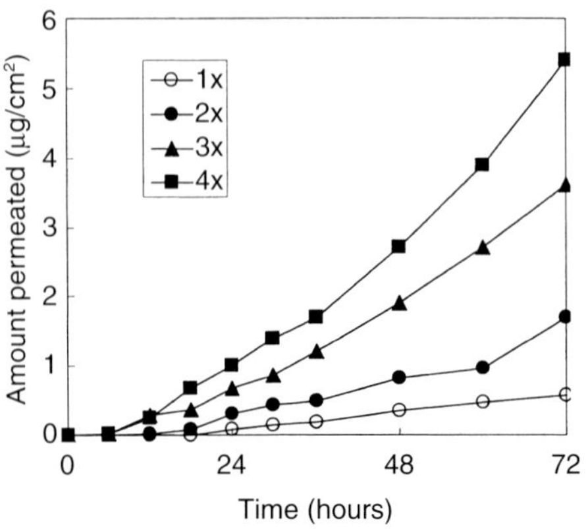

Figure 16.1
The in vitro permeation of piroxicam through human skin showing the effect of the degree of supersaturation. Data adapted from Reference 6.

Enhancer strategies

Diffusion effects

Excipients can be incorporated into the topical formulation that will co-diffuse into the skin with the drug. If they have the correct physicochemical properties, they can intercalate into the structured lipids of the intercellular channels. Their presence will disorder the packing of the lipids and the diffusional barrier can be reduced (i.e. D is increased in Equation 16.1). Typically, these enhancers have a polar head group and a long alkyl chain (often 12 carbon atoms is the ideal length). They are therefore often surfactants and care needs to taken that they do not also have irritant properties. Their interaction with the skin lipids has been investigated using a variety of biophysical techniques, such as Fourier transform infrared (FTIR) spectroscopy,[7] Raman,[8] X-ray diffraction,[9] fluorescence spectroscopy,[10] electron spin resonance (ESR),[11] and nuclear magnetic resonance (NMR).[12] Their mechanism of action is becoming increasingly understood and it is possible to see design elements within the molecular structure that confer the enhancer activity.[13] Subtle changes in the structure can alter the molecule such that its activity is removed or even reversed, i.e. it becomes a penetration retarder. This is seen in the structures given in Figure 16.2. Azone[T] is a well-known penetration enhancer, its sulphur analogue is inactive and the structure with the 5-membered ring (N-0915) is a permeation retarder.[13]

Partition effects

Other excipients can diffuse into the skin and alter its solubility properties. If this is in a favourable direction for the permeant, partition into the

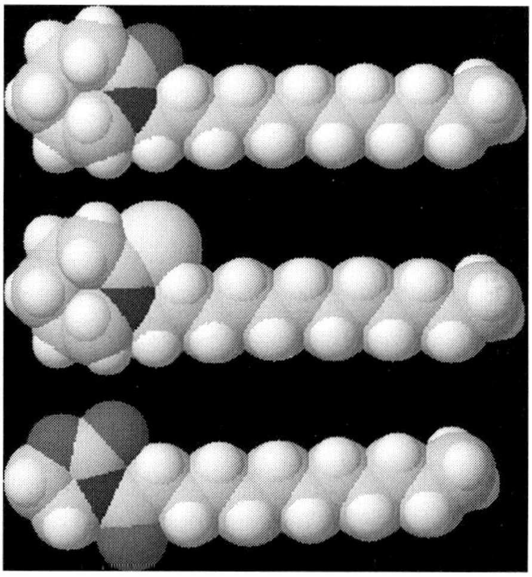

Figure 16.2

Molecular graphics representations of (from top) Azone[T] (a penetration enhancer), the sulphur analogue of Azone[T] (inactive as an enhancer), NO915 (a penetration retarder).

skin is essentially increased (K is increased in Equation 16.1). There have been a number of attempts to rationalize the effects of solvents on the solubility properties of the skin. These have attempted to use solubility parameter as the physicochemical determinant. However, the various studies have not produced any conclusive way of showing how the presence of small solvent-type molecules, such as propylene glycol, affect the partition of the permeant. This is due, in part, to the complex nature of the problem. The degree to which the partition behaviour is influenced depends on the amount of the solvent in the skin. Few studies have measured the uptake of formulation excipients into the skin. Secondly, the excipients could affect more than one parameter; for example, they could also influence the diffusion properties. It is difficult to deconvolute the effects. A typical diffusion experiment involves measurement of the steady state flux (J). The applied concentration, c, is known, which means that it is trivial to calculate the permeability coefficient (= KD/h). However, separating this into D and K is more complex. One way that this can be achieved is using attenuated total reflectance (ATR)–FTIR methodology[14] and a saturated solution of the permeant (this removes any activity effects, which would further complicate data deconvolution). This technique has shown the distinct mechanisms of action of Azone[T] (affects D) and Transcutol[T] (affects K).

Another type of data analysis involves measuring the steady-state flux and, at the end of the experiment, determining the amount of permeant in the skin (C_{skin}). The skin is pre-treated with a solvent for a set period (typically 30 minutes) and, then, an aqueous solution of the permeant is placed on the skin surface.[2,15] The flux values should lie on a line defined by the origin of the J versus C_{skin} plot and the co-ordinates of the control (no solvent pre-treatment). The distance from point (0,0) is a measure of the increase in partition effect caused by the solvent. Points above the line indicate an increase in D, induced by the solvent; those below the line represent a decrease in barrier properties. A typical graph, with tritiated water as the permeant, is shown in Figure 16.3. There are no points significantly below the line and most solvents act by changing the partition behaviour.

Solvents, which show maximum effect above the line, are mixtures (e.g. propylene glycol–decanol). It is possible that these act by skin lipid fluidization or by the mixed solvent extracting the skin lipids.

Lipid extraction

Skin lipids are integral to barrier function; hence their extraction can have profound effects. Treatment of the skin with methanol and chloroform mixtures extracts the lipids and the barrier properties are destroyed. It is difficult to separate the effects of the solvent. It could be affecting D or K, or extracting part of the lipid matrix. This question can be addressed using a tape-stripping technique coupled with ATR–FTIR.[16] The solvents

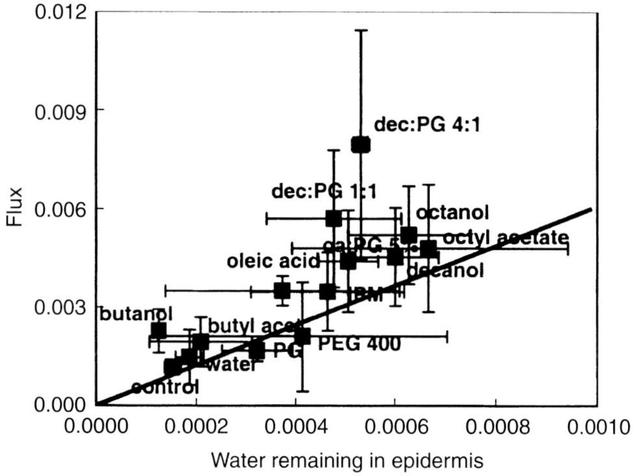

Figure 16.3

The flux of water as a function of water remaining in the skin, at steady state. The skin was pre-treated with nothing (control) or solvents for 30 minutes. These are labelled on the graph. The line is drawn through the origin and the control point. Data adapted from Reference 15.

are perdeuterated so that their signal can be distinguished from the CH stretch of the skin lipids. It is then possible to examine the effect of the solvent on the skin lipid mobility, lipid extraction and solvent uptake simultaneously. In initial experiments, simple alkanols were chosen. n-hexanol and n-octanol extract some of the intercellular lipids, whereas n-decanol does not. The uptake of n-decanol was higher than the other two alkanols, all of which increased the disorder of the skin lipids (change in CH stretch frequency), which was in proportion to the uptake. An example of this is shown in Figure 16.4.

Conclusions

It is possible to employ a number of techniques to improve dermal bioavailability. The main strategies are to co-formulate a drug with an enhancer that will improve D or K (or both) in the stratum corneum. Simple inspection of Equation 16.1 shows that, if both approaches can be used at the same time, that synergy is possible. A modest increase in D (e.g. 3-fold) coupled with one for K (e.g. 3-fold) will have an almost 10-fold effect on the amount of drug that permeates.[17] If supersaturation is also used, even greater effects can be achieved.[18] If rational drug and formulation design is used for dermal delivery, it should be possible to optimize dosage regimens. It should be possible to lower the dose

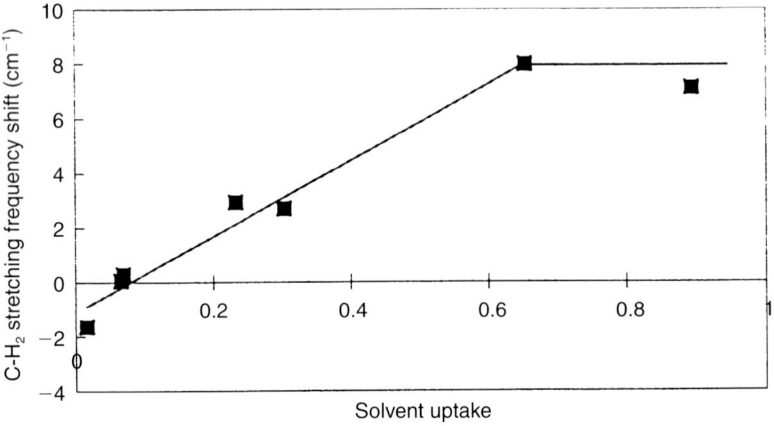

Figure 16.4

The relationship between hexanol uptake (normalized C-D peak area) and the C-H frequency shift after 30 min of exposure to D-hexanol. Data adapted from Reference 16.

applied to the patient and minimize unwanted systemic side-effects. Dose titration, as seen routinely in oral therapy, also becomes a possibility.

References

1. Hadgraft J. Skin, the final frontier. Int J Pharmaceut 2001; 224:1–18.
2. Hadgraft J. Modulation of the barrier function of the skin. Skin Pharmacol Appl Skin Physiol 2001; 14:72–81.
3. Lippold BC, Schneemann H. The influence of vehicles on the local bioavailability of betamethasone-17-benzoate from solution-type and suspension-type ointments. Int J Pharmaceut 1984; 22:31–43.
4. Hadgraft J, du Plessis J, Goosen C. The selection of non-steroidal anti-inflammatory agents for dermal delivery. Int J Pharmaceut 2000; 207:31–7.
5. Pellett MA, Roberts MS, Hadgraft J. Supersaturated solutions evaluated with an in vitro stratum corneum tape stripping technique. Int J Pharmaceut 1997; 151:91–8.
6. Pellett MA, Davis AF, Hadgraft J. Effect of supersaturation on membrane-transport. 2. Piroxicam. Int J Pharmaceut 1994; 111:1–6.
7. Ongpipattanakul B, Burnette RR, Potts RO et al. Evidence that oleic acid exists in a separate phase within stratum corneum lipids. Pharmaceut Res 1991; 8:350–4.
8. Williams AC, Edwards HGM, Barry BW. Fourier-transform Raman-spectroscopy – a novel application for examining human stratum corneum. Int J Pharmaceut 1992; 81:R11–14.
9. Bouwstra JA, Gooris GS, van der Spek JA et al. Structural investigations of human stratum corneum by small-angle X-ray scattering. J Invest Dermatol 1991; 97: 1005–12.
10. Garrison MD, Doh LM, Potts RO et al. Effect of oleic acid on human epidermis: fluorescence spectro-

scopic investigation. J Control Release 1994; 31:263–9.

11. Gay CL, Murphy TM, Hadgraft J et al. An electron spin resonance study of skin penetration enhancers. Int J Pharmaceut 1989; 49:39–45.
12. Fenske DB, Thewalt JL, Bloom M et al. Models of stratum corneum intercellular membranes: ^{2}H NMR of macroscopically oriented multilayers. Biophys J 1994; 67: 1562–73.
13. Hadgraft J, Peck J, Williams DG et al. Mechanisms of action of skin penetration enhancers retarders: Azone and analogues. Int J Pharmaceut 1996; 141:17–25.
14. Harrison JE, Watkinson AC, Green DM et al. The relative effect of Azone® and Transcutol® on permeant diffusivity and solubility in human stratum corneum. Pharmaceut Res 1996; 13:542–6.
15. Rosado CBF. *Formulation Strategies in Transdermal Delivery.* Cardiff University; 2000.
16. Dias MM. *Facilitated Percutaneous Penetration.* Cardiff University; 2001.
17. Hadgraft J. Passive enhancement strategies in topical and transdermal drug delivery. Int J Pharmaceut 1999; 184:1–6.
18. Pellett MA, Watkinson AC, Brain KR et al. Synergism between supersaturation and chemical enhancement in the permeation of flurbiprofen through human skin. In: Brain KR, James VJ, Walters KA, eds. *Perspectives in Percutaneous Penetration.* Vol 5b. Cardiff: STS Publishing; 1998:173–6.

17
Lipid organization and barrier function

J-L Lévêque

Introduction

We have known for years that skin barrier function is mainly ensured by the stratum corneum (SC). Both the nature of its components and its structural organization explain its efficacy in limiting the penetration of xenobiotics into the skin and in controlling the dehydration of the biological milieu. Numerous studies have illustrated the role of the different SC components (lipids, protein materials, water-soluble materials, etc.) on transepidermal water loss (TEWL), which is considered a valuable index for checking the functionality of SC.[1] Clearly, epidermal lipids, and particularly ceramides, the most polar fraction, play a key role in the diffusion process through SC.[2] Influence of SC proteins has been investigated far less, but the weakening of SC barrier function after treatment by detergents is unlikely to be related to lipid extraction alone.[3]

Irrespective of the physical and chemical nature of SC components, it is of interest to consider the influence of the structural organization of SC. This 'organization' may be considered according to different levels of examination: macroscopic (as viewed in histology, in the micron range), microscopic (electron microscopy, hundreds of nanometers' range) or at the molecular and supra-molecular level, some nanometers by means of X-ray diffraction.

We know that lipids are mainly located in the intercorneocyte spaces, forming bilayers, as viewed by transmission electron microscopy (TEM), following proper preparation of ultra-thin SC sections.[4] These bilayers appear under two different types of organization: as either regular or irregular alternations of clear and dark bands (Figure 17.1). A chemical model, which may represent and explain the peculiar geometry of some of these bilayers, has been previously presented.[5]

The exact three-dimensional geometrical arrangement of these lipids was characterized through X-ray diffraction studies, taking advantage of the strong brightness and flux of the very thin X-ray beam generated by synchrotron sources.[6] In brief, SC bilayers could be characterized by two reticular distances, at 6.5 and 4.5 nm, this second figure being probably the third order of a 13.5-nm reticular distance.[6,7] The lateral packing of

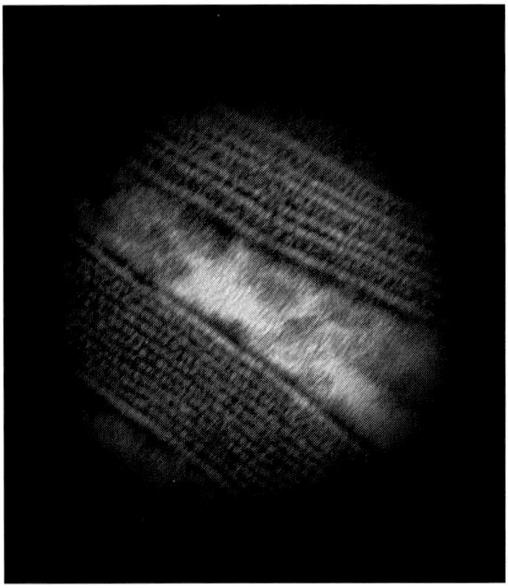

Figure 17.1

Densitometric profiles of the SAXD pattern according to hydration.

the aliphatic chains of the lipids forming these bilayers was also determined.[8]

This short presentation illustrates the relationship between the organization of lamellar lipid bilayers and TEWL through SC, according to three different experimental situations: effects of water, thermal treatment, and SC extension.

The influence of water

Water molecules markedly change all the physical properties of the keratinized tissues and particularly increase the diffusion coefficient.

Differential scanning calorimetry (DSC) studies of SC samples at different water content show that the temperature of the second peak representing the epidermal lipid fusion (Tm2) is decreased from about 78 to 70°C[9] when SC is hydrated from 0% to 70% RH. This 'fluidification' of the aliphatic chains is in agreement with an electron spin resonance (ESR) study showing some disordering of the chains.[10]

X-ray diffraction studies carried out at small angles (SAXD) demonstrated that there is no swelling of the bilayers. No change in the location of the diffraction peaks and shoulder, corresponding to 13.4, 6.5 and 4.5 nm, respectively, can be detected.[7,11] Moreover, Ribaud[11] found a clear thinning of the 45-nm shoulder, indicative of a better organization of the periodic molecular assembly (Figure 17.2). In any case, these results support a model of SC hydration into which water molecules would disorganize the periodic arrangement of the intercellular lipids.

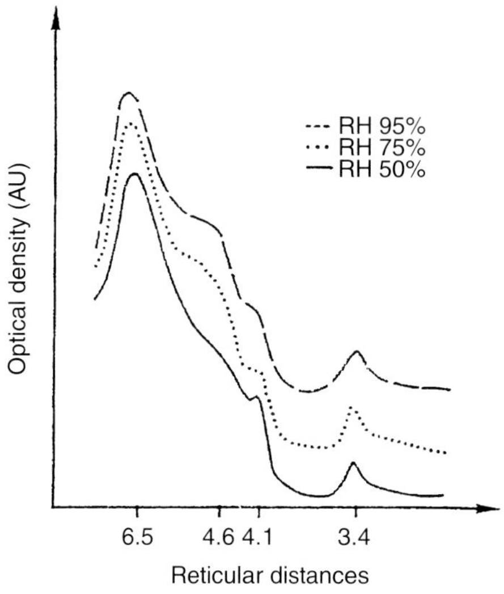

Figure 17.2

Influence of the temperature of successive heating of a stratum corneum sample on the relative increase of the water vapour diffusion coefficient.

TEM studies of fully hydrated SC samples show that water is able to disrupt the structure, shifting lamellar bilayers by creating amorphous intercellular lipid zones.[12] Using a freeze-etching technique, we also confirmed the existence of water voids in the intercellular spaces (Figure 17.3). These studies support the view that water can be highly damaging for SC structure. Such a situation corresponds, however, to a fully hydrated SC (for at least 2 hours), which hardly represents the actual situation. As described later, liquid water hardly modifies lipid bilayers.

These results (DSC, X-ray diffraction, TEM) show that water would have two different types of effect, according its concentration. In the intermediary stages, probably when water molecules are bound to proteins (up to 34%), they have a structuring effect on the lamellar bilayers, although, at saturation, they totally swell SC membrane, damaging both cells and intercellular spaces; these damages, however, appear to be reversible. Water molecules would be located between the 'polar' head of the same lipid layer, inducing some fluidity to the chains and making the diffusion process easier.[11]

The influence of thermal treatment

It is very interesting to look at the effects of successive thermal treatments of SC, known to increase skin penetration. Progressively preheating SC samples from 75 to 90°C increases SC permeability to alcanol.[13] Diffusion, through porcine SC, of tritiated water vapour is also enhanced after preheating the sample to 75°C.[9]

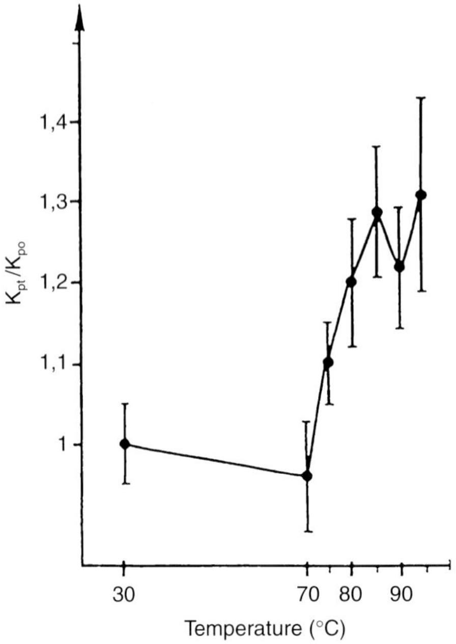

Figuro 17.3
Morphology of a fully hydrated stratum corneum after freeze-etching processing of the sample (courtesy of AM Minondo, L'Oréal).

X-ray diffraction studies, carried out on SC sheets at SAXD, show that preheating the sample to 90°C markedly smoothes the densitometry profile of the diffraction pattern. The features located at 6.5 and 4.6 nm, representing the periodical arrangement of lamellar bilayers, are less clearly marked.[14] In the same study, these authors found a progressive decrease in temperature of the second DSC peak, and a correlative increase of the permeability constant of water (Figure 17.4). In such an experimental situation, disorganization of lipids (in terms of supramolecular arrangement and chain fluidity) corresponds to a weakening of the barrier function of SC.

The influence of SC deformation

SC is subjected to numerous deformations generated by body movements. On the forearm, for example, these deformations can reach 40%, by simply opening out the arm.[15] On other sites, such as the face, this figure could be overcome. Would such strong deformations disorganize SC lipids and, therefore, alter skin barrier function? Only two studies have addressed this important question. The first,[16] conducted in vivo on humans, showed no increase in TEWL on the forearm after 8% and 16% extension. Inversely, a more recent study,[17] carried out on pig SC in vitro,

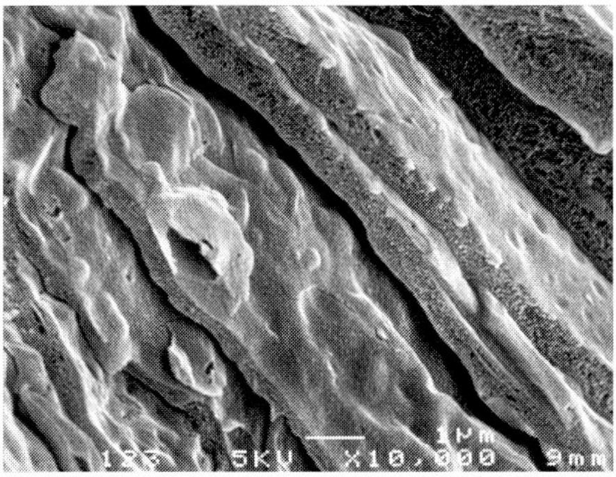

Figure 17.4
Aspect of the two types of lamellar bilayers present in the intercellular spaces of stratum corneum (courtesy of F Fiat, L'Oréal).

concluded a strong increase of TEWL (about twofold) following an 8% extension. Ultra-structural changes in SC during extension were followed by TEM. Results show that the structure of lamellar bilayers is progressively disrupted, resulting in a perturbed barrier function. We recently revisited this question by combining in vivo measurement of TEWL and in vitro investigation of SC structure, through TEM and X-ray diffraction.[18]

Diffraction studies at SAXD of human SC under extension do not exhibit any marked differences in the location and intensity of the main peak at 6.5 nm.

TEM studies, carried out on samples fixed and contrasted under extension, showed that the main damage caused by extension is the disruption of the corneocyte cell membrane from the lipid bilayer. In very rare places, bilayers, as well as some corneodesmosomes, appeared broken, leading to a general aspect of a loose, but somewhat intact, structure.

In vivo measurement of TEWL under skin extension demonstrated no statistical increase of TEWL. These results are in line with those published by Takahashi and Marks,[16] but in complete disagreement with those obtained in vitro by Rawlings et al.[17] According to our results, skin deformation does not alter either the lipid organization or the barrier function.

Conclusion

The "brick-and-mortar" model only schematically described the SC as a composite material where lipids and proteins are segregated. This is both untrue and oversimplified. Today, more subtle models attempt to take into account the cohesion of the cells, and the structural, diffusion and thermal properties of this important epidermal layer.[19] If the importance of ceramides and other polar lipid moieties on the diffusion property of SC is no longer disputed, the influence of the molecular organization of lipids begins to be fairly well documented. For example, results, dealing with the effects of water, heat, sodium lauryl sulfate, and penetration enhancers on their diffusion properties through SC, illustrate the importance of this parameter.

Our recent studies, carried out on stretched SC, demonstrate that the supra-molecular organization of the intercellular lipids is maintained and that no increase of TEWL can be recorded after deformation. The presence of the skin micro-relief likely explains why bilayers are not altered after strong deformations. Unfolding of this 'deformation reservoir' would appear to be an adaptive capacity of the skin to its necessary and repeated deformations.

References

1. Lotte C, Rougier A, Wilson DR et al. In vivo relationship between TEWL and percutaneous penetration of some organic compounds in man: effect of anatomic site. Arch Dermatol Res 1987; 279:351–6.
2. Mao Qiang M, Elias PM, Feingold KR. Fatty acids are required for epidermal permeability barrier function. J Clin Invest 1993; 92: 791–8.
3. Lévêque JL, de Rigal J, Saint-Léger D et al. How does sodium lauryl sulfate alter the skin barrier function in man? A multiparametric approach. Skin Pharmacol 1993; 6:111–15.
4. Landman L. Epidermal permeability barrier. Transformation of lamellar granule-disks into cellular sheets by a membrane-fusion process, a freeze-fracture study. J Invest Dermatol 1986; 87:202–9.
5. Schwarzendruber DC, Werz PW, Madison KC et al. Evidence that corneocyte has a chemically bound envelope. J Invest Dermatol 1987; 88:709–13.
6. Garson JC, Doucet J, Lévêque JL et al. Oriented structure in human stratum corneum revealed by X-ray diffraction. J Invest Dermatol 1991; 96:43–9.
7. Bouwstra JA, Gooris GS, Van der Speck JA et al. Structural investigations of human stratum corneum by small angle x-ray scattering. J Invest Dermatol 1991; 97:1005–12.
8. Bouwstra JA, Gooris GS, Salmon de Vries MA et al. Structure of human stratum corneum as a function of temperature and hydration: a wide angle x-ray scattering. J Invest Dermatol 1992; 84:205–16.
9. Golden GM, Guzek DB, Harris RR et al. Lipid thermotropic transitions in human stratum corneum. J Invest Dermatol 1986; 86:255–9.
10. Alonso A, Meirelles MC, Tabak M. Effect of hydration upon the fluidity of intercellular membrane of stratum corneum: an EPR study. Biochem Biophys Acta 1995; 1237:6–15.
11. Ribaud Ch. Pharmacy Thesis, Université de Paris-Sud, 1994.
12. Warner RR, Boissy YI, Spears MJ et al. Water disrupts stratum corneum lipid lamellae: damage is similar to surfactants. J Invest Dermatol 1999; 113:960–6.
13. Al Saidan SM, Winfield AJ, Selkirk AB. Effect of preheating on the permeability of neonatal rat stratum corneum to alkanols. J Invest Dermatol 1986; 89:430–3.
14. Ribaud Ch, Garson JC, Doucet J et al. Organisation of stratum corneum lipids in relation to permeability: influence of sodium lauryl sulfate and preheating.

Phamaceutical Res 1994; 11: 1414–18.

15. Corcuff P, de Lacharrière O, Lévêque JL. Extension-induced changes in the microrelief of the human volar forearm: variations with age. J Gerontol 1991; 46: 223–7.
16. Takahashi M, Marks R. Conformational and functional changes in the stratum corneum after forced extension. Bioeng Skin 1985; 2:39–48.
17. Rawlings AV, Watkinson A, Harding CR et al. Changes in stratum corneum lipid and desmosome structure together with water barrier function during mechanical stress. J Soc Cosmet Chem 1995; 46:141–51.
18. Lévêque JL, Hallegot Ph, Doucet J et al. Structure and function of human stratum corneum under deformation. 2002 in press.
19. Norlen L. Skin barrier structure and function: the single gel phase model. J Invest Dermatol 2001; 117:830–6.

18

Structure of multi-phasic dermatological formulations and the influence of the structure and of vehicle evaporation on transdermal drug permeation

D Hummel and G Imanidis

Introduction

The majority of dermatological formulations contain components that are not mutually miscible, thus forming separate phases. These phases are intermixed, producing macroscopically homogeneous systems, on the microscopic level; however, they form distinct structures that may influence, among other characteristics, the distribution and the transport of the active ingredient(s). Phospholipids are one class of components that can form liposomal structures in the formulation, which are thought to positively affect skin permeation of the drug by interacting with the lipids of the stratum corneum.

In the present work, formulations consisting basically of phospholipid, triglyceride, emulsifier surfactant and water, were investigated. These formulations had the potential to form colloidal liposomal dispersions, (O/W) emulsions and possibly other systems. The phases formed, constituting the dispersed fraction of the formulation, were studied as a function of its percentile composition. The effect of the phase structure on drug release and drug permeation through stratum corneum (SC) and the skin was assessed and a physicochemical model describing these processes was developed. As a model drug, S-Ibuprofen, a non-steroidal anti-inflammatory agent, was incorporated in the formulations. Finally, the evaporation of volatile components of the formulation during the time of application and its influence on skin permeation of drug were determined.

Materials and methods

The compositions of the formulations used are shown in Table 18.1. NAT

Table 18.1 Composition of formulations (in weight-%).

	Study formulations			Reference formulations	
	1	2	3	O/W Emulsion	Liposomal dispersion
S-Ibuprofen	1.0	1.0	1.0	1.0	1.0
Purified water	69.4	59.4	57.4	72.4	80.0
Ethanol 96%	13.4	13.4	13.4	15.0	12.1
NAT 8539®	3.6	3.6	3.6		6.8
Triglyceride	10.0	20.0	20.0	10.0	
Tween 80	2.0	2.0	4.0	1.0	
Tocopherol	0.1	0.1	0.1	0.1	0.1
Xanthan gum	0.5	0.5	0.5	0.5	

8539® (Nattermann-Rhone Poulenc Rorer; Cologne, Germany) consists of 75% Phospholipon 80®, which is a soybean phospholipid with 80% phosphatidylcholine, and 25% ethanol. A medium-chain triglyceride containing 95% saturated fatty acids with C-8 and C-10 chains, was used (Stearinerie Dubois & Fils; Ciron, France). Tween 20 (Polysorbate 20) (Seppic; Paris, France) is an O/W emulsifier; tocopherol (Eastman; Klagsport, TN, USA) was used as antioxidant, xanthan gum as a thickener to increase physical stability, and ethanol was added in the appropriate amount to guarantee that the final ethanol content of all formulations was the same. S-Ibuprofen (>99%) was purchased from Ethyl Corporation (Orangeburg, SC, USA).

Formulations were prepared by mixing NAT 8539®, tocopherol and S-Ibuprofen with the ethanol, adding the mixture to the water and homogenizing for 5 minutes with an Ultra-Turax T25 (Janke+Kunkel; Staufen, Germany) at 15 000–20 000 rpm. Subsequently, the premixed triglyceride with Tween 20 were added and the product was homogenized once again, as above. For the O/W emulsion, ethanol, tocopherol and S-Ibuprofen were mixed with the triglyceride and the Tween 20, before being added to the water and homogenized. Xanthan gum was added at the end. Formulations were equilibrated for at least 48 hours before use.

To identify the kind of dispersed phases formed in the formulations, these were fractionated by means of ultracentrifugation for 2 hours at 222 000–450 000 g. The isolated fractions were studied by transmission electron microscopy (TEM), which was preceded by freeze fracture and preparation of replicas. Also, the chemical composition of the fractions was determined. S-Ibuprofen was assayed by high performance liquid chromatography (HPLC), ethanol by gas chromatography (GC), water by Karl–Fischer titration, and phospholipid by colorimetric determination of phosphate. The results of the study formulations were compared with those of the reference formulations, for which the type of dispersed phases formed was, to a large extent, foreseeable. No xanthan gum was contained in the centrifuged formulations, to facilitate fractionation.

Release of drug from the formulations was measured in Franz-type glass diffusion cells at 32°C, using a hydrophilic Polysulfon membrane (Supor-450, Gelman Sciences; Ann Arbor, MI, USA) to separate the formulation from the receiver medium, which was aqueous at pH 7.4. Skin permeation was studied using full-thickness pig-ear skin, under the same conditions as above. A practically infinite dose of formulation (290 mg/cm^2) was applied. The evaporation of water and ethanol from the formulation during application was measured in separate experiments using custom-made apparatus.

Results and discussion

Structure

Figure 18.1 shows an electron micrograph of the complete, i.e. non-fractionated, study formulation 1. Level structures depict oil droplets, while protruding and depressed structures depict phospholipid vesicles, as this is verified by comparison with the reference formulations. Thus, in this formulation, liposomal, i.e. liquid crystalline, and bulk triglyceride phases coexisted. Figure 18.2 shows the chemical composition of the

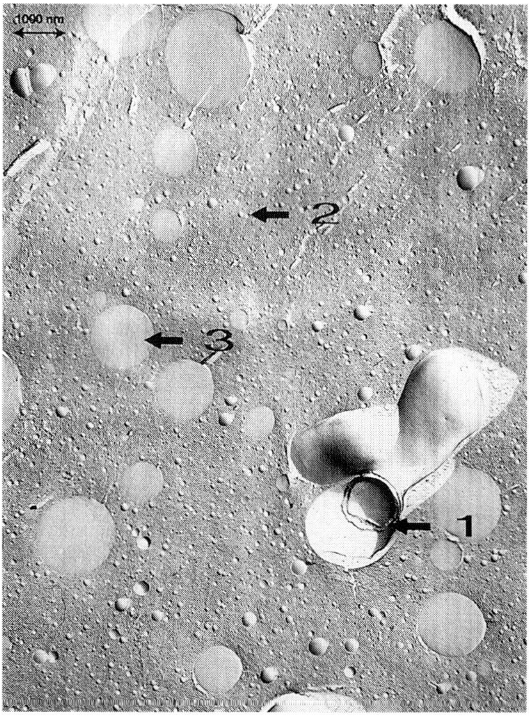

Figure 18.1

Electron micrograph of the complete study formulation 1. 1: large vesicle; 2: small vesicle; 3: oil droplet.

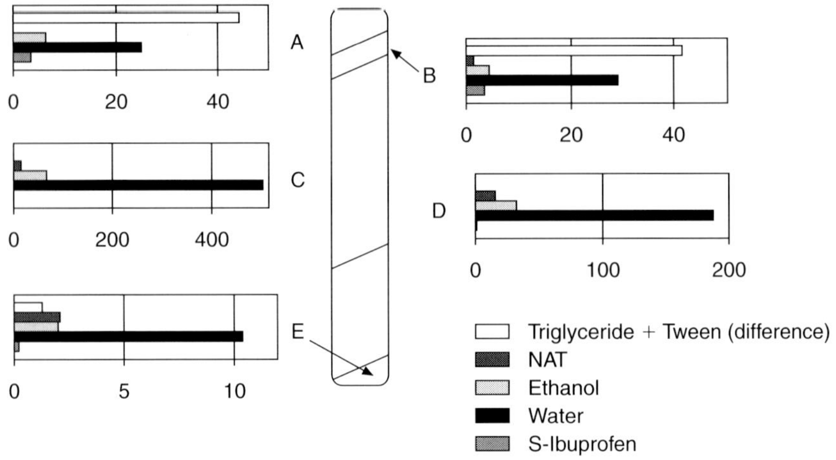

Figure 18.2

Fractions (A–E) of study formulation 1 after ultracentrifugation and their chemical composition in mg/g of formulation.

fractions of study formulation 1, obtained by ultracentrifugation. Triglyceride was present almost exclusively in fractions A and B, which contained oil droplets (micrograph not shown). A small amount of phospholipid was present in these fractions, possibly being associated in part with the oil droplets, which, in this formulation, were smaller in size than the droplets of the reference O/W formulation. A large portion of phospholipid was present in fraction D, which contained vesicles similar in appearance to those of the reference liposomal formulation, but considerably smaller in size (results not shown). Fraction C was similar to fraction D, in that it contained a lot of water and a marked portion of phospholipid; very few vesicles, however, were visible in it by TEM. The phospholipid could be present in the form of mixed micellar aggregates, constituting the third coexisting dispersed phase in the system.

Study formulation 3 contained no vesicles at all. In addition to oil droplets in fractions A and B, the presence of structures < 20 nm was evident by TEM in its fraction C. Thus, the increase of the triglyceride and surfactant content caused the liposomal phase to disappear in this formulation and the phospholipid to form mixed aggregate structures, probably with portions of the surfactant and the triglyceride. This example demonstrates how a change in composition can affect the formation of the dispersed phases, and points out that liposomes do not always exist alongside oil droplets when phospholipids are present in the system.

Transdermal permeation

The apparent skin permeability coefficients of S-Ibuprofen for study formulation 1 and the reference O/W and liposomal formulations were 1.08×10^{-7} cm/s, 1.78×10^{-7} cm/s and 2.62×10^{-7} cm/s, respectively. Drug release for these formulations followed the same rank order.

In the above investigation, the drug was found to reside almost exclusively in the dispersed phases, i.e. oil droplets, vesicles and mixed aggregates, which is consistent with its low water solubility. For the interpretation of the permeation results, it is postulated that the concentration of the drug in the continuous phase of the formulation governs its transport kinetics. This concentration is given by Equation 18.1:

$$C_D^{II} = \frac{C_D^{tot}}{\phi^I (K_{I/II} - 1) + 1} \qquad (18.1)$$

where, C_D^{II} is the drug concentration in the continuous phase (phase II) of the formulation, C_D^{tot} is the total drug concentration, ϕ^I is the total volume fraction of the dispersed phases (phase I), and $K_{I/II}$ is the drug partition coefficient between the dispersed and the continuous phase.

To test this hypothesis, the measured (apparent) permeability coefficients were plotted against C_D^{II} in Figure 18.3. The excellent correlation obtained supports the validity of the hypothesis. These results, therefore, demonstrate that, with the present systems, only the volume of the dispersed phase(s) plays a role in transdermal permeation, while the kind of structure of this phase is inconsequential for this matter.

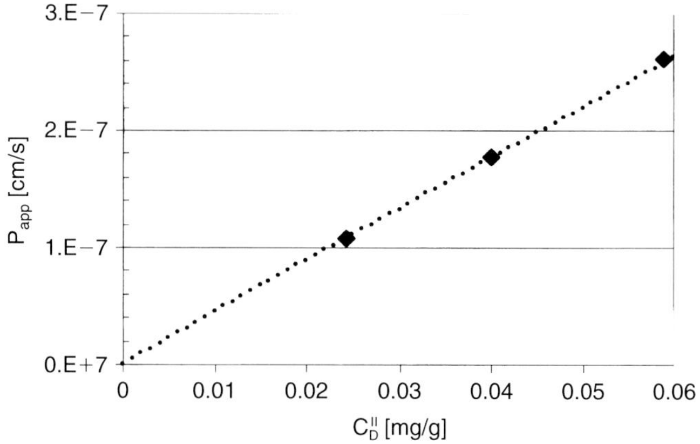

Figure 18.3

Apparent skin permeability of drug as a function of the concentration in the continuous phase of formulations.

Loss of water and ethanol, due to evaporation, took place rapidly in the first hour and reached 85% of the initial content for water and 100% for ethanol after 8 hours. This loss causes a change in the volume fraction of the phases of the formulation which, in turn, changes the drug concentration in the continuous phase. This concentration change is given by Equation 18.2:

$$\frac{C_{D,0}^{II}}{C_{D,t}^{II}} = \frac{(K_{I/II} - 1) + \dfrac{1}{\phi_t^I}}{(K_{I/II} - 1) + \dfrac{1}{\phi_0^I}} \qquad (18.2)$$

in which the subscripts 0 and t denote concentration and volume fraction at time zero and t, respectively.

Equation 18.2 shows that, when the partition coefficient $K_{I/II}$ is quite high, the drug concentration in the continuous phase stays constant, even if the volume fraction of the dispersed phase changes considerably. Therefore, in this case, evaporation does not affect the transdermal permeation rate, as long, of course, as the continuous phase is not entirely depleted.

19

Comparison of cutaneous bioavailability of cosmetic preparations containing caffeine or α-tocopherol applied on human skin models or human skin ex vivo at finite doses

F Dreher, F Fouchard, C Patouillet, M Andrian, J-T Simonnet and F Benech-Kieffer

Introduction

Whereas the determination of percutaneous penetration using human skin ex vivo is a widely-accepted alternative method for evaluating cutaneous bioavailability of topically-applied ingredients, the use of human skin models for performing such studies still needs further investigation and validation. Although human skin models were shown to be more permeable than human skin ex vivo, they seemed to correctly predict the permeability rank order of compounds having different physico-chemical properties when they were applied in simple vehicles at infinite doses.[1] However, only a few studies have been reported on human skin models dealing with vehicle effects on percutaneous penetration. Apart from a comparative study carried out on a simple emulsion versus a multiple emulsion containing caffeine applied at infinite dose,[2] most reports relate to the influence on percutaneous absorption of simple vehicles, such as water or petrolatum. The present study was performed on the human skin models EpiDerm™ (MatTek Inc, Ashland, MA, USA) and Episkin® (Episkin SNC, Lyon, France) in order to investigate the influence of cosmetic vehicle on skin bioavailability of caffeine and α-tocopherol. The preparations were applied at a finite dose as commonly done when applying cosmetic products. The data were then compared with those obtained on human skin ex vivo under similar experimental conditions.

Material and methods

Preparations

Four cosmetic preparations were selected which contained [^{14}C]-caffeine or [^{14}C]-α-tocopherol. A (w/o)-emulsion, an (o/w)-emulsion, and an alcohol-containing hydrogel were selected to formulate both ingredients. For α-tocopherol, a liposome dispersion was made as the fourth preparation, whereas a simple aqueous solution was chosen for caffeine instead.

Diffusion system

The diffusion system was composed of In-Line cells (PermeGear Inc., Hellertown, PA, USA)[3] having an 8-mm diameter, corresponding to an application area of 0.5 cm^2. Phosphate buffered saline containing 0.25% Tween 80 served as receptor solution and was pumped at a flux rate of 3 ml/h. The human skin models as well as the dermatomed human skin were mounted as recently described.[4]

Product application

After 1 hour equilibration time, the preparations were applied at a dose of 10 mg/cm^2 using a small plastic spatula having a rectangular bent top or a 10-μl micro-pipette. The actual amount administered was determined by subtracting the amount remaining on the spatula or in the pipette after application from the weight of the preparation either put onto the bent part of the spatula or contained in the pipette, respectively.

Sample preparation and analysis for solute content

The receptor fluid was collected every hour for 24 hours. Thereafter, the skin surface was extensively washed and the diffusion cell dismantled. Then, the reconstructed epidermis of human skin models was separated from the support membrane using forceps. In the case of human skin, the stratum corneum (SC) was removed by sequential stripping with adhesive tape (Scotch™ no. 810, 3M, St Paul, MN, USA). Afterwards, the human epidermis was removed from the dermis by heat separation. Analysis for solute content in the various compartments was performed using liquid scintillation counting.

Data analysis

Mass balance was calculated using the applied dose of [^{14}C]-caffeine or of [^{14}C]-α-tocopherol corresponding to 100%. If the overall recovery of the test solute did not reach $100 \pm 15\%$, the data were excluded.

Results

The permeation profiles of [^{14}C]-caffeine or [^{14}C]-α-tocopherol from the respective preparations through the reconstructed skin models, or through human skin ex vivo, into the receptor solution are shown in Figures 19.1 and 19.2. The permeation profiles are given as permeation rates (%/h, corresponding to the percentage of applied solute permeating within 1 hour) and as cumulated amounts (%) of solute permeated as a function of time after product application. Irrespective of the formulation, [^{14}C]-caffeine permeated human skin ex vivo to a much higher extent as compared to [^{14}C]-α-tocopherol. This permeation rank order, as well as the clear distinction between these two actives having known different skin penetration properties, were also obtained on both human skin models. Human skin was shown to be less permeable for [^{14}C]-caffeine and [^{14}C]-α-tocopherol as compared to both human skin models under finite dose conditions. Otherwise, Episkin® was slightly less permeable than EpiDerm™ for both solutes studied.

On human skin, the selected cosmetic preparations influenced skin bioavailability of [^{14}C]-caffeine and [^{14}C]-α-tocopherol only a little. With the exception of α-tocopherol hydrogel, no significant differences in skin bioavailability were observed between the preparations for either solute. As compared to the results obtained on human skin ex vivo, the cosmetic vehicle affected skin bioavailability in human skin models differently. For instance, in contrast with the findings in human skin ex vivo, [^{14}C]-α-tocopherol absorption from the hydrogel into EpiDerm™ or Episkin® was similar to, or even lower than, the other α-tocopherol-containing preparations studied.

Conclusion

This study indicated that solute permeability rank order can also be correctly predicted when applied at finite dose using human skin models, such as EpiDerm™ or Episkin®, at least for compounds having far different physico-chemical properties, such as caffeine and α-tocopherol. Slight effects of cosmetic vehicles on skin bioavailability were, however, less predictable using these models. In particular, alcohol-containing formulations seem to act differently on both EpiDerm™ and Episkin®. The less pronounced barrier properties, due to different composition and organization of intercellular SC lipids, the increased hydration of superficial stratum corneum layers, as well as other still unknown factors, may explain the observed differences in human skin models as compared to human skin.

Improved human skin models were obtained when cultured in the presence of vitamin C.[5] For instance, vitamin C plays a key role in the

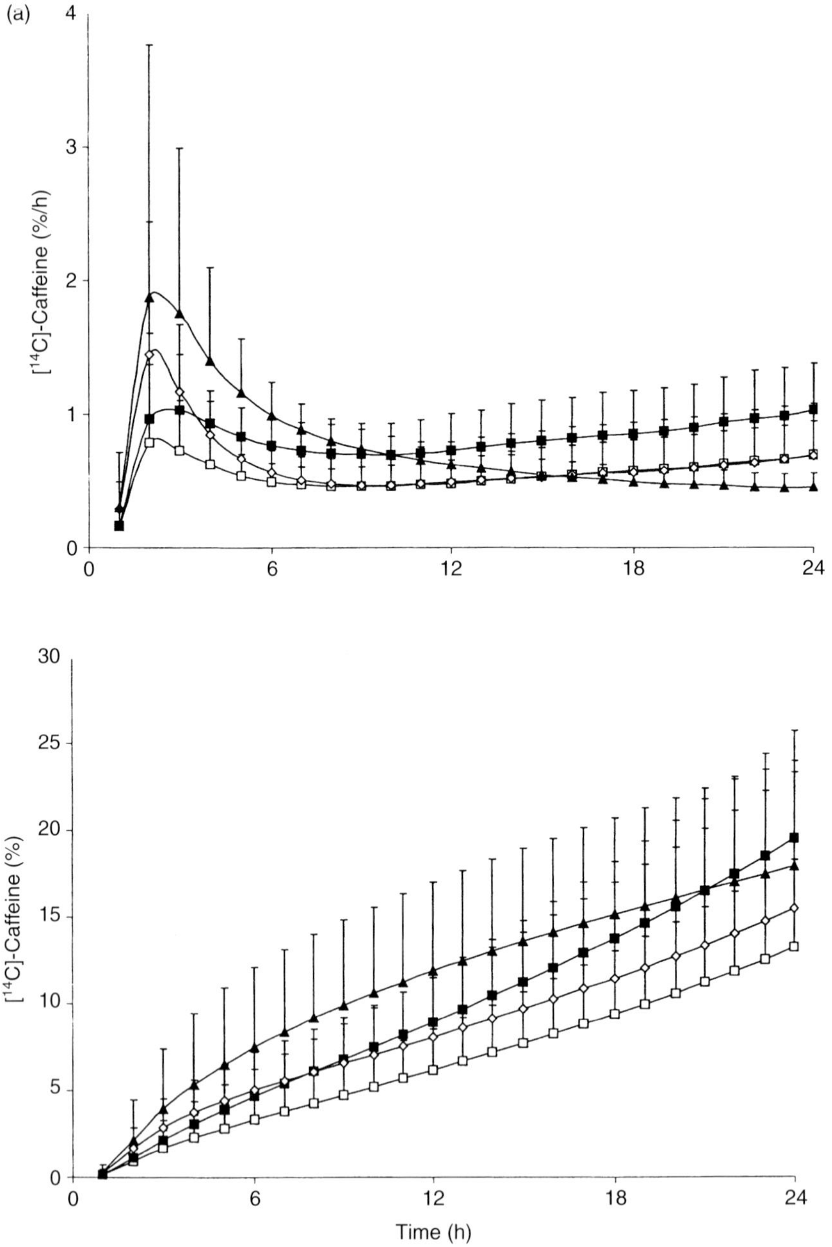

Figure 19.1

Skin penetration rates (%/h) and cumulated penetrated amounts (%) of [^{14}C]-caffeine. Penetration through (a) human skin, (b) EpiDerm™ and (c) Episkin® into the receptor solution as a function of preparation: (□) o/w-emulsion, (■) w/o-emulsion, (◇) aqueous solution, (▲) hydrogel. Mean ± SD of percentages of the applied dose are shown; only positive error given.

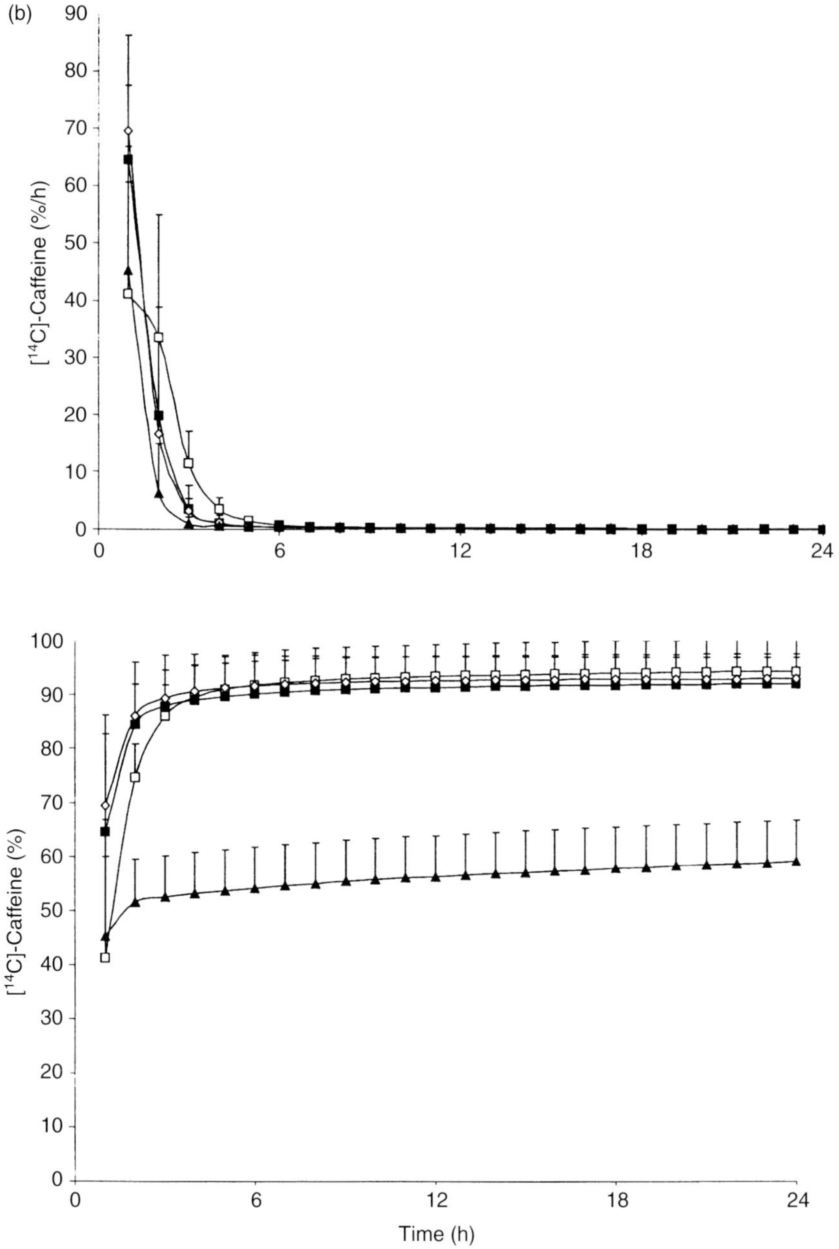

Figure 19.1
Continued

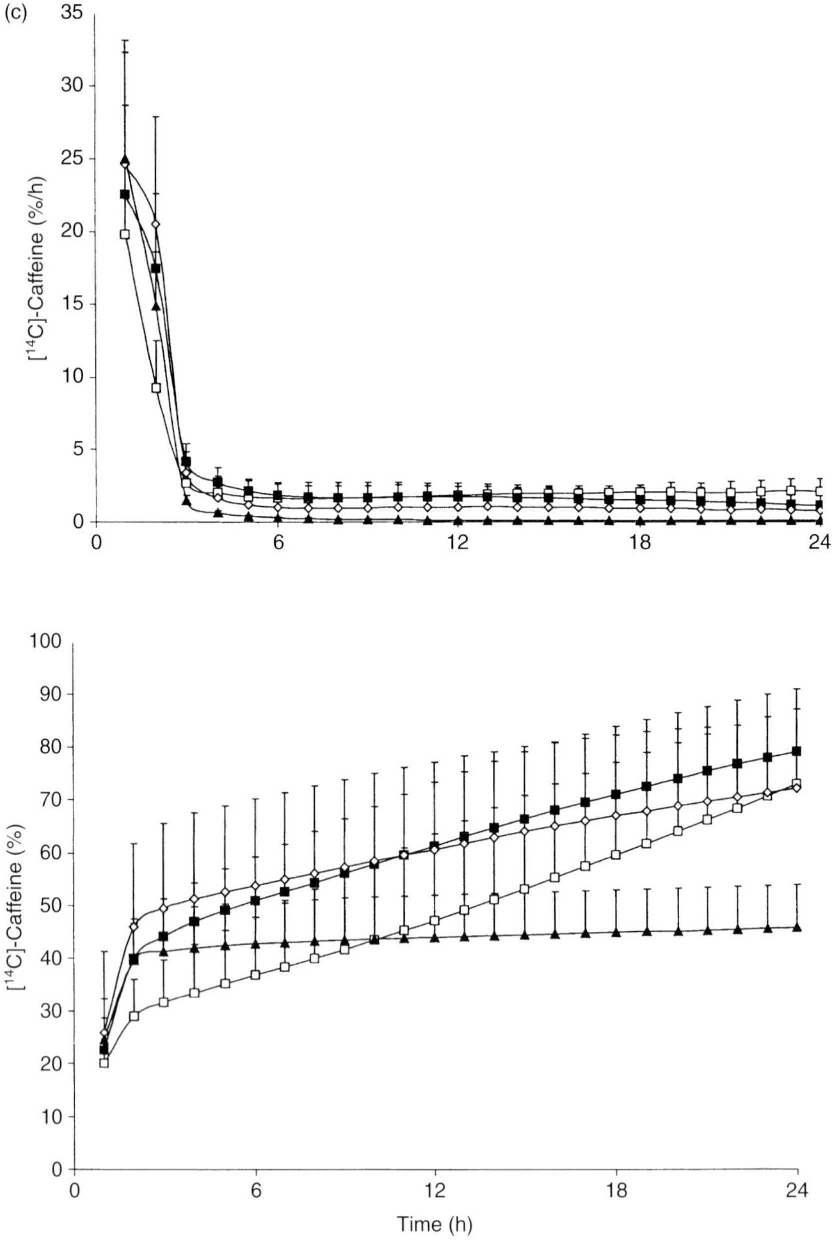

Figure 19.1
Continued

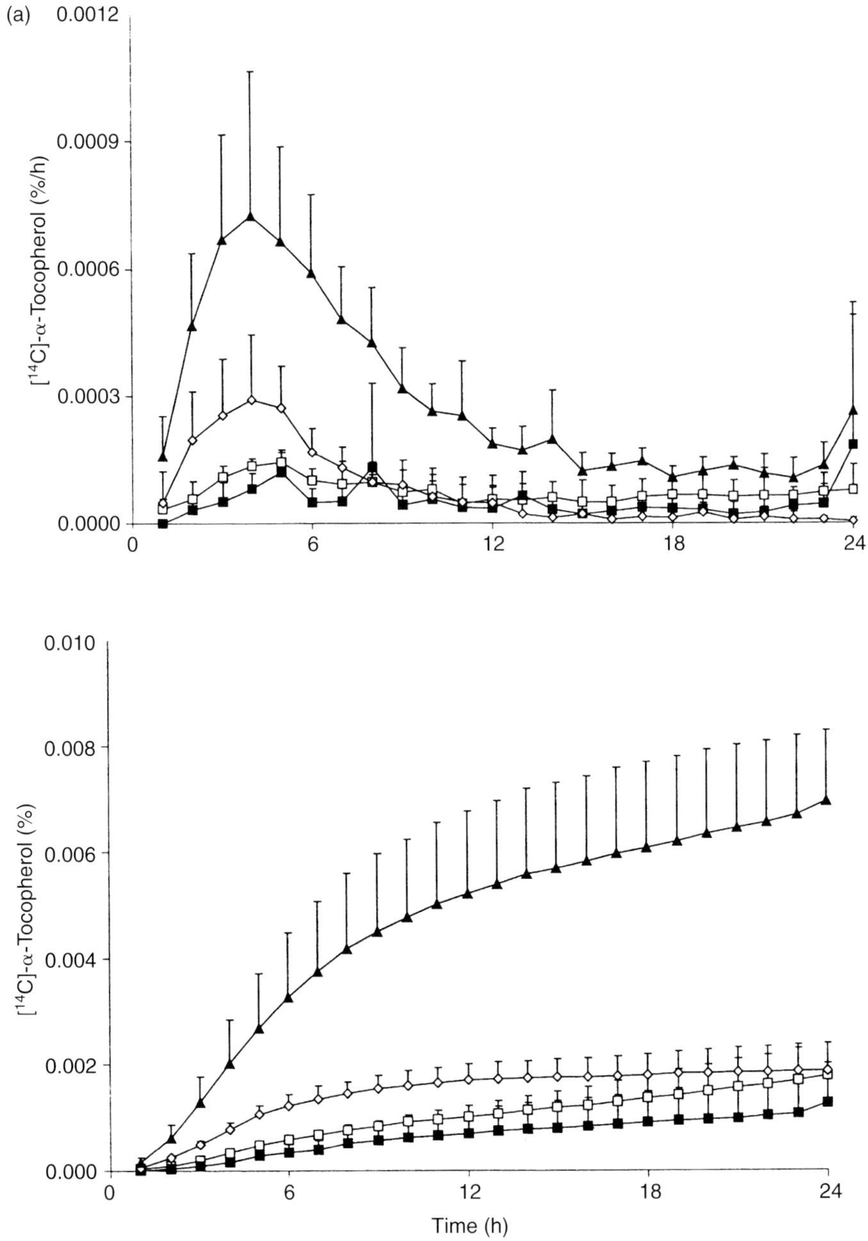

Figure 19.2

Skin penetration rates (%/h) and cumulated penetrated amounts (%) of [^{14}C]-α-tocopherol. Penetration through (a) human skin, (b) EpiDerm™ and (c) Episkin® into the receptor solution as a function of preparation: (□) o/w-emulsion, (■) w/o-emulsion, (◇) liposomes, (▲) hydrogel. Mean ± SD of percentages of the applied dose are shown; only positive error given.

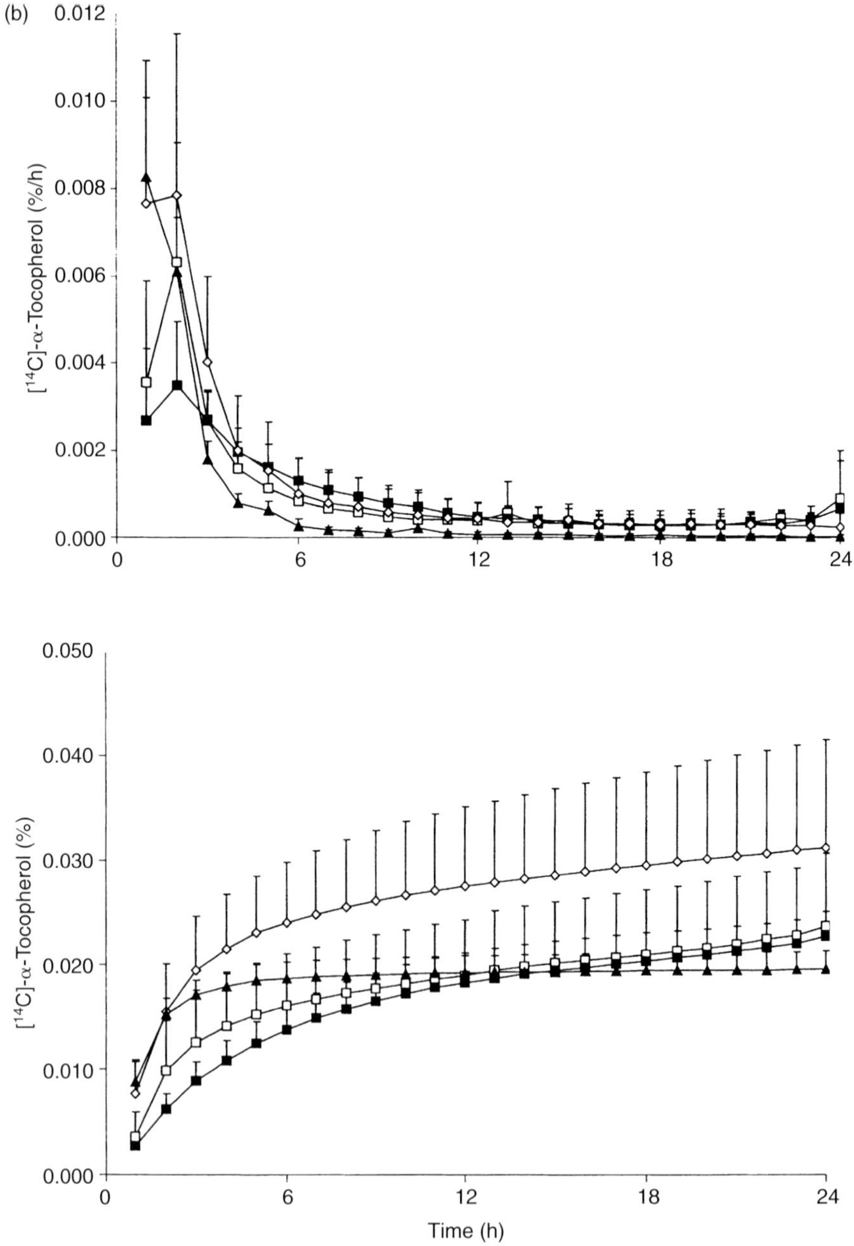

Figure 19.2
Continued

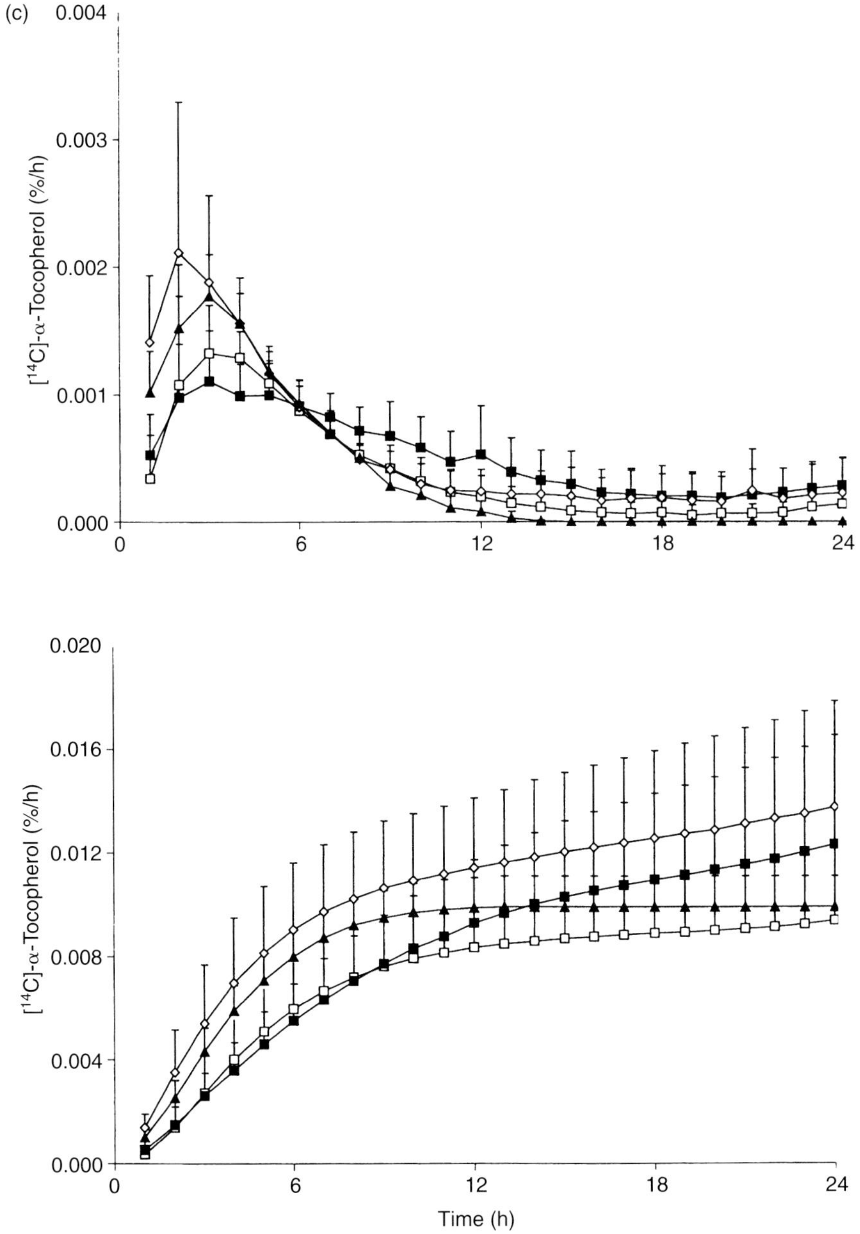

Figure 19.2

Continued

formation of SC barrier lipids in human skin models and was shown to increase the barrier properties of Episkin®.[6] Consequently, more detailed investigations are needed to further clarify the influence of cosmetic preparations on skin bioavailability of actives in human skin models, particularly with respect to the improvement of available skin models.

Acknowledgements

This work was performed within the program of the European project 'Standards, Measurements and Testing SMT4-CT97-2174', which is dedicated to the 'Testing and improvement of reconstructed skin kits in order to elaborate European standards', and was partially granted by the European Commission (DG XII). R Roguet (L'Oréal) and the partners of this project, H Beck, M Bracher, C Faller (Wella–Cosmital SA, Marly, Switzerland), U Pfannenbecker (Beiersdorf AG, Hamburg, Germany), and M Ponec (University of Leiden, Leiden, Netherlands) are gratefully acknowledged for excellent cooperation and constructive discussions.

References

1. Gay R, Swiderek M, Nelson D et al. The living skin equivalent as a model in vitro for ranking the toxic potential of dermal irritants. Toxicol in Vitro 1992; 6:305–15.
2. Doucet O, Ferrero L, Garcia N et al. O/W emulsion and W/O/W multiple emulsion: physical characterization and skin pharmacokinetic comparison in the delivery process of caffeine. Int J Cosm Sci 1998; 20:283–95.
3. Squier CA, Kremer M, Wertz PW. Continuous flow mucosal cells for measuring the in vitro permeability of small tissue samples. J Pharm Sci 1997; 86:82–4.
4. Dreher F, Patouillet C, Fouchard F et al. Improvement of the experimental setup to assess cutaneous bioavailability on human skin models: dynamic protocol (submitted for publication).
5. Ponec M, Weerheim A, Kempenaar J et al. The formation of competent barrier lipids in reconstructed human epidermis requires the presence of vitamin C. J Invest Dermatol 1997; 109: 348–55.
6. Castiel-Higounenc I, Ferraris C, Guey C et al. Ascorbic acid and derivatives improve 6-hydroxysphingenin synthesis and barrier function of human reconstructed skin via a distinct non-anti-oxydant related activity [abstract]. 29th Annual Meeting of the European Society for Dermatological Research, Montpellier, France; 1999.

20

Quantification of vitamin E-acetate (cosmetic formulations) in the stratum corneum of an in vitro model by tape-stripping, UV-spectroscopy and HPLC

P Lampen, W Pittermann, HM Heise, H Jungmann and M Kietzmann

Introduction

The cosmetic emulsions of today's market usually contain bioactive ingredients, such as vitamins, for ameliorating the protective and regulating function of the skin. However, the release of vitamins from the cosmetics into the stratum corneum (SC) depends on the topical application conditions.[1,2] During exposure, the formulations undergo a dramatic change due to evaporation processes which may influence the SC penetration capability. Formulations using microparticles as transport vehicles can increase the bioavailability of the active compounds within the surface skin layer, as well as diminish the exposure period needed for cutaneous penetration.[3–5] Depth profiling for absorbed substances can be easily carried out by repeated adhesive tape-stripping and subsequent analysis.[6]

The follicular skin of the isolated perfused bovine udder skin (BUS-model) was employed as a viable in vitro substitute for our recent penetration efficiency studies.[7] The applicability of a study design using vitamin E-acetate-loaded adhesive tape strips has been tested. The spectrometrically obtained results are compared with those derived from a costly and time-consuming high performance liquid chromatography (HPLC) method, usually considered for such studies. Ultraviolet (UV)-spectroscopy is well suited for a fast, quantitative determination of trace amounts of vitamin E-acetate, owing to its strongly absorbing chromophore.

Methods and materials

The chosen galenic formulations possessed similar physicochemical characteristics. The basic oil/water (O/W) cream (LC; lamellar type) contained vitamin E-acetate, which was dissolved in the natural oil phase (2.0%, in wt% for the active substance; Roche, Switzerland). For the other two creams, the vitamin E-acetate (10%) was found either in liposomes (RS, Rovisome®) or in microparticles (RP, Roviparts®).

The latter particles, supplied by ROVI GmbH (Germany), are vesicles composed of phospholipids, in particular, phosphatidylcholine, surrounding an inner fluid compartment. The liposomes consisted of an aqueous inner compartment, and the lipophilic vitamin is therefore found in the lipid bilayer, in contrast to the case of the microparticles, which have an oily compartment surrounded by only one layer of lipids. Both types of vesicles with a size of 150 nm are used for cosmetics, due to their permeation ability to transport active ingredients into the skin and to stabilize sensitive components.[4]

The various emulsions were topically applied to bovine udder skin, with a surface density of 3–4 g/100 cm^2, in three independent studies after maintaining the udder perfusion for a certain period. The high dosage was aimed at preventing any depletion of the vitamin concentration during exposure. After a lapse of 30 minutes after starting the application, the residual cream was carefully removed with a dry paper towel (finite dose).

Adhesive tape-stripping, using Tesa R, type 4204 from BDF (Germany), was utilized to remove the SC successively. After each topical application, two parallel series, consisting of 15 adhesive tape strips with an area of 1.9 cm × 10 cm (= 19 cm^2) for corneocyte layer removal, were peeled off. The tape samples were analysed for vitamin E-acetate, either by the conventional HPLC method or UV/VIS spectroscopy, and the results were calculated as μg/cm^2 per tape strip.

For the UV/VIS-spectroscopic investigation, spectra of the adhesive tapes loaded with corneocytes were measured in transmission, as sketched in Figure 20.1. The UV light of a deuterium lamp was projected by a mirror through the adhesive tape. Above the adhesive tape, a fibre-optic probe was used to collect and guide the transmitted light to a mini-spectrometer containing a diode-array for detection (Ocean Optics, Inc; Dunedin, FL, USA). Spectroscopic data were recorded within the range of 260–525 nm. A Cary 5G scanning dispersive spectrometer with a double monochromator (Varian; Darmstadt, Germany) was also used for recording reference spectra of different cream components.

In contrast to the HPLC method, only five visually controlled spots on each tape (1–15) and several unloaded tapes (controls) were included. The spots chosen were identical to highly packed sections covered by corneocytes, and tape areas with a low content were strictly avoided. For

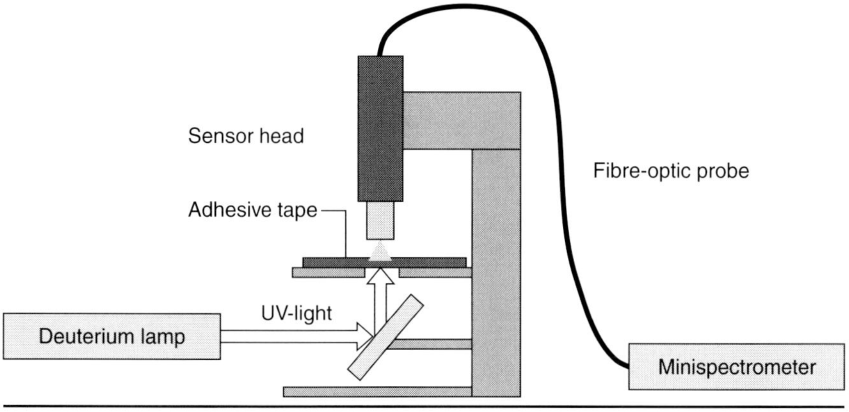

Figure 20.1

Experimental set-up used for UV-transmission spectroscopy of adhesive tapes.

spectral evaluation, a reference spectrum of vitamin E-acetate and that of a representative corneocyte's measurement, as well as a linear baseline, were sufficient as fitting components for modeling the loaded tape spectra. A special mathematical criterion, i.e. the matrix condition number, was applied, so that the optimal spectral interval between 265 and 350 nm was exploited for quantitative analysis.[7]

Results

After an exposure period of 30 minutes, the total amount of vitamin E-acetate (strips 1–15), analysed either by HPLC or UV-spectroscopy, was comparable for the samples taken after LC or RP application. However, for the RS cream, a significant difference was observed (Figure 20.2A). The difference between the results obtained by the two methods is completely reduced when the total amount is calculated without the values of the first-taken adhesive strip (Figure 20.2B). The detailed analysis shows a substantial similarity of the means and the standard deviations obtained by both analytical methods, with the exception as discussed.

The different kinetics as found for the formulations studied were estimated from the results using two different exposure periods. A ratio (see Table 20.1) can be defined from the respective total amounts of vitamin E after the exposure periods of 1.5 hours and 0.5 hours.

Regarding the total amount penetrated, a steady state was nearly reached after an exposure period of 0.5 hours for the LC- and RP-treated skin. The liposome-based RS cream had a different penetration efficiency

Table 20.1 Natural and supplemented amount of vitamin E (μg/cm[2] tape) and ratio determined as obtained from accumulated HPLC-results from strips 1–15.

Formulation	Exposure period 0.5 h	Exposure period 1.5 h	Ratio $m_{1.5\,h}/m_{0.5\,h}$
Tocopherol (natural amount)	0.06	not determined	–
LC (vitamin E-acetate)	30.0	34.6	1.15
RP (20% Roviparts®)	17.6	24.0	1.36
RS (20% Rovisome®)	45.4	20.2	0.44

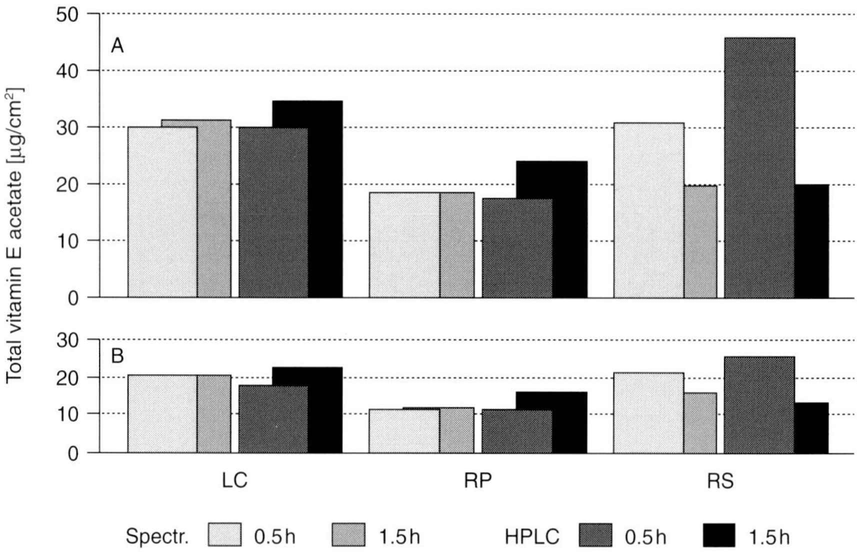

Figure 20.2

Analytical results for total penetrated vitamin E acetate by UV-spectroscopy and an HPLC method at exposure periods of 0.5 hours and 1.5 hours, respectively. Total amount in the horny layer of bovine udder skin with (A) and without (B) the amount obtained on the first tape strip after LC, RP, and RS cream applications.

for vitamin E-acetate, because a severe decrease in the total amount was observed, as based on the ratio calculation.

The Rovisome®-based formulation released a significant amount of the vitamin, within the short exposure period of 30 minutes, into the horny layer. Compared to the other two formulations, the RS cream only enables the penetration of vitamin E-acetate into the lower epidermal layers after an additional exposure period (Figure 20.3).

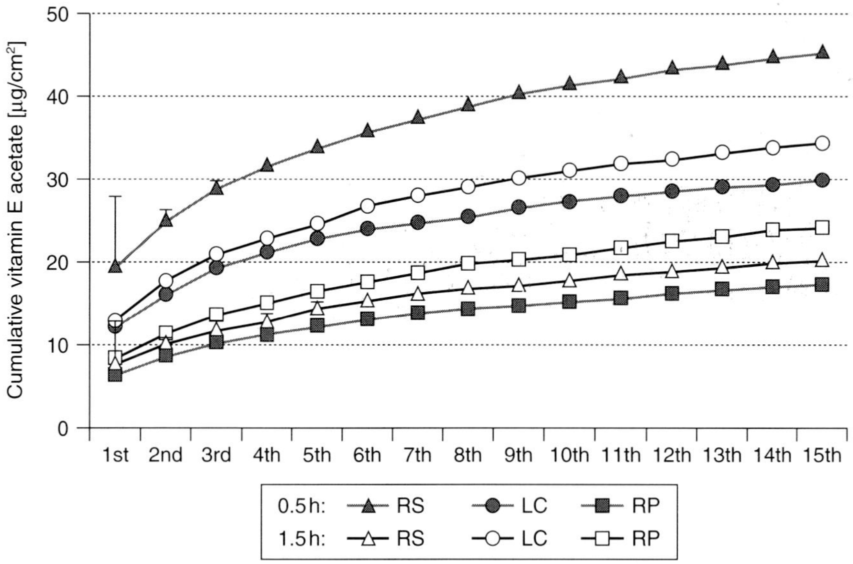

Figure 20.3

Cumulative HPLC-results for vitamin E-acetate within the horny layer, obtained from strips 1–15 (µg/cm² tape) after LC, RP, and RS cream applications with exposure periods of 0.5 h and 1.5 h, respectively.

Conclusions

Compared to our HPLC method, UV/VIS spectroscopy is a fast and economic analytical method for evaluating large numbers of samples of the horny layer taken by the tape-stripping method. The latter is an established tool for depth profiling of substances within the SC.

The Rovisome®-formulated (RS) cream was most successful in vitamin E-acetate delivery into the horny layer, which can be explained by an alteration in the corneal plasticity (reservoir capacity) and by opening an additional pathway through follicular penetration during the early exposure time.

References

1. Förster Th, Pittermann W, Schmitt M et al. Skin penetration properties of cosmetic formulations using a perfused bovine udder model. J Cosmet Sci 1999; 50:147–57.
2. Förster Th, Jackwerth B, Pittermann W et al. Properties of emulsions: structure and skin penetration. Cosmetics & Toiletries 1997; 112: 73–82.
3. Schaefer H, Redelmeier Th. *Skin Barrier – Principles of Percuta-*

neous Absorption. Basel: Karger 1996.

4. Blume G, Pittermann W, Waldmann-Laue M et al. Rovisome – a carrier system for vitamins. EURO-COSMETICS 2000; 3-2000:30–2.

5. Cordech L, Oliva M, Pons M et al. Percutaneous penetration of liposomes using tape stripping technique. Int J Pharm 1996; 139: 197–293.

6. Beebe KR, Pell RJ, Seasholtz MB. *Chemometrics: A Practical Guide*. New York: John Wiley & Sons, 1998.

7. Kietzmann M, Löscher W, Arens D et al. The isolated perfused bovine udder as an in vitro model of percutaneous drug absorption. Skin viability and percutaneous absorption of dexamethasone, benzoyl peroxide and etofenamate. J Pharm Toxicol Meth 1993; 30:75–84.

21

Influence of in vivo iontophoresis on the skin barrier and percutaneous penetration

R Lambrecht, P Clarys, K Alewaeters and AO Barel

Introduction

Iontophoresis is a technique used to enhance the transdermal delivery of a drug by means of an electric current. The iontophoretic transport is influenced by several factors, such as concentration, size, ionic strength and the Ip of the drug and pH of the solvent, and also by the applied intensity and shape of the current and the application time.[1]

The enhancement of the transdermal delivery is usually explained by the repulsion due to electric forces. The primary flux is followed by a secondary flux of ions, called electroosmosis, as a consequence of the osmotic pressure that was developed.[2] The electrical force seems to be the most important factor in the iontophoretic delivery.

Several authors were able to demonstrate a substantial contribution of the follicular and the sebaceous route during iontophoretic transport, because of its low electrical resistance.[3] The effect of the current on the barrier properties needs to be considered equally. A reorganization of the lipid bilayer has been described,[4,5] as well as an elevated hydration[6] and a stimulated microcirculation.[7] Because changes in hydration and perfusion of the microcirculation are linked with an altered percutaneous absorption behavior of molecules, we were interested to see whether these changes are intensity dependent. Therefore, we compared several physical parameters in vivo at two current intensities.

In a second in vivo approach, we followed the passive penetration of lipophilic hexyl- and hydrophilic methyl-nicotinate with and without a direct current pretreatment. In this part, we were interested in whether the percutaneous absorption of a lipophilic and a hydrophilic molecule was influenced by a current pretreatment.

Materials and methods

Volunteers

Two groups of twelve young, healthy volunteers, males and females (age group 1 = 23.3 years ± 2.2 years, and group 2 = 22.7 years ± 2.4 years) were selected for this study.

Experimental conditions

All experiments were carried out in a climatized room (T = 20°C ± 2°C, relative humidity = 45% ± 5%). Prior to the measurements, the volunteers underwent an acclimatization period of 30 minutes.

Instruments

The Minolta Chromameter CR 2000 was used as a colour analyser. In this study, we evaluated the a* parameter, which is situated in the red area of this 3-dimensional colour system.

Transepidermal water loss (TEWL) was measured with the Tewameter TM 210®. The probe was placed on the adjacent skin area for 15 minutes, before measurements were taken to obtain thermal equilibrum with the skin.

Hydration of the skin was determined with the capacitance method, using the Corneometer CM 825 PC. The mean of three adjacent measurements was calculated.

The perfusion of the microcirculation was used for the quantification of related erythema, but equally as an indication of bloodflux. Perfusion of the skin microcirculation was monitored with laser Doppler flowmetry, using the Periflux PF3.

The pH of the skin was followed using a skin electrode – the Metler Toledo, Inlab 426. We followed the temperature of the skin with the Testoderm 9010.

Application method

Influence of intensity

For the first set of measurements, direct currents at two intensities of 0.13 and 0.26 mA/cm^2, respectively, were compared for all measured parameters. The application was performed on both forearms. A randomization was used to avoid regional influences. The current was applied for 20 minutes, using wet sponges with a diameter of 3 cm. The current was generated by an instrument used for electrophysiotherapic treatment, the Duo 410, Gymna. Data were evaluated every 2.5 minutes over 65 minutes' post current application.

Influence on the barrier properties

In the second experiment, the skin was pretreated with a direct current with an intensity of 0.2 mA/cm^2 for 20 minutes. The cathode was used as the active electrode. After current pretreatment, we performed a nicotinate test with methyl- and hexyl-nicotinate (0.005 mol/l). Saturated paper filter disks were applied for 30 seconds on the pretreated skin. As nicotinate evokes a vasodilatation of the superficial microvessels, the penetration was followed with laser Doppler measurements and the accompanied redness was examined with colorimetric measurements. The response was followed for 2 hours' post application. These values were compared with the control values, obtained after application of the nicotinates on a skin site which was covered with the electrode only.

Normality was tested using the Kolmogorov Goodness of Fit test ($p = 0.05$). As all data were normally distributed, we used a Multiple Anova Of Variance procedure for further analysis.

Results

Influence of intensity

Application of a current for 20 minutes provokes an important increase in the superficial microcirculation measured by laser Doppler flowmetry (Figure 21.1a). This increase was current dependent, since the highest intensity provoked higher values. The increased perfusion of the microcirculation was accompanied by a significant increase in redness (Figure 21.1b), indicating that the current provokes an important erythema of the skin. The values of the 0.26-mA curve tend to be higher than those of the 0.13-mA intensity curve, but the differences were not significant. There was also an important increase in the TEWL and hydration values after 20 minutes' current application (Figures 21.1c and 21.1d). No differences were detected between the two intensities, indicating that the occlusive effect of the sponges is probably the predominant factor. When evaluating the temperature of the skin (Figure 21.1e), we could only observe a slight increase in skin temperature with the 0.26-mA intensity. A secondary cooling-down effect of the skin was observed for both intensities. The pH value (Figure 21.1f) increased from 5.2 before current application to 6.8 post application. Return to baseline values was not reached completely after 65 minutes. No significant differences could be detected between the two intensities.

Influence on the barrier properties

When observing the vascular response, as an indication for percutaneous penetration of the lipophilic hexyl-nicotinate and the hydrophilic methyl-nicotinate without a current pretreatment, higher maximum values are observed for hexyl-nicotinate (Figures 21.2c and 21.2d). Higher maximum values and shorter lagtimes were also observed for the hexyl- and methyl-nicotinate when a current pretreatment was performed compared to passive penetration after 20 minutes' sponge application (Figures 21.2a and 21.2b) with laser Doppler. Similar results were obtained when using skin color measurements as an indication for percutaneous penetration.

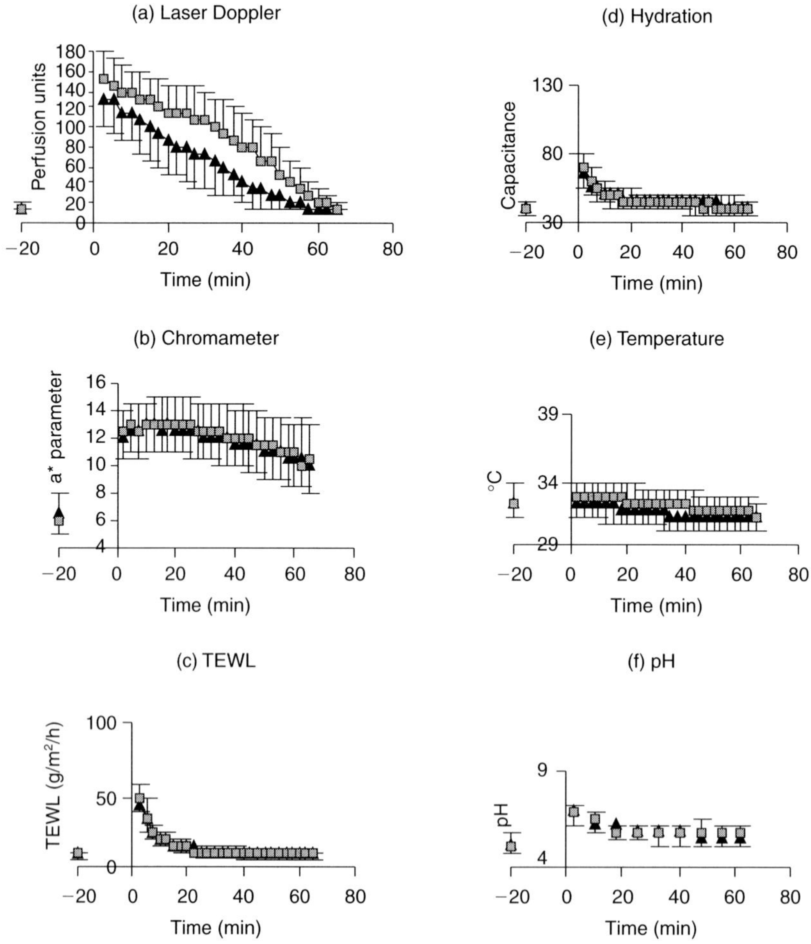

Figure 21.1

Influence of current intensity (0.13 mA/cm² and 0.26 mA/cm²) on the measured parameters: (a) Laser Doppler flowmetry; (b) a* parameter; (c) TEWL; (d) hydration; (e) temperature; (f) pH of the skin.

When comparing the skin-color response after application of the two molecules and current application, we can observe that the shapes of the two curves are similar, for both the microcirculation and the a* parameter. No differences in lagtime or maximum values could be observed between the hydrophilic and the lipophilic molecules (Figures 21.3a and 21.3b).

Discussion

It has already been pointed out that the properties of the skin are changing temporally when it is submitted to a direct current.[1] By the use of non-

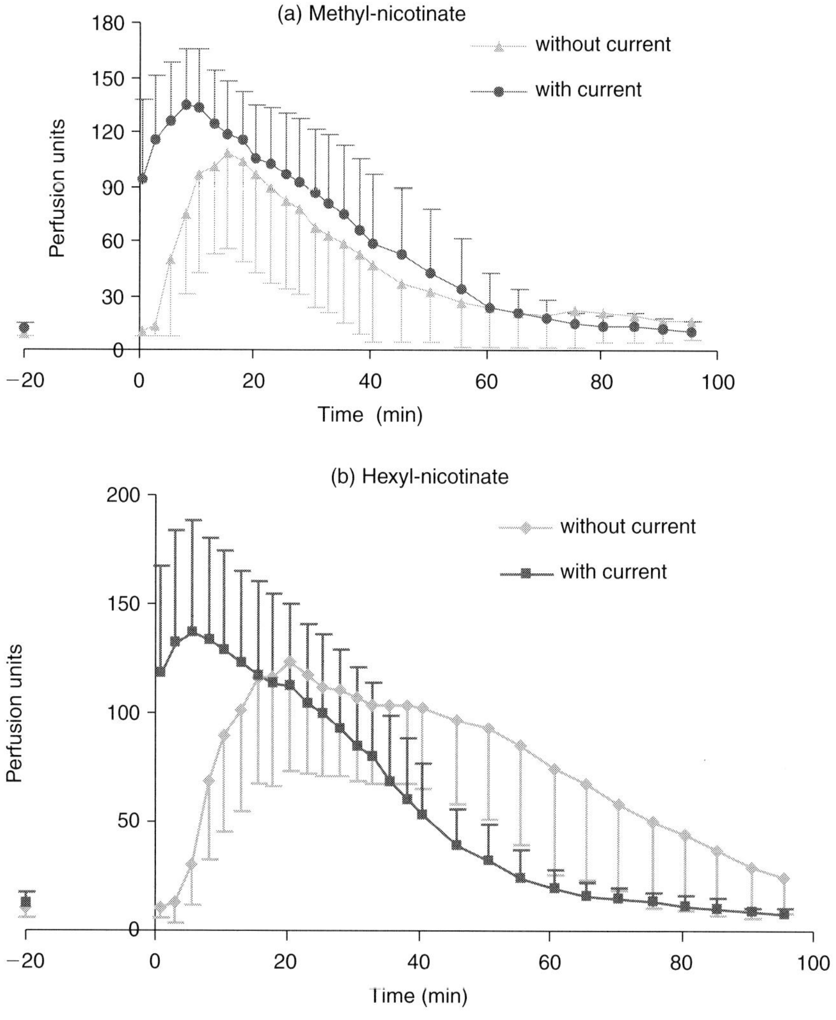

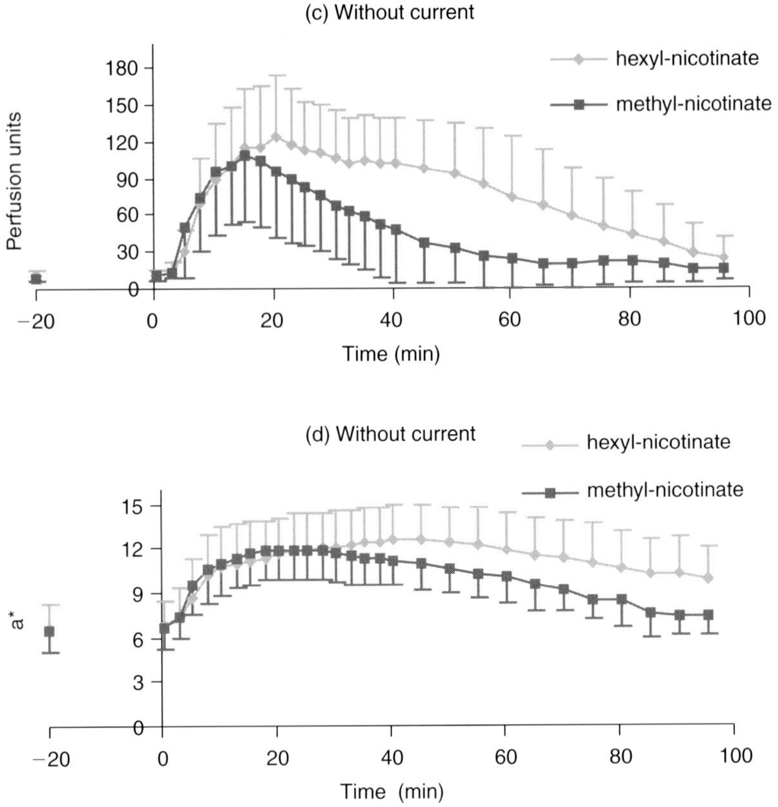

Figure 21.2

Passive penetration of methyl- and hexyl-nicotinate without current pretreatment for (a) laser Doppler and (b) a* parameter, and passive penetration of (c) hexyl-nicotinate and (d) methyl-nicotinate, with and without current pretreatment for laser Doppler data.

invasive bioengineering methods it should be possible to have an idea about the extent of these changes. If we argue on the assumption that the skin properties are altered as a function of the current intensity, it should be possible to discriminate these effects with physical parameters. The use of non-invasive bioengineering methods to measure current-influenced skin properties is very attractive but it has some limitations. The use of TEWL, the favorite parameter to demonstrate barrier changes, did not show any current-dependent changes. Due to the occlusive effect of the wet sponges, it is very difficult to discriminate between the effect of the current and the effect of the occlusion. Few studies were able to demonstrate the effect of current on TEWL.[8] When performing hydration measurements, we encountered similar problems.

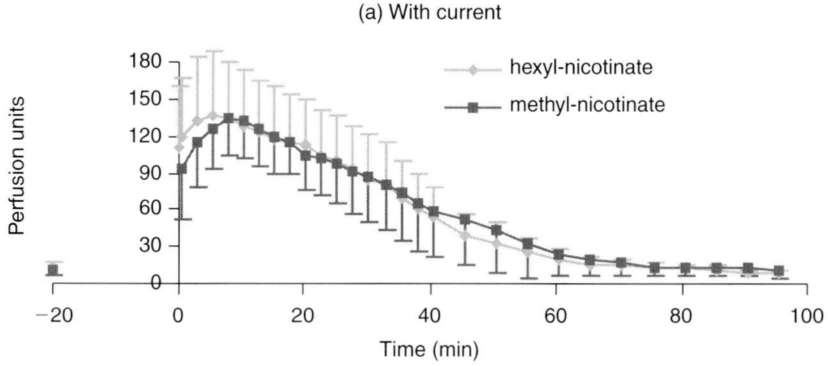

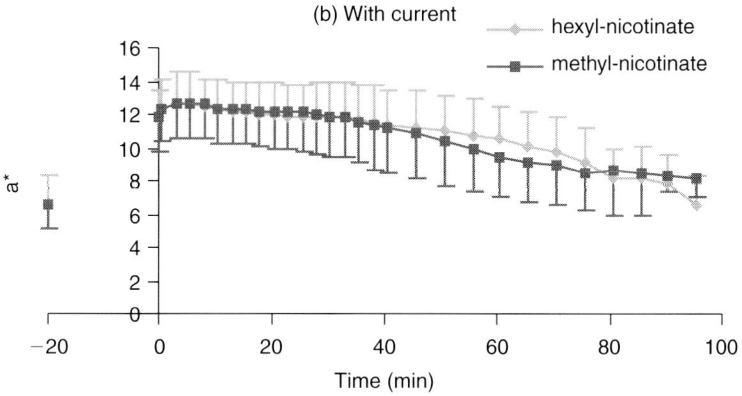

Figure 21.3

The passive absorption of methyl- and hexyl-nicotinate after current pretreatment for (a) laser Doppler and (b) a* parameter.

Other methods, such as laser Doppler and color and temperature measurements, seemed to be useful to discriminate current effects. These bioengineering methods are equally useful for studying the effects of current application on the barrier properties of the skin. We were able to demonstrate that the passive penetration of hexyl- and methyl-nicotinate is influenced by a current pretreatment. Our results indicated that the effect of the current caused an enhanced penetration, for both molecules. This was shown by a decrease in the lagtimes and the time-to-peak height. Obviously, the erythema caused by the electric current has to be kept in mind when interpreting the results. The passive penetration of the two molecules was different, as demonstrated by higher time-to-peak values for the lipophilic hexyl-nicotinate. After current pretreatment, the curve of the lipophilic molecule was the same shape as the curve of the hydrophilic molecule. This implies that the lipophilic substance acted like a hydrophilic one, and this may indicate that the reservoir formation of hexyl-nicotinate decreased. A possible explanation is given by the theory of Menon and Elias.[4] A reorganization of the intercellular lipid structure was described, together with the formation of dilatated lacunae. This lacunae can serve as a pathway for molecules with different properties. Under this condition, a pathway is possibly created for polar and apolar molecules.

The observation that the skin-barrier properties are influenced by current application corroborate again the assumption that the complex properties of living skin need to be considered carefully during current-involved studies.

References

1. Jadoul A, Bouwstra J, Preat V. Effects of iontophoresis and electroporation on the stratum corneum. Review of the biophysical studies. Adv Drug Deliv Rev 1999; 35:89–106.
2. Pikal MJ. The role of electoosmotic flow in transdermal iontophoresis. Adv Drug Deliv Rev 1992; 9: 201–37.
3. Cullander C, Guy RH. Visualising the pathways of iontophoretic current flow in real time with laser-scanning confocal microscopy and the vibrating probe electrode. In: Scott RC, Guy RH, Hadgraft, Bodde HE, eds. *Prediction of Percutaneous Penetration Methods, Measurements, Modelling*. London: IBC Technical Services, 1991; 2:229–37.
4. Menon GH, Elias PM. Morphologic basis for a pore-pathway in mammalian stratum corneum. Skin Pharmacol 1997; 10:235–46.
5. Chesnoy S, Durand D, Doucet J et al. Effect of iontophoresis in combination with ionic enhancers on the lipid structure of the stratum corneum: an X-ray-diffraction study. Pharmaceut Res 1996; 13: 1581–5.
6. Green RD, Hadgraft J. FT-IR investigations into the effect of iotophoresis on the skin. In: Brain KR, James VJ, Walters KA, eds. *Prediction of Percutaneous Penetration*. STS Publishing Ltd, 1993; 3B:37–43.
7. Preat V, Thijsman S, Van Neste D. Evaluation of human skin after iontophoresis with noninvasive methods. In: Brain KR, James VJ, Walters KA, eds. *Prediction of Percutaneous Penetration*. STS Publishing Ltd, 1993; 4B:406–9.
8. Thysman S, Van Neste D, Préat V. Non-invasive investigation of human skin after in vivo iontophoresis. Skin Pharmacol 1995; 42:165–73.

22
Transdermal iontophoresis of leuprolide in vitro under constant voltage and constant current conditions: physicochemical modelling and the effect of adjuvants

C Kochhar and G Imanidis

Introduction

The stratum corneum (SC) functions as an effective permeation barrier, preventing chemicals and other constituents of the environment from entering the body by way of the skin. This property of the SC, however, also represents an obstacle to the endeavour of delivering drugs systemically to the organism across the skin. This mode of delivery is desirable for certain drug classes, since it offers the possibility of delivery at a constant rate for long periods of time and circumvents the gastrointestinal tract and the detrimental effects its juices may have on drug molecules. Therefore, methods are developed that specifically enhance the transport of drugs through the SC in order to allow delivery of therapeutically relevant doses by the transdermal route. Iontophoresis is a technique with which the transdermal permeation rate of drug molecules is increased by the application of an electric field.

Leuprolide is a peptide analogue of the leutinizing hormone releasing hormone that is used in combination therapy for the treatment of hormone-related cancers. Based on its enzymatic instability and its pharmacodynamic profile, leuprolide is a good candidate for transdermal iontophoretic delivery. In the present work, the mechanisms governing the transport of leuprolide across SC in the presence of an electric field are investigated and a physicochemical model is presented that allows quantifying the effect of relevant parameters of the process. Based on the insights gained, adjuvants are developed which, when included in the drug formulation, can augment the impact of iontophoresis in terms of skin permeation enhancement of the drug. Finally, the feasibility of the delivery of leuprolide by this technique from the point of view of dosing is discussed.

Materials and methods

Leuprolide, a nonapeptide with the sequence Pyr-His-Trp-Ser-Tyr-D-Leu-Leu-Arg-Pro-NHEt was kindly donated by Bachem AG (Bubendorf, Switzerland). Skin permeation experiments were carried out in vitro at 37°C using heat-separated epidermis from human cadaver skin (supplied by the Department of Pathology, University Hospital, Basel, Switzerland). The epidermal membrane was mounted vertically in a two-chamber diffusion cell, that was symmetrical about the membrane and each chamber was outfitted with a pair of voltage and reference Ag/AgCl electrodes connected to a direct current (DC) supply unit (Institute of Physics, University of Basel). The anode was placed in the donor compartment of the diffusion cell containing the drug at a concentration of 5 mg/ml.

Drug permeation through the membrane was measured consecutively under passive, iontophoretic and again passive conditions, the drug being assayed in withdrawn samples by high performance liquid chromatography (HPLC). Experiments were carried out in aqueous buffer systems at pH 4.5 and 7.2, at which the drug had an average net ionic valence of 1.98 and 1.09, respectively. Iontophoresis was performed under constant voltage conditions using voltages of 250, 500, 750 and 1000 mV and under constant current conditions using current densities of 0.5, 1, 1.5 and 2.3 $\mu A/cm^2$. In the constant voltage studies, acetyl-leucine-leucinolyl-phosphate (LLP), a negatively charged dipeptide (synthesized and donated by Bachem AG) was used as an adjuvant at a concentration of 2.4 mg/ml. In the constant-current studies, polymaleic acid (PMA) (Polysciences, Inc, Warrington, USA), a macromolecular polyelectrolyte with molecular weight between 800 and 1200 was used to replace the universal citrate-phosphate-borate buffer system otherwise employed.

Results and discussion

Constant voltage

In the experiments with constant voltage application, iontophoretic enhancement factor, E, was calculated with Equation 22.1.

$$E = \frac{P_{total}^{\Delta\psi}}{P_{total}^{passive}} \tag{22.1}$$

where, P is permeability coefficient, the subscript 'total' refers to permeation through both lipid and aqueous domains of the SC, and the superscripts '$\Delta\Psi$' and 'passive' refer to iontophoresis and passive conditions, respectively.

Enhancement increased with increasing voltage (Figure 22.1). For a

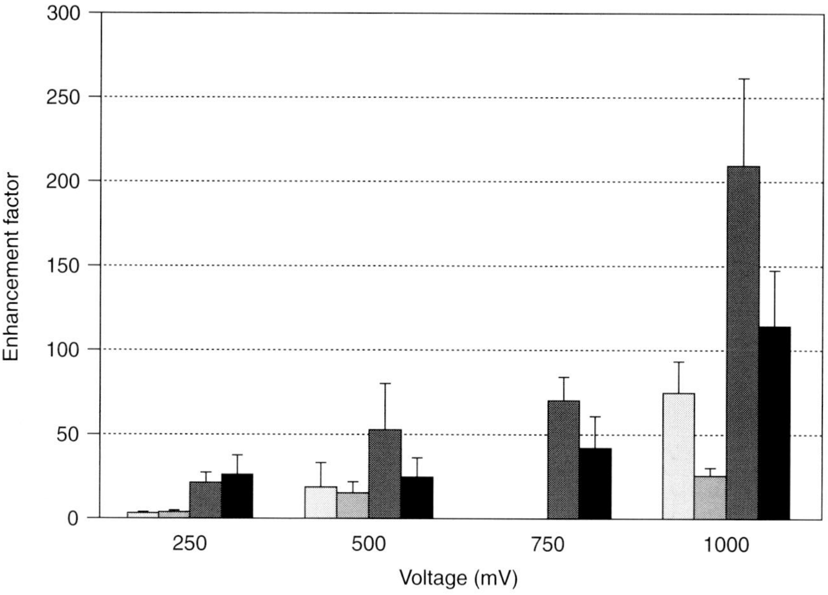

Figure 22.1

Iontophoretic enhancement factors of leuprolide obtained with constant voltage application. For each voltage, first and second bar from the left denote pH 4.5, and third and fourth bar denote pH 7.2 (for 750 mV, only pH 7.2 is shown). First and third bar indicated calculation based on baseline passive permeability co-efficient, and second and fourth bar indicate calculation based on post-iontophoretic passive permeability coefficient.

voltage larger than approximately 500 mV, enhancement factors calculated on the basis of the baseline (pre-iontophoretic) passive permeability coefficient were higher than those on the basis of the post-iontophoretic passive permeability coefficient. This indicates that, while below 500 mV, the application of the electric field induced no alterations to the epidermal membrane; it did so at voltages above 500 mV. Enhancement at pH 7.2 was greater than at pH 4.5 despite the fact that at the former the ionic valence of the drug was lower than at the latter.

To gain a better understanding of the factors governing iontophoresis and quantitatively assess the contribution of relevant parameters, a model describing the process on a mechanistic basis was developed and used to analyse the experimental results. This model starts from the modified Nernst-Planck equation, which takes into account the electric field force on ions and the electroosmotic flow, and is extended to distinguish between the contribution of the aqueous and the lipid pathway of the stratum corneum to drug permeation and to include the change of the volume fraction of the aqueous domain (expressed as porosity) induced by the electric field. Based on this model, the following expression for the enhancement factor (E) is derived.

$$E = \frac{\frac{\epsilon'}{\epsilon}(-\bar{z}_{ad}B + Pe)}{1 + \left(\frac{P_{ld}}{P_{ad}}\right)^{passive}} \tag{22.2}$$

with

$$B = \frac{F\Delta\Psi}{RT} \text{ and } Pe = \frac{vh}{D_{ad}} \tag{22.3}$$

where, ϵ' and ϵ are the fractions of aqueous pathway during iontophoresis and passive permeation, respectively, $\bar{z}_{ad}$ is the weighted average net ionic valence of the drug in the aqueous domain, P_{ld} and P_{ad} are the passive permeability coefficients for the lipid and the aqueous domains, respectively, $\Delta\Psi$ is the applied potential difference, Pe is peclet number, v is electroosmotic flow velocity, D_{ad} is drug diffusion coefficient in the aqueous domain, F is the Faraday constant, R is the gas constant and T is absolute temperature.

Values of the parameters of Equation 22.2 were determined that provided the closest fit of the calculated to the experimental enhancement factors considering simultaneously all enhancement factors obtained based on the baseline passive permeability coefficient (Table 22.1). The estimated parameters describe very well the experimental results. These parameters indicate firstly, that a small fraction of permeation (≈20%) under passive conditions takes place through the lipid domain which seems reasonable considering the relative lipophilicity of the drug molecule. This fraction is not affected by iontophoresis. Secondly, there is a

Table 22.1 Estimated parameter values of the model and enhancement factors.

pH	Voltage (mV)	$(P_{ld}/P_{ad})^{passive}$	Pe	ϵ'/ϵ	E	
					calculated	observed
4.5	250	0.24	−10.4	1.00	6.52	3.83
4.5	500	0.24	−20.8	1.44	18.9	18.9
4.5	1000	0.24	−41.6	2.86	74.5	75.0
7.2	250	0.24	12.7	1.00	18.4	21.6
7.2	500	0.24	25.4	1.44	53.3	53.0
7.2	750	0.24	38.1	1.28	70.8	70.7
7.2	1000	0.24	50.8	2.86	210.3	210.1

voltage dependent increase of the porosity of the membrane which reaches almost a factor of three at 1000 mV. Thirdly, due to the sign of Pe, the electroosmotic flow takes place from the donor to the receiver compartment, i.e. anode to cathode, at pH 7.2 and in the opposite direction at pH 4.5, the magnitude of this flow in absolute terms being similar at both pH values. This can be explained by an adsorption of leuprolide to the epidermal membrane, which at pH 4.5 (at which leuprolide has two positively charged groups) turns the bound skin charge from negative (prevailing under physiological conditions) to positive, thus reversing the direction of the electroosmotic flow.

The addition of LLP to the solution at pH 4.5 increased the enhancement factor of leuprolide for 250 mV from 3.83 to 8.13. This corresponds to a decrease of the magnitude of the electroosmotic flow, which has a negative sign at this pH. This decrease is attributed to the addition of negatively charged sites to the tissue because of binding of the added LLP. Thus, it is demonstrated that the adjuvant used augments the permeation enhancing effect of iontophoresis under these conditions.

Constant current

With the application of constant current, a positive, nearly linear relationship between the iontophoretic permeability coefficient and current density was obtained (Figure 22.2), showing that a current-regulated drug delivery rate could be achieved. Transference number, T_n, was calculated according to Equation 22.4.

$$T_n = \frac{\bar{z}_{ad} F dQ/dt}{M_r I} \qquad (22.4)$$

where, dQ/dt is the transported amount per time during iontophoresis, M_r is the drug molecular weight and I is the total current.

Permeability at pH 7.2 was higher than at pH 4.5 and the transference number was approximately the same (≈0.6%) despite the lower ionic valence at the former pH compared to the latter. This is probably because of the direction of the electroosmotic flow being positive at pH 7.2 and negative at pH 4.5 as demonstrated by the above model analysis of the constant voltage data.

When the low molecular weight universal buffer system of a concentration of 24.8 mmol/l was substituted with a low concentration (0.6 mmol/l) of the high molecular weight buffer polymaleic acid, drug permeability was increased two-fold at comparable pH values (Figure 22.3). The transference number was likewise increased to about 1%, showing that by this substitution of the background electrolyte the efficiency of iontophoresis could be improved.

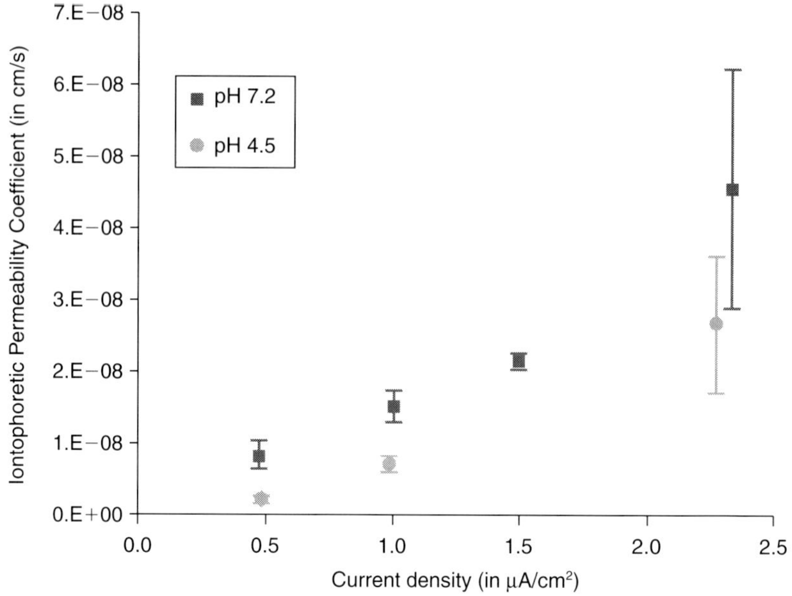

Figure 22.2

Iontophoretic permeability coefficient of leuprolide as a function of the applied current density at two pH values using the universal buffer system. Points and bars indicate mean ± standard error margin.

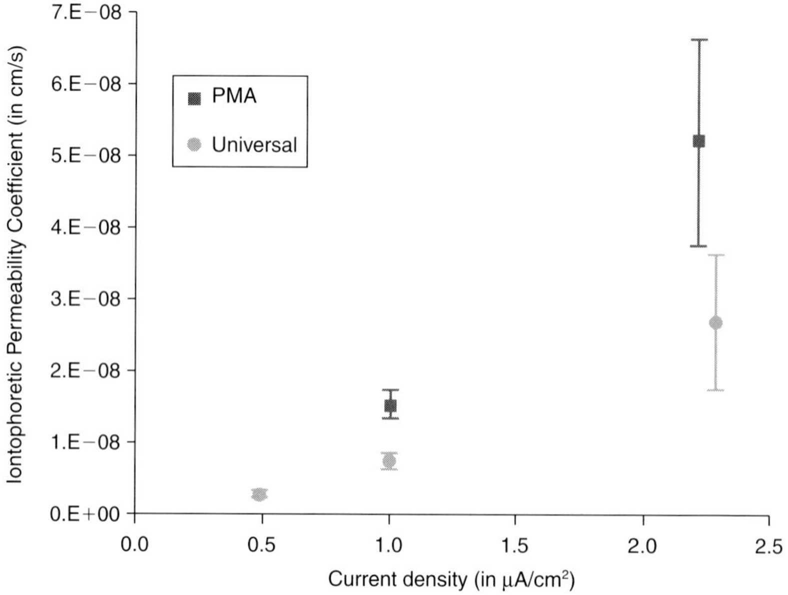

Figure 22.3

Iontophoretic permeability coefficient of leuprolide as a function of the applied current density with universal buffer system at pH 4.5 and polymaleic acid (PMA) at pH 5.1. Points and bars indicate mean ± standard error margin.

From the measured permeation rates it is extrapolated that a total current of at least 26 μA is required to deliver 8.4 μg of drug per hour, at which rate a therapeutic dose is reached within 24 hours of continuous delivery. The required current can be applied using current densities well below the maximum safe value (i.e. 0.5 mA/cm^2) and leaves room for adjustment if other dose regimens are desirable. Thus, the delivery of therapeutic doses of leuprolide by iontophoresis appears to be feasible.

Acknowledgements

Financial support was provided by Bachem AG, Bubendorf, Switzerland and Asulab SA, Marin, Switzerland. Human skin biopsies were supplied by the Institute of Pathology, University of Basel, Prof. J Torhorst.

23
In vitro systems to characterize dermal permeation and penetration

U Bock, S Schmitz and E Haltner

Aims

Permeation and penetration studies are of importance in the development of topical formulations in the pharmaceutical industry. The cosmetics and chemical industries, however, are more interested in demonstrating non-absorption of actives or ingredients. In vitro techniques are used to determine the absorption into the skin (penetration) and through the skin (permeation).

Methods

Biological membrane

Human abdominal skin of female or male patients who had undergone plastic surgery was used. Immediately after excision, the subcutaneous fatty tissue was removed and the skin was stored at –24°C until use. In permeability studies, it can be used as full skin, dermatomized, heat-separated skin, or isolated stratum corneum (SC) membranes.

Model drugs and formulations

Caffeine was chosen as a model drug to study the integrity of the skin under all experimental conditions. A topical caffeine formulation was taken from a local pharmacy.

Analytics

High-performance liquid chromatography (HPLC) analysis was performed using a Waters Alliance 2690 system with a Photodiode Array Detector. Fast linear gradients on reversed-phase columns were performed

Permeation

Diffusion experiments were performed under infinite-dose conditions at 32°C using Franz diffusion cells (diffusion area 3.08 cm^2 and an acceptor volume of 20.0 ml). The receptor medium consisted of Krebs–Ringer buffer (pH 7.2) spiked with 0.05% NaN_3. Samples at different time points up to 48 hours were drawn from the receptor compartment for quantitative HPLC analysis.

Penetration

A detailed description of the model can be found in Wagner et al.[1] The cavity of a teflon punch was filled with the drug preparation. This punch was applied on the surface of the full skin and optimal contact of skin and drug preparation was achieved by placing a weight of 0.5 kg on top of the punch for 2 minutes. This weight was subsequently removed and the punch was fixed in its position at 32°C during study time.

Adhesive tape-stripping

After application of the drug preparation, removal of the skin was successfully performed by stripping, using 20 pieces of adhesive tape (Multifilm Kristallklar; Beiersdorf AG, Germany), and extracted for analytical purposes.[1,2]

Cryosection

Immediately after stripping, the skin was rapidly frozen to –24°C and, in order to evaluate the depth of penetration of the drugs into the skin layers, it was separated by cryo-cuts of 25 µm. These cuts were pooled according to a fixed scheme, extracted and analysed by HPLC.[1]

Results

All permeation studies (P_{app}) showed a clear dependence on the skin specimen used as membrane. The P_{app} for caffeine was independent of the thickness of the membrane (f, d, h, t). The permeation rates of caffeine from solution or creme were comparable (Table 23.1).

The penetration of caffeine showed marked differences between the SC and the deeper skin layers, depending on incubation time. Therefore, both techniques can be qualified by this marker molecule and allow reproducible and standardized in vitro studies (Figure 23.1).

Table 23.1 Permeability coefficients (P_{app}) for marker substrate caffeine on different human skin membranes in vitro. The values are mean values from experiments performed in parallel (n = 3, mean ± SD) for permeability studies. The thicknesses of the membranes and the stratum corneum were determined tenfold (n = 10, mean ± SD).

Skin number	Age	Gender	Membrane (μm) [1]	P_{app} (cm/s) [2]	P_{app} (cm/s) [3]	SC thickness (μm) [4]
003-01-0500	43	F	2147 ± 209, f	5.80E-8 ± 1.40E-8	–	–
004-01-0500	51	M	1834 ± 284, f	1.20E-7 ± 4.80E-8	–	–
005-01-0800	69	M	1732 ± 192, f	5.10E-8 ± 2.40E-8	–	–
047-01-1100	21	F	2303 ± 131, f	1.90E-7 ± 2.03E-7	–	–
047-01-1100	21	F	514 ± 162, d	2.10E-7 ± 1.10E-7	–	–
062-01-0701	53	F	614 ± 45, d	5.34E-8 ± 9.58E-9	1.15E-7 ± 2.19E-8	11.30 ± 0.70
064-01-0801	18	M	509 ± 40, d	3.84E-7 ± 6.82E-8	4.90E-7 ± 1.30E-7	10.38 ± 0.70
065-01-0901	33	F	514 ± 121, d	8.95E-7 ± 1.65E-8	1.30E-7 ± 2.89E-8	12.75 ± 1.56
067-01-0901	35	F	486 ± 35, d	6.52E-8 ± 1.31E.8	1.15E-7 ± 2.65E-8	13.80 ± 2.32
068-01-0901	32	F	617 ± 62, d	5.15E-8 ± 1.37E-8	1.18E-7 ± 3.00E-8	10.13 ± 1.69
069-01-0901	39	F	490 ± 36, d	4.90E-8 ± 2.41E-9	1.48E-7 ± 1.52E-8	19.13 ± 3.44
074-01-1101	35	F	668 ± 46, d	1.08E-7 ± 6.66E-8	1.86E-7 ± 3.04E-8	20.48 ± 2.95
065-01-0901	33	F	59.44 ± 11.07,h	3.60E-8 ± 4.80E-10	–	12.75 ± 1.56
067-01-0901	35	F	89.83 ± 4.65, h	5.80E-7 ± 2.70E-8	–	13.80 ± 2.32
055-01-0501	31	F	26.91 ± 8.92, t	2.90E-7 ± 3.60E-8	–	25.00 ± 4.23
065-01-0901	33	F	22.86 ± 2.59, t	1.80E-7 ± 2.60E-8	–	12.75 ± 1.56

f full-thickness skin, d: dermatomized skin, h: heat separated skin, t: stratum corneum isolated with 0.1% trypsin solution.

[1] thickness of the skin membrane determined by Haidenhain thickness measurement apparatus at the start of the experiment;

[2] 10 mg/ml caffeine in Krebs–Ringer bicarbonate buffer (pH 7.2);

[3] hydrophilic ointment (unguentum emulsificans aquosum) containing 0.86% caffeine;

[4] determined by microscope.

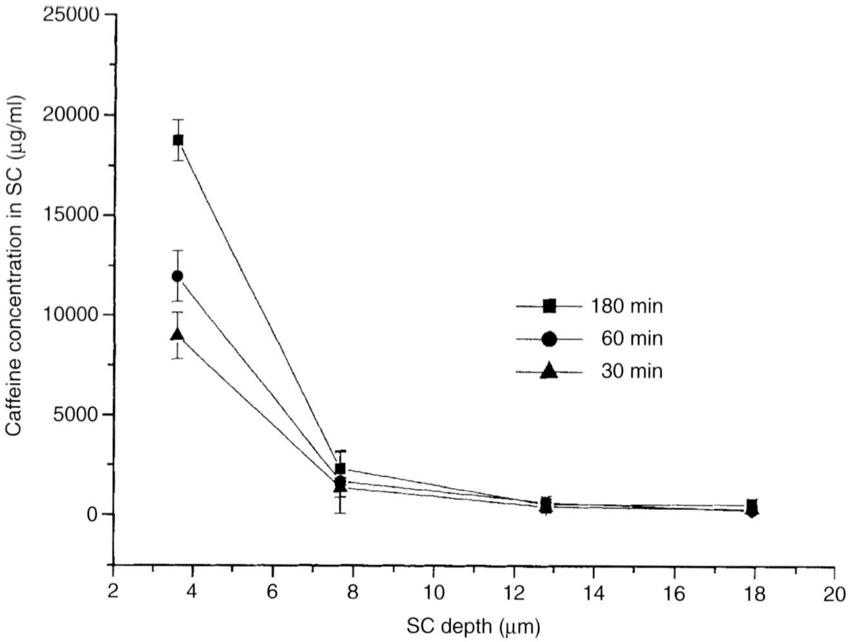

Figure 23.1

Penetration characteristics of caffeine from topical formulation after 30, 60 and 180 minutes' incubation time in full-thickness skin specimen 074-01-1101 in the SC. The values are mean values from experiments performed in parallel (n = 3, mean ± SD).

Conclusion

The above-described in vitro methods are useful tools in predicting cutaneous or percutaneous absorption in drug development processes, penetration-enhancing concepts prior to clinical trials, or safety evaluation in cosmetic and chemical science.

References

1. Wagner H, Kostka K-H, Lehr C-M et al. Drug distribution in human skin using two different in vitro test systems: comparison with in vivo data. Pharm Res 2000; 17: 1475–81.
2. Shah VP, Glynn GL, Yacobi A et al. Bioequivalance of topical dermatological dosage forms – methods of evaluation of bioequivalance. Pharm Res 1998; 15: 167–71.

24
Permeation and sorption studies of water transport in stratum corneum

ThA Steriotis, GCh Charalambopoulou, AK Stubos and NK Kanellopoulos

Aims

The equilibrium and diffusional properties of water in stratum corneum (SC) are of great importance, since hydration affects its appearance, flexibility and, most of all, its barrier function to chemical transport.[1] In the present work, permeability and diffusion coefficients of water, in dry and H_2O-loaded SC, were determined experimentally, by employing permeation and sorption techniques, respectively. Both human and porcine SC samples were examined.

Methods and results

The permeability experiments were performed on a home-made rig that consisted of a high- and a low-pressure section, separated by the membrane, aiming to investigate the effect of varying hydration on water transport through the SC.

The measurements for porcine samples pre-equilibrated at certain relative humidities (RH) ranging from 0% to 99% were performed at 23°C. The results suggest that water induces certain structural changes, which lead to a significant increase of H_2O permeance, from 3.67×10^{-4} cm/s for the dry sample, to 23.30×10^{-4} cm/s for the fully hydrated SC. The corresponding values in the case of human samples were found in the range between 2.23×10^{-4} cm/s and 5.30×10^{-4} cm/s (Figure 24.1a). The structural changes are also supported by relative permeability experiments, in which an inert gas, such as helium, passes through hydrated SC. In this case, the permeance values for the porcine SC samples were between 4.57×10^{-6} cm/s and 11.76×10^{-6} cm/s, while for the human SC samples, they were between 1.34×10^{-6} cm/s and 3.47×10^{-6} cm/s (Figure 24.1b).

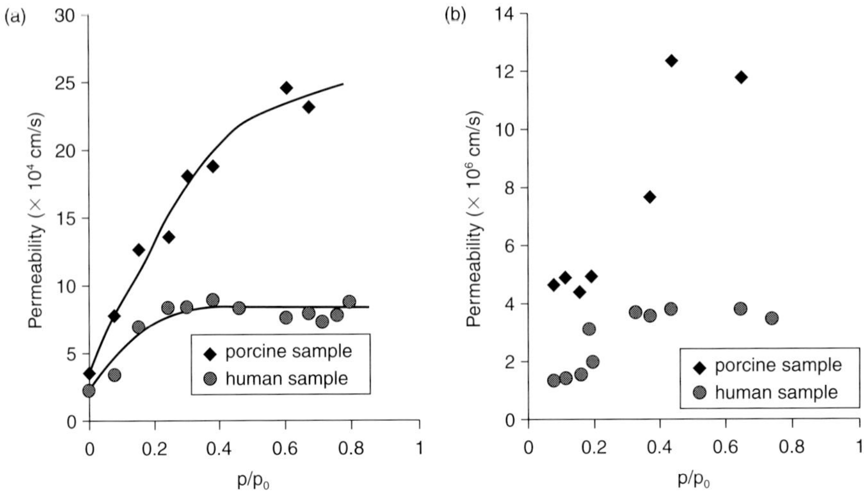

Figure 24.1

(a) Effect of SC water content on water permeability at 23°C. (b) Effect of SC water content on He permeability at 23°C.

Apart from directly measuring the local concentration gradient and the resulting steady state flux, the mobility of water molecules in the SC matrix can be studied by transient state, sorption kinetic experiments. In this case, SC samples are exposed to a certain H_2O pressure and the mass change is recorded versus time, until equilibrium is attained. The data obtained at 23°C showed that the porcine SC-water absorption isotherm is characterized by a straight line, starting at equilibrium RH = 20%, and extending to about RH = 60%, followed by an upward curve, which indicates that water gain is significantly enhanced at increased relative humidities (Figure 24.2a). This trend is in good agreement with similar bibliographic data.[2] The water content per gram of dry tissue of the fully hydrated sample was found to be ~0.35 g. The comparison of the absorption isotherms obtained from the measurement of intact and delipidized samples revealed significant differences at high RH values, indicating that intercellular lipids do indeed affect the capability of SC to retain water.

Additionally, the absorption kinetic curves were analysed and the corresponding diffusion coefficients (D) were derived by fitting the kinetic data to the solution of the Fick's diffusion equation for plane sheets.[3] The results (Figure 24.2b), in agreement with bibliographic data,[4,5] showed that initially, water diffusivity increases, changing from 0.18×10^{-10} cm²/s at RH = 10%, to 2.1×10^{-10} cm²/s at RH = 60%. Beyond this RH value, diffusion does not seem to be affected by the amount of water uptake. This behaviour can be explained as follows. At low hydration levels, water

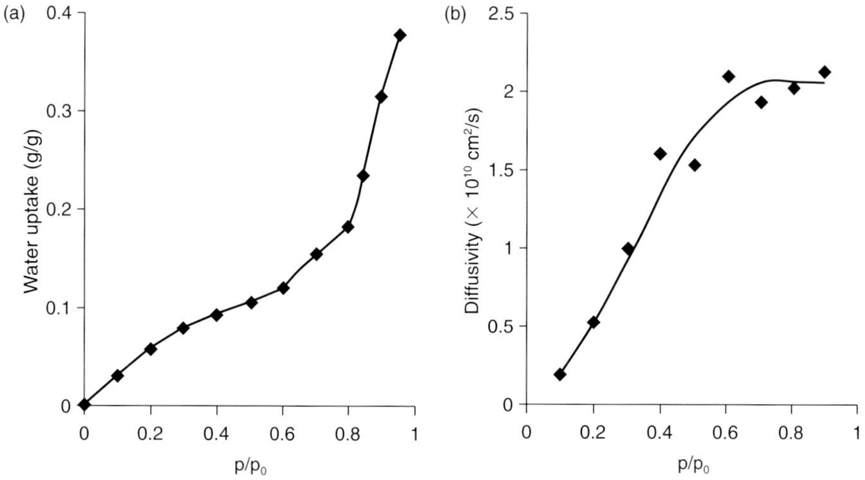

Figure 24.2

(a) Porcine SC–water sorption isotherm at 23°C. (b) Effect of porcine SC water content on the diffusion coefficients in the water sorption process.

molecules must overcome diffusion barriers, set by the well-ordered lipid bilayers, and subsequently reach specific sorption sites, associated with the polar lipid heads. Since the molecules are firmly bound to these sites, restricted mobility is expected. As a result, small D values are obtained. As hydration increases, the intercellular lamellar structure is distorted by water-rich regions, which eventually form conductive pathways, while the interaction of the water molecules with the polar heads weakens, leading to higher mobility. The overall effect is the observed increase of D values. Finally, at RH beyond 60%, a phase of 'loose' water is formed and constant D values are obtained.

References

1. Roberts MS, Walker M. Water, the most natural penetration enhancer. In: Walters K, Hadgraft J, eds. *Pharmaceutical Skin Penetration Enhancement.* 1st edn. New York: Marcel Dekker 1993: 1–29.
2. Liron Z, Clewell HJ, McDougal JN. Kinetics of water vapor sorption in porcine stratum corneum. J Pharm Sci 1994; 83:692–8.
3. Crank J. *The Mathematics of Diffusion*, London: Oxford University Press 1975.
4. Scheuplein RJ, Blank IH. Permeability of the skin. Physiol Rev 1971; 51:702–47.
5. Blank IH, Moloney H, Alfred BS et al. The diffusion of water across the stratum corneum as a function of its water content. J Invest Dermatol 1984; 82:188–94.

25
A random walk model of stratum corneum diffusion

HF Frasch

Introduction

A mathematical model has been developed that is based on the molecular mechanism of diffusion and that explicitly incorporates the non-uniform structure of the stratum corneum (SC).[1] The model is used to predict permeability coefficients of chemicals based on their molecular weight (MW) and octanol-water partition coefficient (P).

Methods

Diffusion through the heterogeneous SC is modeled as a random walk process. Particles of a diffusing substance are placed on the surface of a model SC membrane and undergo two-dimensional random walks through the transverse section of the biphasic (lipids and corneocytes) membrane. From any current location, a molecule moves randomly to a new location. The movement of molecules within the membrane is determined by two independent variables: relative diffusivity within the corneocytes and lipids, and instantaneous partitioning of the chemical between lipid and corneocyte phases.

Two variables are calculated from the random walk simulations: effective diffusivity (D^*) and effective path length (l^*). These are defined as the diffusivity and thickness of a homogeneous membrane having identical diffusion properties as the heterogeneous SC for a specific chemical. These are derived by examining the behavior of many diffusing particles under identical input conditions.

Steady-state permeability (k_p) is given by: $k_p = K_{mv}D/l$, where K_{mv} is the membrane-vehicle partition coefficient. Thus, we use D^* and l^* to estimate permeability coefficients. All variables are reduced to simple algebraic functions of MW and P.[1] Values for four variable parameters were found by non-linear regression of the model with the Flynn[2] database of 94 permeability measurements.

Results

Figure 25.1 shows a comparison between the model predictions of k_p and experimental values reported by Flynn.[2] The correlation coefficient (R^2) is 0.84. Diameters of the circular symbols are proportional to molecular weights of the compounds. Also shown is the line of identity.

For comparisons among different models, identical regression analyses were performed on five published models that predict k_p as a function of MW and P (Table 25.1).

Discussion

The random walk model of diffusion through the SC has advantages over other approaches: this model is based on first principles – the molecular basis of diffusion – and it permits diffusion calculations in a morphologically realistic, heterogeneous SC membrane.

In this model, lipids and corneocytes are considered distinct phases with different diffusivities and different chemical affinities. Consequently, neither diffusivity nor diffusional path length of the SC membrane is a simple constant. However, comparison of model results with an appropriate solution to the classic diffusion equation for a homogeneous membrane permits the identification of an effective diffusivity (D*) and an effective path length (l*). These chemical-specific quantities are used to

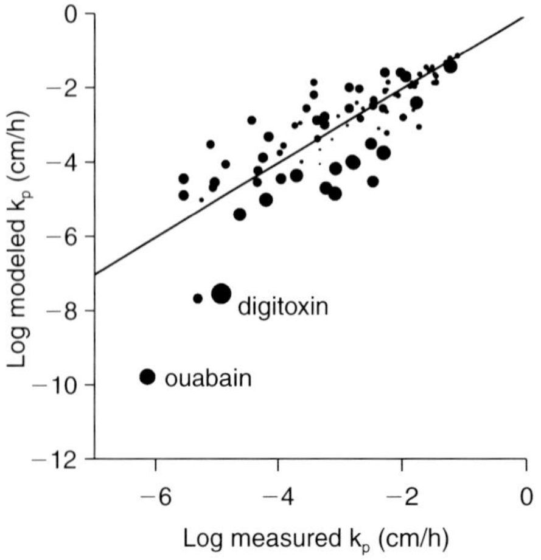

Figure 25.1

Modeled skin permeability k_p compared with experimental measurements reported by Flynn.[2] Diameters of symbols are proportional to the MW of the compounds. The two compounds with the largest MW (ouabin, digitoxin) have the largest residual differences. Line of identity is also shown.

Table 25.1 Regression statistics for six models. The models were fitted to the Flynn database[2] of 94 measurements. np: number of fitted parameters of model; R^2: correlation coefficient; SE: standard error of the model estimate; F: measure of the predictive value of the independent variables (higher F statistic indicates greater predictive value).

Model (reference)	np	R^2	SE	F
Frasch[1]	4	0.84	0.008	154
Modified Robinson[3]	4	0.80	0.009	116
McKone and Howd[3,4]	5	0.80	0.009	87
Cleek and Bunge[5]	3	0.78	0.009	158
Modified Potts and Guy[3]	3	0.73	0.653	120
Potts and Guy[3,6]	3	0.68	0.704	96

predict steady-state permeability of chemicals in an aqueous vehicle. All variables are reduced to simple algebraic functions of MW and P.

In conclusion, we have presented a novel mathematical model of skin permeation. The model is based on the fundamental molecular mechanism of diffusion and accounts for the structural and chemical heterogeneity of the SC. It provides mechanistic insight into the process of skin permeation and has excellent predictive capacity.

References

1. Frasch HF. A random walk model of skin permeation. Risk Analysis 2002; 22:265–76.
2. Flynn GL. Physicochemical determinants of skin absorption. In: Garrity TR, Henry CJ, eds. *Principles of Route-to-route Extrapolation for Risk Assessment.* New York: Elsevier 1990:93–107.
3. Wilschut A, ten Berge WF, Robinson PJ et al. Estimating skin permeation. The validation of five mathematical skin permeation models. Chemosphere 1995; 30: 1275–96.
4. McKone TE, Howd RA. Estimating dermal uptake of nonionic organic chemicals from water and soil: I. Unified fugacity-based models for risk assessment. Risk Analysis 1992; 12:543–57.
5. Cleek RL, Bunge A. A new method for estimating dermal absorption from chemical exposure. 1. General approach. Pharm Res 1993; 10:497–506.
6. Potts, RO, Guy RH. Predicting skin permeability. Pharm Res 1992; 9:663–9.

26
Stratum corneum lipid composition as a predictive tool for permeability?

T Schmidt, N Widler, F Gafner and G Imanidis

Theory

This theory envisages a linear correlation between the logarithm of the steady-state flux and the exchange cohesive energy between the permeating molecule and the lipid compounds of the stratum corneum (SC).[1] The latter cohesive parameter is obtained from solubility parameter calculations and an attempt is made to verify the theoretical approach with experimental permeability data.

Summary

The passive permeability of beta-blocking substances of different lipophilicity/polarity through shed snake skin was investigated from aqueous buffered solutions. Organic solvents were avoided, to minimize the influence on the natural lipid pattern of the skin.

A low-receiver volume flow-through cell system with automated fraction collector was used in the experimental part.

The partial solubility parameters, according to Hansen, were calculated for each lipid compound found in *Bothrops atrox*, as well as for the test substances. The latest Beerbower compilation of fragmental group molar attraction constants comprised almost all functional groups relevant for the investigated beta-blockers and lipid compounds.[2] After Bagley projection and determination of the exchange cohesive energy, the latter was finally correlated with the permeability coefficient found for each test substance.

As expected, a significant correlation could not be shown from the theory, despite two possible outliers, preventing a final conclusion about a linear correlation as yet. It should be mentioned that the literature data and theory are based on calculated permeability values.[1]

Materials and methods

Sample and skin preparation

The beta-blocking substances were selected according to their ability to form aqueous solutions. As mentioned earlier, a possibly low depletion effect of lipids from the SC into donator or receiver medium was thus expected. Low-volume flow-through cells (Laboratory Glass Apparatus; Bageley, USA) were constantly kept at a temperature of 32°C, by means of an air bath. Fresh sheddings (mainly SC) were obtained from female adult *B. atrox* species, kept at Pentapharm's serpentarium in Aesch, Switzerland. All dorsal-skin samples were hydrated in the receiver solution for 1 hour, prior to excision of the required skin circles.[3]

At this point, the circles were mounted onto the cells and the receiver medium was circulated for a reasonable period of time, until tightness of all the cells could be ascertained. Transepidermal water loss (TEWL) was also measured, using a Tewameter® TM 210 (Courage + Khazaka Electronic GmbH).

Passive water flow across the barrier membrane was assumed to be negligible, since donator and receiver solutions were both buffered at pH 7.2 and the osmolarity was adjusted to 300 mOsmol/kg in both cases.

Permeation experiments

The donator solutions were applied and the donator cell compartments covered; meanwhile, the flow rate of the receiver medium was monitored. The receiver medium was collected in test tubes, in hourly fractions.

Analytical part

The pH and osmolarity of the receiver fractions were measured directly after each experiment, using a standard pH electrode and a micro-osmometer. Thereafter, one could easily determine irregularities in the experiments, e.g. unstable flow of receiver, evaporation or leaks. Donator and receiver solutions were analysed by high performance liquid chromatography (HPLC) and ultraviolet (UV) photometer.

Solubility parameter, Bagley diagram, exchange cohesive energy

From the previous work of Widler (unpublished work), the lipid composition was adopted. The molecular formulae of all compounds were established and the Hansen parameter successively calculated, on the basis of the Beerbower fragmental approach. The general equations to determine the Hansen parameter and exchange cohesive energy (ECE, Equation 26.5) were as follows:

$$\delta_d = \frac{\Sigma F_{d,i}}{\Sigma V_i}$$

(Equation 26.1)

$$\delta_p = \frac{\sqrt{\Sigma F^2_{p,i}}}{\Sigma V_i}$$

(Equation 26.2)

$$\delta_h = \frac{\sqrt{\Sigma F_{h,i}}}{\Sigma V_i}$$

(Equation 26.3)

$$\delta_d = \sqrt{\delta_d^2 + \delta_p^2}$$

(Equation 26.4)

$$d^2 = \Delta^2\delta_M = \Delta\delta_h^{\ 2} + \Delta\delta_v^{\ 2}$$

(Equation 26.5)

F is the respective group molar attraction constant, broken down into dispersion, polar and hydrogen bond portions. The latter is divided by the molar volume of the respective functional group.

The so-called Bagley diagram (Figure 26.1) shows a plot of δ_h (Equation 26.3) over δ_v (Equation 26.4).

The exchange cohesive energy ($\Delta^2\delta_M$) is derived for each lipid-beta-blocker pair, expressed through their squared distances in the Bagley projection (Equation 26.5, Figure 26.1), and finally correlated with the permeability coefficient P (Equation 26.6).

$$P = \frac{dm}{dt} \cdot \frac{1}{S \cdot c_D}$$

(Equation 26.6)

P describes the flux of a substance (m) per time (t) and surface area (S), independent of the donator concentration (c_D). It is derived from Fick's Law of Diffusion. Equation 26.6 is valid under perfect sink conditions and the decrease in c_D is negligible, as proved by experimental data.

Results

The pH and osmolarity remained almost constant during the experiment. If the osmolarity of any fractions showed striking differences after the experiment, the data were discarded.

If $\Delta^2\delta_M$ is plotted against lnP, e.g. Figure 26.2, the result shows a certain dependency of permeability on the exchange cohesive energy.

Exchange cohesive energies for all lipid compounds were finally plotted against the lnP and P of the tested substances. The results are shown and summarized below (Table 26.1).

Discussion

The applied methods allow reliable determination and clear differentiation of the permeability of beta-blocking substances with different functional

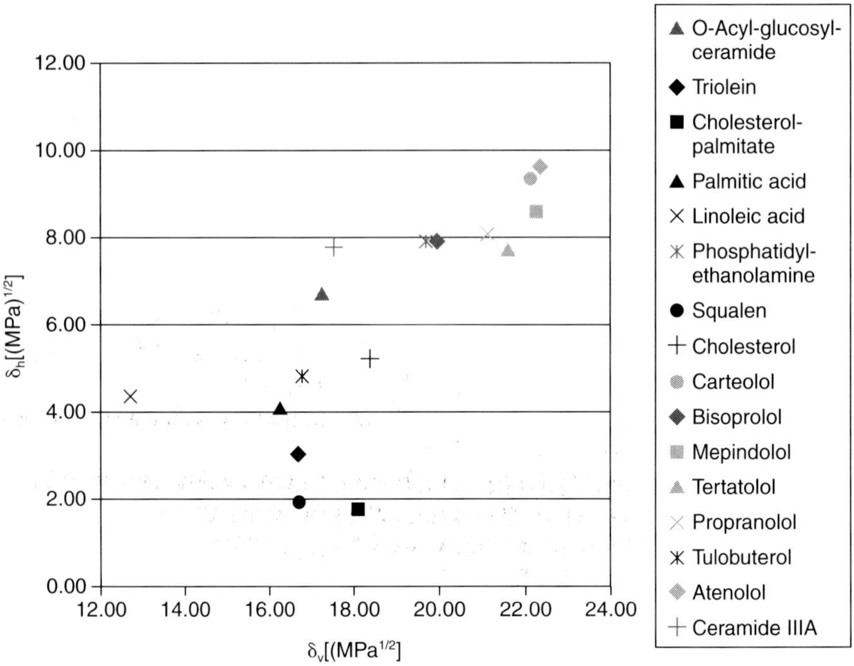

Figure 26.1

Bagley diagram

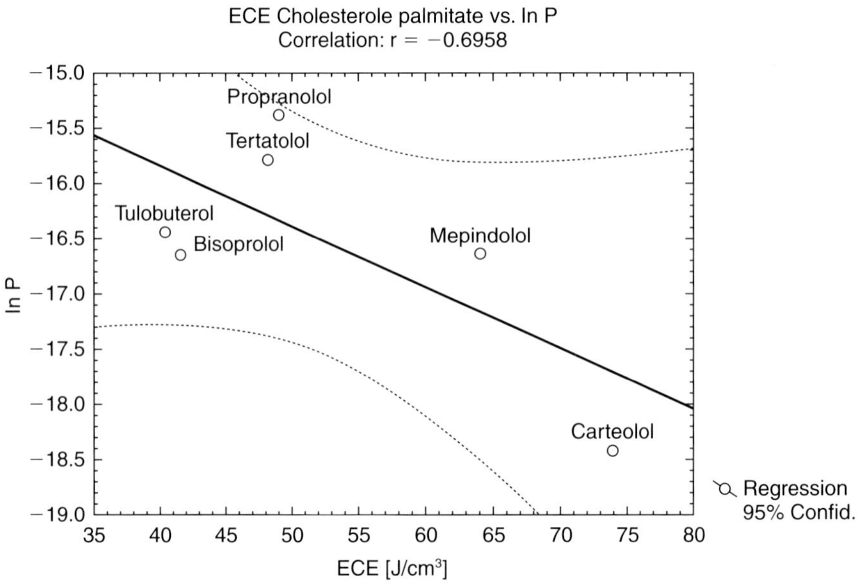

Figure 26.2

Correlation of permeability against exchange cohesive energy.

Table 26.1 Correlations of permeability versus different lipids' ECE.

Plot *P vs.* $\Delta^2\delta_M$	**r(X,Y)**	**rV**	**t**	**p**	**N**
O-Acylglycosyl ceramide	−0.253	0.064	−0.524	0.628	6
Ceramide IIIA	−0.201	0.040	−0.411	0.702	6
Triolein	−0.356	0.127	−0.763	0.488	6
Cholesterol palmitate	−0.450	0.203	−1.009	0.370	6
Palmitic acid	−0.313	0.098	−0.659	0.546	6
Linoleic acid	−0.220	0.049	−0.452	0.675	6
Phosphatidylethanolamine	−0.310	0.096	−0.652	0.550	6
Squalen	−0.382	0.146	−0.825	0.455	6
Cholesterol	−0.382	0.146	−0.826	0.455	6
Plot *In P vs.* $\Delta^2\delta_M$					
O-Acylglycosyl ceramide	−0.476	0.227	−1.082	0.340	6
Ceramide IIIA	−0.411	0.169	−0.902	0.418	6
Triolein	−0.598	0.357	−1.492	0.210	6
Cholesterol palmitate	−0.696	0.484	−1.938	0.125	6
Palmitic acid	−0.550	0.302	−1.316	0.258	6
Linoleic acid	−0.451	0.203	−1.010	0.370	6
Phosphatidylethanolamine	−0.544	0.296	−1.298	0.264	6
Squalen	−0.626	0.392	−1.605	0.184	6
Cholesterol	−0.616	0.380	−1.565	0.193	6

Level of significance for r at $\alpha = 5\%$, n = 6: 0.811

groups attached to the constant pharmacophore. For all structures, the solubility parameter could be calculated and the Bagley projection was deduced. The correlation postulated in the literature, between ECE and permeability, based on *calculated* permeability data, was focused on a certain ceramide. The goal of this work was to verify this postulated correlation with experimental data and to check with other lipid compounds. The correctness of the correlation between P or lnP and the exchange cohesive energy could not be demonstrated definitively. The minimum r for significant data correlation with $\alpha = 5\%$, n = 6, is 0.811, and was not reached herein. The special situation of Bisoprolol needs to be further elucidated, as the molecule apparently does not fully dissociate from its counter ion fumarate, which was disregarded during the calculation of the solubility parameter. On the other hand, the influence of hydrogen bridges on permeability is currently being investigated in a separate approach.

Compared to far more common models, such as prediction via lipophilicity,[4,5] this method does not remarkably improve or ease the selection process of new drug candidates for transdermal application, as yet.

References

1. Gröning R, Braun FJ. Three-dimensional solubility parameters and their use in characterising the permeation of drugs through the skin. Die Pharmazie 1996; 51:337–41.
2. Barton AFM. *CRC Handbook of Solubility Parameters and Other Cohesion Parameters*. Boca Raton, Ann Arbor, Boston, London: CRC Press, 1991.
3. Itoh T, Xia J, Magavi R et al. Use of shed snake skin as a model membrane for in vitro percutaneous penetration studies: comparison with human skin. Pharm Res 1990; 7:1042–7.
4. Potts RO, Guy RH. Predicting skin permeability. Pharm Res 1992; 9:663–9.
5. Itoh T, Magavi R, Casady RL et al. A method to predict percutaneous permeability of various compounds: shed snake skin as a model membrane. Pharm Res 1990; 7:1302–6.

27

Evaluation of a direct spectrophotometric method for percutaneous bioavailability studies

T Tassopoulos, S Maeder, G Imanidis, V Figueiredo, EW Smith and C Surber

Introduction

Treffel and Gabard[1] demonstrated the ability of ultraviolet (UV) filters to act on the skin surface and within the stratum corneum (SC). For maximum sun protection and minimal UV filter permeation, the penetrated amount must remain in the outer layers of the SC.

Tape-stripping is a technique that has been found useful in dermatological research for selectively and, if performed correctly, exhaustively removing the SC. In recent years, the technique has gained appreciable significance in dermatopharmacokinetic research. Currently, xenobiotics (e.g. drugs, sunscreen agents) are extracted from single or combined tapes and the concentration in the extracted solution is determined. The amount of xenobiotic is expressed per square centimetre area of adhesive tape (e.g. μg/cm^2) or by other adequate means (e.g. μg/protein content or μg/weight of removed SC). These methods are laborious and susceptible to analytical artefacts. Based on recent investigations of Weigmann et al,[2] we evaluated a spectroscopic method where the concentration of a xenobiotic in an SC layer and the amount of SC removed by tape-stripping can be determined simultaneously (Figure 27.1, Equation 27.1). The amount of xenobiotic determined by a direct spectrophotometric method was verified by subsequent quantification using high performance liquid chromatography (HPLC).

$$A_{\text{xenobiotic}} = A(\lambda 1) - \frac{[A(\lambda 2) - A(\lambda 3)](\lambda 1 - \lambda 3)}{(\lambda 2 - \lambda 3)} - A(\lambda 3)$$

Equation 27.1

Baseline correction by three-wavelength analysis.

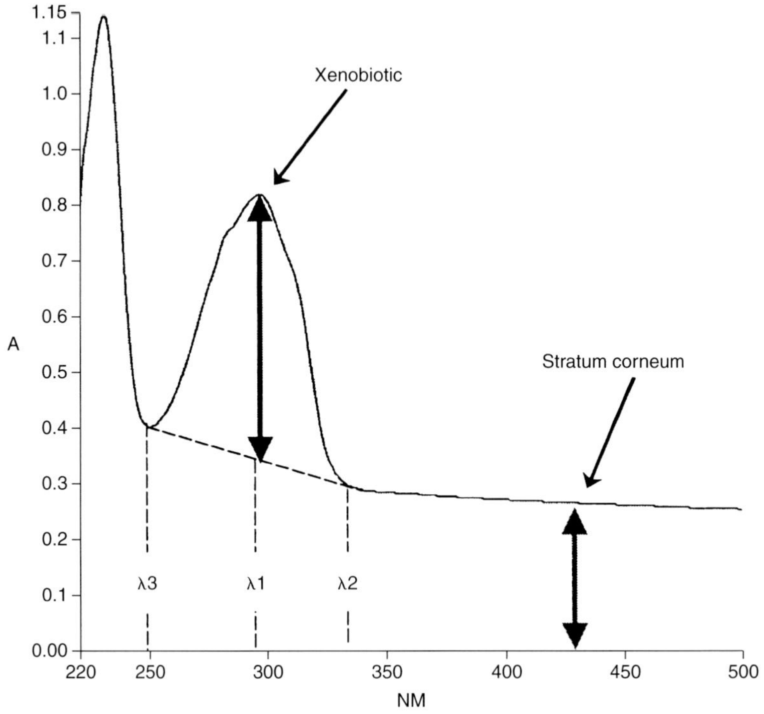

Figure 27.1

UV spectrum of a tape strip removed from skin treated with MBC formulation.

Methods

We determined the penetration of 4-methylbenzylidene camphor (MBC) (2% and 4%) into SC from a standard vehicle by tape-stripping. Preparation of the test area (volar aspect of the forearm), vehicle application and tape-stripping procedure (use and form of template, tape material and adhesive capacity, tape application and roll-on pressure) as well as environmental conditions were standardized (see Table 27.1).

MBC concentration and SC thickness were determined simultaneously with a spectrophotometer, modified to monitor a rectangular beam of 1 cm^2 in each tape removed. The spectra were recorded between 220 and 500 nm. MBC concentration in each single tape was verified by reversed phase (RP)-HPLC. The HPLC-assay for MBC was validated according the ICH guidelines. For the spectrophotometric determination of MBC a calibration curve was established over a wide range. The limit of detection, limit of quantification, linearity, specificity, precision and accuracy were determined directly on the tape matrix.

Table 27.1 Parameters and defined values for tape-stripping standardization.

Parameter	Defined value
Environmental conditions	20 ± 1°C (temperature) 38 ± 5% (rel. humidity)
Washing procedure of the skin	distilled water
Dose applied	2 mg/cm² with a saturated glove finger
Tape characteristics	Tesa 57315 Beiersdorf width of 1.9 cm
Template	1.3 cm × 3.3 cm
Pressure applied on tape strips	140 g/cm²
Time interval between tape-stripping and measurement	24 h

Results and conclusion

A statistically significant correlation was found between MBC concentrations determined by the spectrophotometric evaluation and by the HPLC assay ($r^2 > 0.9$) (Figure 27.2). Therefore, the spectrophotometric determination appears to be feasible as a stand-alone method for topical bioavailability determinations and should accelerate bioavailability and bioequivalence studies.

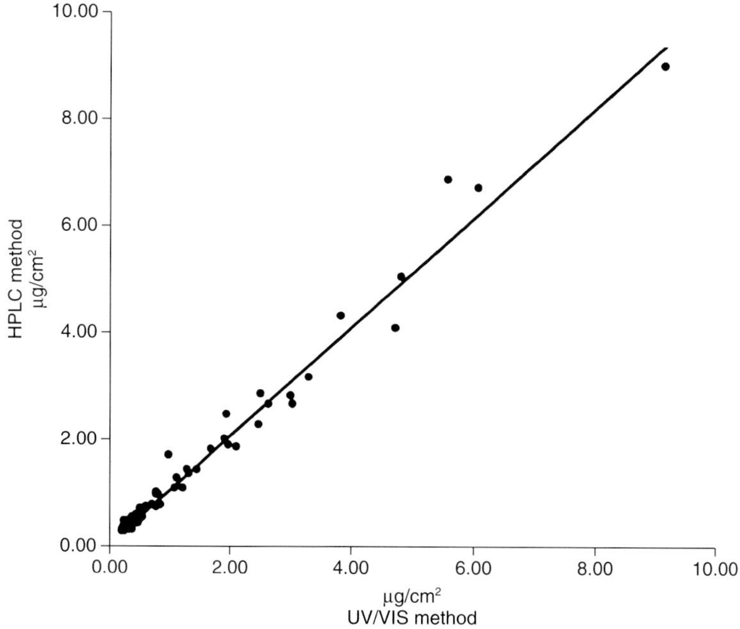

Figure 27.2

Correlation UV/VIS–HPLC, $y = 1.0178 + 0.0706$, $R^2 = 0.9804$

References

1. Treffel P, Gabard B. Skin penetration and sun protection factor of ultra-violet filters from two vehicles. Pharm Res 1996; 13:770–4.
2. Weigmann H-J, Lademann J, Meffert H et al. Determination of the horny layer profile by tape stripping in combination with optical spectroscopy in visible range as a prerequisite to quantify percutaneous absorption. Skin Pharmacol Appl Skin Physiol 1999; 12:34–5.

28

Penetration enhancement by interaction of the human stratum corneum with externally applied lipids and terpenes

J Lasch and S Zellmer

A number of studies suggest that topically applied lipids act as 'percutaneous permeation enhancers' which weaken the penetration barrier of the stratum corneum. In spite of clear-cut physical and histological evidence of the existence of a penetration barrier consisting of multilamellar intercellular lipid layers (MILLs),[1,2] the intercellular route of topically applied compounds predominates over other routes of percutaneous penetration.

We studied the effect of a number of various topically applied (external) lipids as well as mono- and sesquiterpenes (see Figure 28.1) which interact with the unique lipids of human skin and could thus disrupt their highly ordered structure by changing the fluidity and/or repeat distance and/or hydration of the MILLs. The enhancement of the penetration of 5-fluorouracil and oestradiol by monoterpenes was first reported by Williams and Barry in 1991.[3]

Fresh human skin mounted onto Franz-type diffusion cells and air-interfaced primary cultured keratinocyte layers, derived from foreskin biopsies, grown on permeable supports[4] (reconstructed human epidermis, RHE, Figure 28.2) were used as attractive models for the elucidation of skin penetration enhancement by terpenes. Caucasian breast skin (remnants after surgical intervention) was enzymatically dissected by putting the mamma skin pieces into a 0.1% solution of trypsin in phosphate buffered saline, pH 8.4. After 18 hrs of incubation at 37°C the stratum

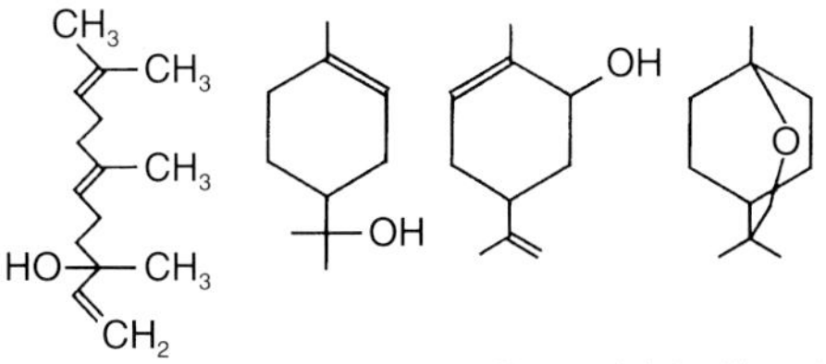

Nerolidol Terpineol Carveol 1,8- Cineol

Figure 28.1
Chemical structures of the terpenes studied.

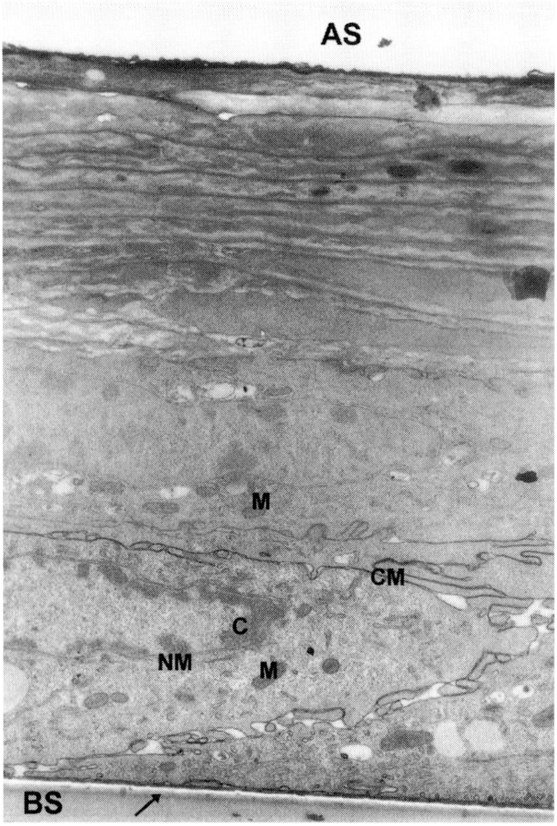

Figure 28.2
Electron microscopic image of air-interfaced supported 3-D reconstituted human epidermis- RHE (reproduced from J. Contr. Release 55 (1998), Zellmer S, Reissig D, Lasch J, Penetration enhancement by interaction of the human stratum corneum with externally applied lipids and terpenes, pp. 271–279, with permission from Elsevier Science). BS, basal support, AS apical site, M mitochondria, NM nuclear membrane, CM cellular membrane, C chromatin.

corneum completely detached from the living cells of the metabolically active strata. These stratum corneum sheets were mounted onto Franz-type diffusion cells.

For reasons of solubility terpenes were handled as terpene liposomes ('terpenosomes') produced by sonication of an appropriate mixture of the compounds. Depending on the type of terpene, up to 40 mol% could be incorporated into egg lecithin liposomes containing traces of rhodamine-phosphatidyl-choline (PC) (Avanti Polar Lipids, Inc, Alabaster, Alabama). The amounts of terpenes incorporated into liposomes were determined after separation of the phospholipids from terpenes by high performance thin layer chromatography (HPTLC), staining of terpenes with anisic aldehyde, scanning with the CAMAG scanner and integration of the peaks of light absorbance measured in the reflection mode. The areas of the peaks were calibrated by scanning runs with appropriate amounts of reference terpenes mixed with PC. The use of these 'terpenosomes' is important because most studies use ethanol [5] or propylene glycol[6] to dissolve terpenes.

Penetration of liposomes through skin models, as measured by the

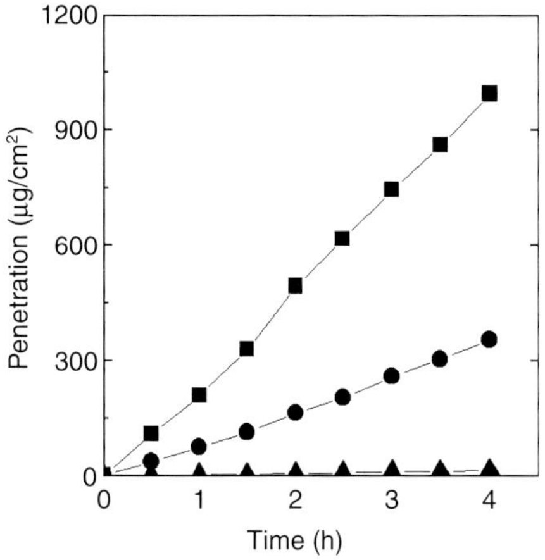

Figure 28.3

Time course of penetration of egg lecithin/carveol 'terpenosomes' through RHE measured by the increase of the hydophobic lipid marker rh-PE in the receiver compartment. ■ 30 mol% carveol, • 10 mol% carveol, ▲ 0 mol% carveol.

time course of appearance of the fluorescent marker rhodamine-phosphatidylethanolamine (PE) (rh-PE) at the receiver side, is a function of terpene density in the lipid vesicles. This is illustrated for carveol with the 3-D culture of reconstructed human skin in Figure 28.3. The penetration rates increase from 0 μg rh-PE/min·cm^2 at 0 mol% carveol to 40 μg rh-PE/min·cm^2 at 10 mol% carveol and 100 μg rh-PE/min·cm^2 at 30 mol% carveol.

Although no clear evidence of bilayer disruption by terpenes could be found by wide-angle diffraction experiments,[6] penetration enhancement by these compounds is found in the present and other [3] studies.

References

1. Madison KC, Schwarzendruber DC, Wertz PW, Downing DT. Presence of intact intercellular lipid lamellae in the upper layers of the strartum corneum. J Invest Dermatol 1987; 88:714–18.
2. Fartasch M, Bassukas JD, Diepgen TL. Structural relationship between epidermal lipid lamellae, lamellar bodies and desmosomes in human epidermis: an ultrastructural study. Br J Dermatol 1993; 128:1–9.
3. Williams AC, Barry BW. The enhancement index concept applied to terpene penetration enhancers for human skin and model lipophilic (oestradiol) and hydrophilic (5-fluorouracil) drugs. Int J Pharm 1991;74:157–68.
4. Zellmer S, Reissig D, Lasch J. Reconstructed human skin as model for liposome-skin interaction. J Contr Release 1998; 55:271–9.
5. Magnusson BM, Runn P, Koskinen L-OD. Terpene-enhanced transdermal permeation of water and ethanol in human epidermis. Acta Derm Venereol 1997; 77:264–7.
6. Cornwell PA, Barry BW, Stoddart CP, Bowstra JA. Wide-angle X-ray diffraction of human stratum corneum: effects of hydration and terpene enhancer treatment. J Pharm Pharmacol 1996; 46: 938 50.

29

Lateral drug diffusion in comparison with an artificial skin construct towards excised human stratum corneum

G Schicksnus and CC Müller-Goymann

Aims

Percutaneous penetration studies are usually performed using excised human or animal skin. The major drawback of this in vitro method is the diversity of skin quality between individuals and body regions, in addition to long running times of the experiments.

As could be shown in recent studies from our group, artificial skin constructs (ASC) may reduce both standard deviation and running time of the permeation studies.[1] The present contribution deals with lateral diffusion in ASC in order to check whether diffusion characteristics are comparable in ASC towards excised human stratum corneum (EHSC).

Methods

The commercial drug formulation Ibutop Creme® (Deutsche Chefaro Pharma GmbH, D-Waltrop) was used for lateral diffusion experiments of ibuprofen acid within EHSC and ASC, respectively. In order to achieve a constant application area (∅5 mm), adhesive reinforcement rings (Avery Dennison Zweckform, D-Holzkirchen) were stuck in the centre of a circular piece (∅24 mm) of either EHSC or ASC. Both systems were placed on a filter membrane on top of an isotonic phosphate buffer medium of pH 7.4. After a variety of different exposure times, the skin systems were frozen at −20°C. After removal of the formulation, the systems were punched in concentric rings (∅0–5, 5–10, 10–15, 15–20, 20–24 mm), which were extracted separately in methanol. The amount of ibuprofen acid in the separate segments was determined by high performance liquid chromatography (HPLC) analysis.

Results

Plotting ibuprofen concentration versus ring distance from the centre, both EHSC and ASC showed a similar graph of ibuprofen acid concentration in the ring segments (Figures 29.1 and 29.2). In the beginning, the concentration of ibuprofen acid in the centre segment (∅0–5 mm) in direct contact with the Ibutop Creme®, rises rapidly. The second ring segment (∅5–10 mm) also shows a quick increase with time, but the concentration of ibuprofen acid is always distinctly lower than in the central section. In the outer areas, only very small amounts of the drug can be found.

Later on, the concentration of drug in the skin area underneath the ointment reaches a maximum. From this time on, a redistribution of ibuprofen acid within the skin can be observed. This results in a decline of drug concentration in the centre section, while the outer ring segments still show an increase in drug concentration.

This process takes less time in ASC compared to EHSC, due to the lower barrier property of the stratum corneum of ASC.

Conclusion

Examining the lateral diffusion of ibuprofen acid in ASC and EHSC, a similar concentration development in both systems was found. Thus, the

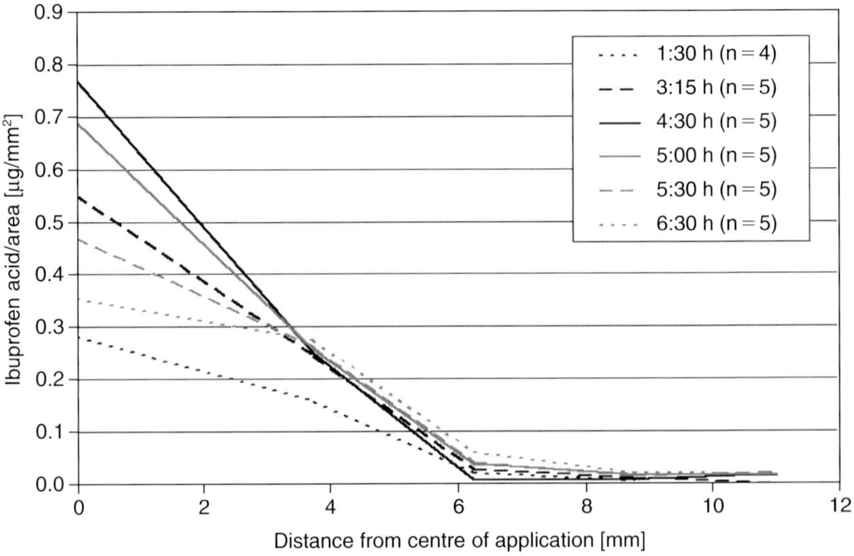

Figure 29.1
Lateral diffusion of ibuprofen acid in EHSC.

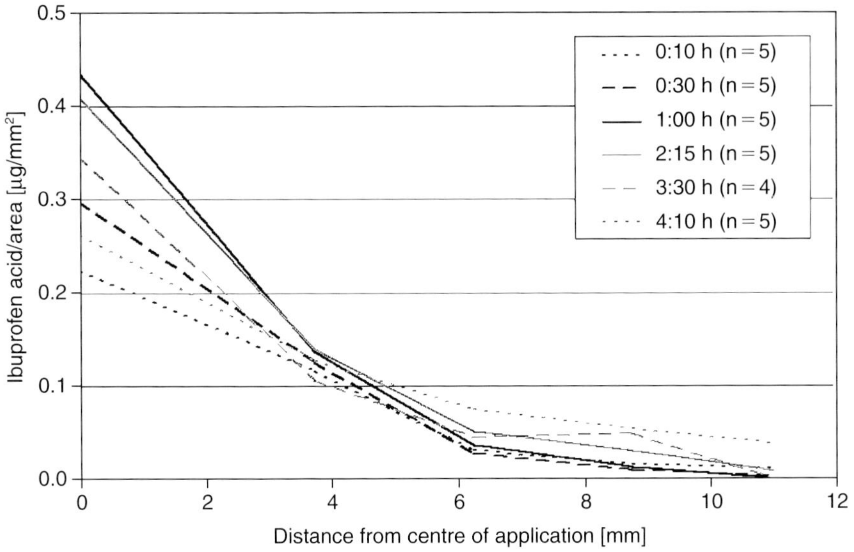

Figure 29.2

Lateral diffusion of ibuprofen acid in ASC.

characteristics in regard to lateral diffusion in ASC and EHSC are comparable. Since the barrier function of ASC is less distinct, a faster development of the diffusion process is explicable.

Reference

1. Wassermann K, Müller-Goymann CC. Arch Pharm Pharm Med. Chem 2000; 333:34.

30
Effect of menthol, a chiral permeation enhancer, on ibuprofen skin permeation

A Casiraghi, P Minghetti, F Cilurzo, L Tosi and L Montanari

Ibuprofen, a chiral phenylpropionic acid derivative, is a non-steroidal anti-inflammatory drug widely used in the treatment of musculoskeletal injuries. Even if the biological activity of ibuprofen resides with the S-enantiomer, the racemate is mostly available on the market. R-enantiomer is therapeutically inactive and, in vivo, there is enantiomeric inversion of R to S.[1]

The inadequate pharmacokinetics of ibuprofen post-oral administration[2] and the localized therapeutic target warrant use as a topical dosage form. In particular, patches are preferred, as they assure a precise dosage and a prolonged release. The success of the transdermal drug delivery system depends on the ability of the drug to penetrate the skin, and, therefore, permeation enhancers could be recommended. Among the chemical enhancers, terpenes such as menthol are used, as they induce low cutaneous irritancy and reversible alterations of skin barrier function.[3] Chirality of menthol may give rise to differences in skin permeation of ibuprofen. Other factors, such as differences in physicochemical properties between enantiomers and racemate of menthol,[4] may also be implicated in enantioselective skin permeation of ibuprofen.

The aim of this work was to evaluate the enhancement effect of menthol on the skin permeation of the ibuprofen enantiomers in solution and in acrylic and siliconic transdermal patches.

Ex vivo permeation profiles of ibuprofen throughout human stratum corneum and epidermis obtained from three different donors were determined for a period of 24 hours using modified Franz diffusion cells.[5] The permeability study was performed using EtOH:H_2O (50/50 v/v) solutions as donor phase. Control solution without menthol and solutions containing menthol, used as racemate and (+) and (–) enantiomers, were tested in order to evaluate the enhancement effect of menthol. Three different types of monolayer self-adhesive patches containing menthol and the corresponding control patches, to which no enhancer was added, were also tested. The matrices were prepared using a methacrylic acid copolymer (Eudragit L100, EuL), an acrylate-vinylacetate polymer (Durotak 387-2287, Dur) and an amine-compatible siliconic adhesive (Bio PSA 4302, Bio PSA). The molar ratio ibuprofen:menthol was fixed at 1:2 for both solutions and patches. The receptor phase was phosphate buffer saline solution.

Ibuprofen high performance liquid chromatography (HPLC) analysis was performed for both racemate and S-enantiomer.

The permeation profiles of ibuprofen in solution indicated that menthol enhanced the drug permeation. The permeated amount of S-enantiomer was over 50%, using both the control solution and the solution containing menthol. In Figure 30.1, the ibuprofen and S-enantiomer permeation profiles of a single donor are reported as an example. The permeation enhancement of ibuprofen by menthol did not seem stereospecific and, therefore, the patches were prepared by adding only the enhancer as racemate.

The ibuprofen permeation profiles obtained with methacrylic and acrylic patches were linear for 24 hours, while those obtained with the siliconic patches were linear only for the first 5 hours (Figure 30.2). The highest flux values of siliconic patches were probably due to a high diffusibility of the drug in these matrices. The skin permeation parameters of the patches containing menthol were not significantly different from those of the patches prepared without menthol.

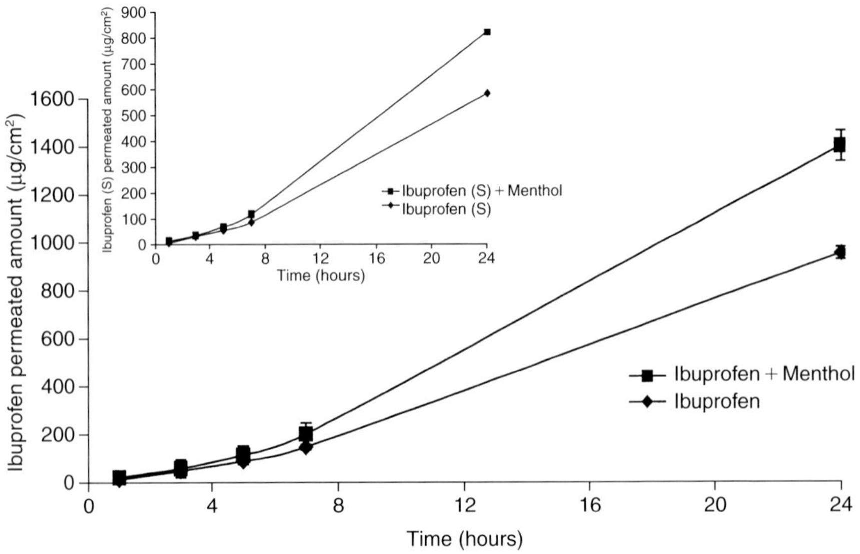

Figure 30.1

Ex vivo permeation profiles of ibuprofen in solution (n = 3; mean ± s.d.)

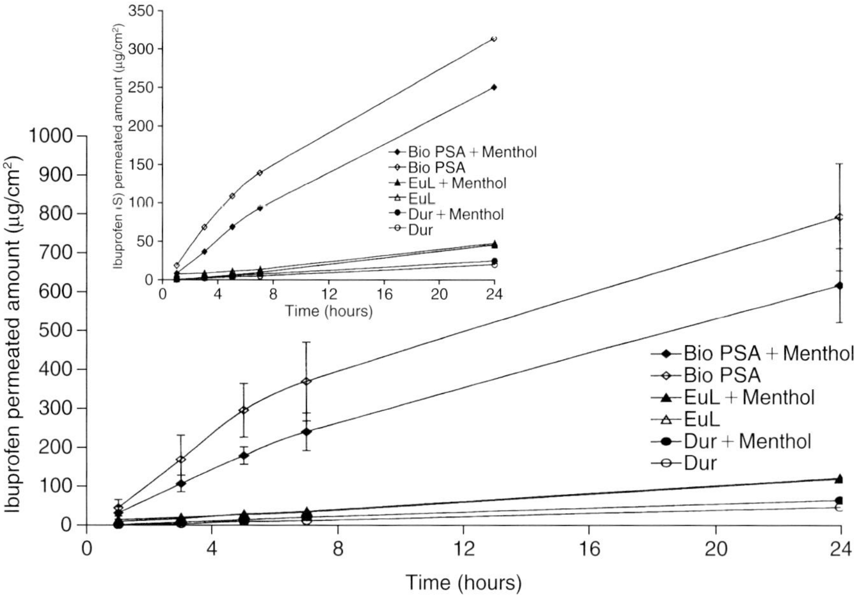

Figure 30.2

Ex vivo permeation profiles of ibuprofen patches (n = 3; mean ± s.d.)

References

1. Jamali F, Singh NN, Pasutto FM et al. Pharmacokinetics of ibuprofen enantiomers in humans following oral administration of tablets with different absorption rates. Pharm Res 1988; 5:40–3.
2. Verbeek RK, Blackburn BW, Loewen GR. Clinical pharmacokinetics of non-steroidal anti-inflammatory drugs. Clin Pharmacokinet 1983; 8:297–331.
3. El-Kattan AF, Asbill CS, Kim N et al. The effect of terpene enhancers on the percutaneous permeation of drugs with different lipophilicities. Int J Pharm 2001; 215:229–40.
4. MacKay KMB, Williams AC, Barry BW. Effect of melting point of chiral terpenes on human stratum corneum uptake. Int J Pharm 2001; 228:89–97.
5. Minghetti P, Casiraghi A, Cilurzo F et al. Comparison of different membranes with cultures of keratinocytes from man for percutaneous absorption of nitroglycerine. J Pharm Pharmacol 1999; 51: 673–8.

31

Influence of phloretin and 6-ketocholestanol on the penetration of 5-aminolevulinic acid through porcine skin

C Valenta, C Kuril and J Hadgraft

Introduction

5-Aminolevulinic acid (ALA) is topically applied in photodynamic therapy of selected percutaneous diseases, including skin cancer. The ALA molecule is hydrophilic and does not penetrate through intact skin in sufficiently high doses. Several attempts have been undertaken to increase the flux, e.g. iontophoresis[1] or addition of DMSO as penetration enhancer.[2] The simple molecule of ALA is, in principle, zwitterionic. With pK_a values of 4.0 and 7.4, it is clear that lowering the pH to 4 will change the ALA to a mainly cationic state. Recently it was shown that pre-treatment of skin with phloretin (PH)-loaded liposomes enhanced the flux of lignocaine hydrochloride (which has a cationic charge at physiological pH) through human epidermis.[3] PH and 6-ketocholestanol (KC) also had a positive effect on the skin permeation of progesterone.[4] The question was whether these two substances also have the potential to increase the ALA flux through porcine skin. The formulations used to incorporate PH or KC were unilamellar vesicles.

Methods

Preparation of unilamellar vesicles (ULVs)

PC (L-α-phosphatidyl-choline) vesicles with PH or KC (each 30 mol%) and controls were prepared using a method that has been previously reported.[4]

ALA diffusion

Permeation of ALA was investigated using Franz-type diffusion cells. The liposomes were applied to the upper, stratum corneum surface of the

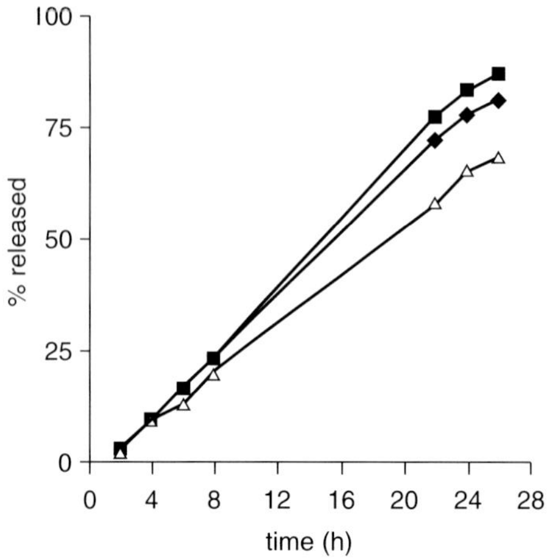

Figure 31.1

Diffusion profiles of ALA through porcine skin at pH 4.0. -■- pre-treated with KC–PC; -◆- pre-treated with PH–PC; -△- pretreated with PC-liposomes (control).

porcine skin. The various pre-treatments were: 150 µl PC-liposomes (control), 150 µl PH-loaded PC-liposomes (PH–PC); and KC loaded PC-liposomes (KC-PC). About 15 hours after application of the liposomes, 1 ml of ALA-buffer solution (ALA concentration: 1.88 mmol/l), adjusted to a defined pH, was applied to the skin surface. The samples from the permeation experiments were analysed for ALA by high performance liquid chromatography (HPLC), according to Oishi et al.[5]

Results and conclusion

At pH 5.0 donor solution, there was no effect of PH and KC on the ALA diffusion. However, at pH 4.0, KC, as well as PH, increased the permeation rates of ALA by a small amount. At pH 4.0, where ALA has a higher cation concentration, the flux was increased about 1.2-fold by PH and about 1.3-fold by KC after 24 hours (Figure 31.1). PH appears to enhance the flux of cations, and KC also had a small positive effect. It would be interesting to see if a more lipophilic counter ion, for example cetylpyridinium, can enhance the ALA flux to a higher extent.

Acknowledgements

This work was supported by Grant P15137 from the Fond zur Förderung Wissenschaftlicher Forschung (FWF) to C Valenta.

References

1. Lopez RFV, Bentley MVLB, Delgado-Charro MB et al. Iontophoretic delivery of 5-aminolevulinic acid (ALA): effect of pH. Pharm Res 2001; 18: 311–15.
2. Casas A, Fukuda H, Di Venosa G et al. The influence of the vehicle on the synthesis of porphyrins after topical application of 5-aminolevulinic acid. Br J Dermatol 2000; 143:564–72.
3. Valenta C, Cladera J, O'Shea P et al. Effect of phloretin on the percutaneous absorption of lignocaine across human skin. J Pharm Sci 2001; 90:485–92.
4. Valenta C, Nowak M, Hadgraft, J. Influence of phloretin and 6-ketocholestanol on the permeation of progesterone through porcine skin. Int J Pharm 2001; 217: 87–100.
5. Oishi H, Nomiyama H, Nomiyama K et al. Fluorimetric HPLC determination of 5-aminolevulinic acid. J Anal Toxicol 1996; 20:106–10.

32

Comparison of the barrier properties of artificial skin constructs and stratum corneum for 5-aminolevulinic acid and its n-butyl ester

A Winkler and CC Müller-Goymann

Aims

5-Aminolevulinic acid (ALA) serves as a pro-drug of protoporphyrin IX (Pp IX). The fluorescence of Pp IX induced by ALA is used for the treatment of skin diseases as well as of cancer of the lung, oesophagus, and bladder, respectively.

Recent investigations have shown an increase of Pp IX concentration in cultivated cells after application of ALA-n-butyl ester (ABE).[1] Franz diffusion cell experiments with stratum corneum (SC) demonstrated a tenfold higher permeability of ABE compared with ALA.[2]

The aim of the present study was to compare SC and artificial skin constructs (ASC) in terms of ALA and ABE diffusion properties. ASC could be an alternative to excised human skin, to minimize inter- and intra-individual variations in permeability between different donors, if Franz diffusion cell experiments with ASC provide a similar increase of permeated ABE towards permeated ALA.

Methods

ASC was cultivated according to Specht et al,[3] with a last-step modification according to Wassermann and Müller-Goymann.[4] A dermis equivalent, containing human dermal fibroblasts, was covered with an epidermis equivalent, using keratinocytes.

The in vitro permeation studies were performed with a modified Franz cell. The donor was Excipial® Fettcreme enriched with ALA (10% (w/w)) or ABE (10% (w/w)) prior to the permeation studies, and the receiver was a phosphate buffer of pH 5.0 (Ph. Helv. 8) to guarantee stability of ALA and ABE.

The permeated amounts of both substances were analysed by high-performance liquid chromatography with fluorometric detection after pre-column derivatization with o-phthalaldehyde.[5]

Results

Permeation profiles of both substances are represented in Figure 32.1. The ascent of the curve became linear after a rapid increase of permeated amounts within the first 3 hours. The permeation coefficient (P) was calculated as the quotient of the linear ascent of the curve as flux and concentration. The permeation coefficient of ABE (4.26×10^{-7} cm/s $\pm 4.19 \times 10^{-8}$) was about 22-fold higher than that of ALA (1.91×10^{-8} cm/s $\pm 1.71 \times 10^{-9}$).

Figure 32.2 shows a comparison for both drugs between permeation data for SC and ASC. Different physicochemical properties of ALA and ABE and differences in structure of SC and ASC could be the reason for these different permeation factors. Permeation studies across ASC were accomplished within one third of the time necessary for SC. Standard deviations were reduced from about 25%, for the diffusion experiments with SC, to 9% for those with ASC.

Conclusion

By using ABE instead of ALA, an increase in percutaneous penetration could be proven with both ASC and SC. Despite its generally higher per-

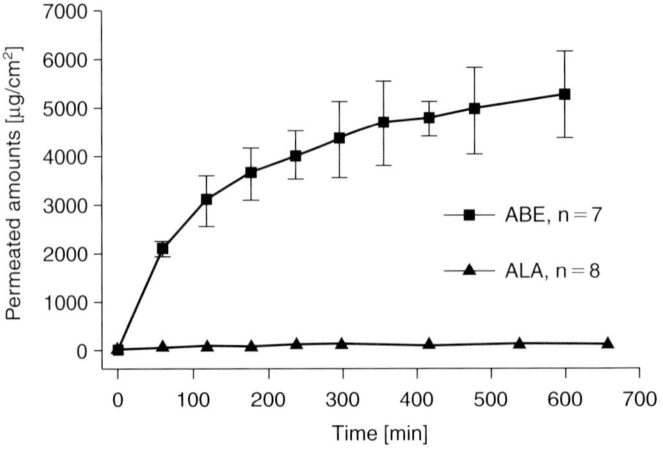

Figure 32.1

Comparison of the permeation profiles of ALA and ABE through ASC.

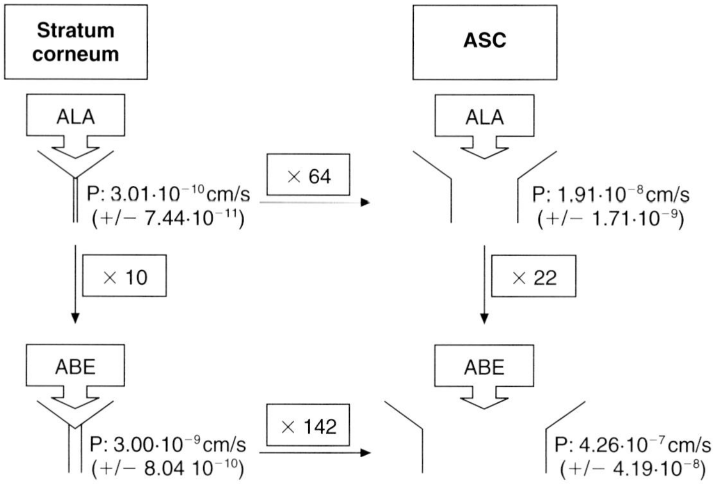

Figure 32.2

Comparison of the permeation properties of ALA and ABE through stratum corneum and ASC, respectively; the respective diameters of the funnels represent differences in permeability (P = permeation coefficient), data for stratum corneum according to Winkler and Müller-Goymann.[2]

meability, ASC is an alternative to excised human SC to reduce running time of permeation studies as well as standard deviation. Differences in drug permeation may be determined even more easily and with higher sensitivity in preclinical screening studies.

References

1. Kloek J, Akkermans W, Beijersbergen van Henegouwen GMJ. Derivatives of 5-aminolevulinic acid for photodynamic therapy: enzymatic conversion into protoporphyrin. Photochem Photobiol 1998; 67: 150–4.
2. Winkler A, Müller-Goymann CC. Comparison of the diffusion properties of d-aminolevulinic acid and its n-butyl ester through human stratum corneum. Arch Pharm Pharm Med Chem 2000; 333:67.
3. Specht C, Stoye I, Müller-Goymann CC. Comparative investigations to evaluate the use of organotypic cultures of transformed and native dermal and epidermal cells for permeation studies. Eur J Pharm Biopharm 1998; 46:273–8.
4. Wassermann K, Müller-Goymann CC. Standardized cultivation of artificial skin constructs for drug permeation studies. Arch Pharm Pharm Med Chem 2000; 333:34.
5. Ho J, Guthrie R. Quantitative determination of porphyrins, their precursors and zinc protoporphyrin in whole blood and dried blood by high-performance liquid chromatography with fluorimetric detection. J Chromat 1987; 417:269–76.

33

Application of hyperosmolar glucose on injured skin: skin bioengineering evaluation during epidermal barrier repair process

SJ Kim, E Jerschow, SJ Yun, JY Kim and YH Won

Introduction

Stratum corneum (SC) and viable epidermis are connected to the local vascular network through the passive diffusion of interstitial fluid which constitutes about 15% of the total epidermal volume,[1] and plays a critical role in keratinocyte metabolism. Previous studies indicated that some ions in the interstitial fluid, particularly potassium and calcium, were actively involved in regulating epidermal barrier functions.[2–4]

The water content of the upper epidermis is modulated by experimental epidermal barrier perturbation reflecting increased transepidermal water loss (TEWL). However, the role of local osmotic gradient applied on the upper epidermal layer after barrier perturbation is unclear. The present study aimed to evaluate the effect of osmotic gradient in the epidermal barrier recovery process by applying hyperosmolar glucose over tape-stripped skin. The distribution of glucose on the upper epidermis was also assessed using a protein assay from stripped-tape discs.

Materials and methods

Nineteen young, healthy volunteers, aged 18–28 years (11 men and eight women), who were free of skin disease on both forearms, participated in the epidermal perturbation experiment. Among them, 10 volunteers were involved in the glucose assay. Treatment sites on the volar forearms of volunteers were assigned in a randomized way. D-glucose (Sigma, St Louis, MO, USA) was prepared as a hyperosmolar solution in deionized water, adjusted to 0.1 mol/l and 1 mol/l.

Results

The concentration of extracted glucose from the tape discs was dependent on the depth of layer – highest in the uppermost then rapidly decreased in the lower portion (Figure 33.1). Adjusted levels of glucose by soluble protein fractions also manifested a similar gradient.

All skin bioengineering data reflected the gradual recovery pattern of the epidermal barrier. Although the trend of barrier recovery for each treatment was similar, the earlier data, measured at day 1, manifested a significant change in the hyperosmolar glucose treatment than in the deionized water treatment or control (Figures 32.2–33.4).

Discussion

Hyperosmolar glucose seems to accelerate barrier recovery, but the mechanism of action was rather difficult to define from this experiment. While carbohydrate compounds (lactose, etc.) are sometimes used as humectants in various cosmetic formulations, the role of the osmotic condition as an effective humectant is unclear. Potassium and calcium are key ions that regulate epidermal barrier repair, and water movement across epidermal layers may also affect the distribution of ions.[3] If the hyperosmolarity affects the passive movement of ions, epidermal barrier recovery under osmotic influence can be speculated as shown here. The hyperosmolar condition of 1 mol/l of glucose is 100 times more concentrated than the capillary glucose level, which is expected to cause a rapid fluid shift. Although our results suggest the osmotic influence on

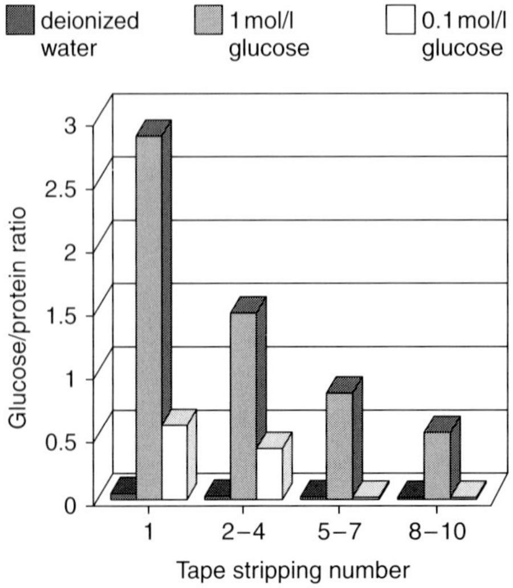

Figure 33.1
Penetration gradient of glucose in the stratum corneum.

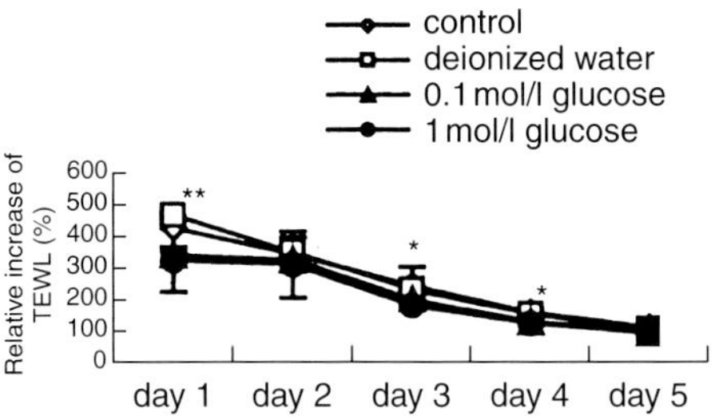

Figure 33.2

The level of TEWL values during the barrier recovery course following 24 hour patch application. Significant differences were observed between deionized water and 1 mol/l glucose at day 1, day 3 and day 4. (* $p<0.05$, ** $p<0.005$).

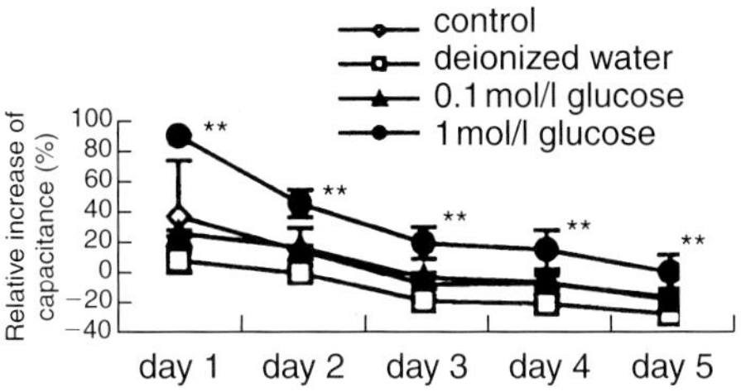

Figure 33.3

The level of capacitance values during the barrier recovery course following 24 hour patch application. Significant differences were observed between treatment groups: control or deionized water vs. 1 mol/l glucose from day 1 to day 5. (** $p<0.005$).

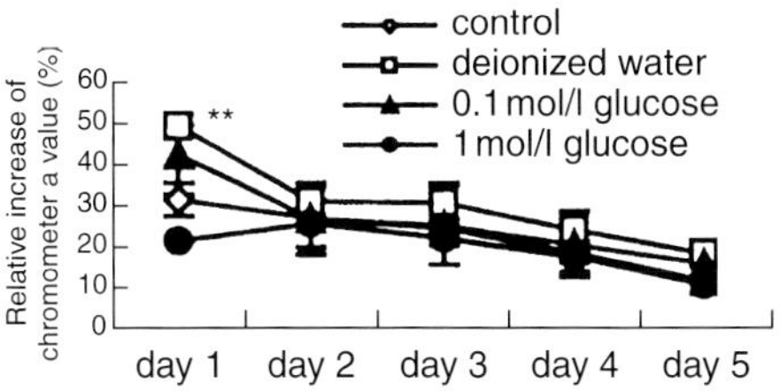

Figure 33.4

The level of colorimetric values during the barrier recovery course following 24 hour patch application. Significant differences were observed between treatment groups: deionized water or 0.1 mol/l glucose vs. 1 mol/l glucose at day 1. (** $p<0.005$).

barrier homeostasis, further study is necessary to define the role of hyperosmolarity.

References

1. Halprin K, Ohkawara A, Adachi K. Glucose entry into the human epidermis. I. The concentration of glucose in the human epidermis. J Invest Dermatol 1967; 49:315–19.
2. Ahn SK, Hwang SM, Jiang SJ et al. The changes of epidermal calcium gradient and transitional cells after prolonged occlusion following tape stripping in the murine epidermis. J Invest Dermatol 1999; 113:189–95.
3. Lee SH, Elias PM, Proksch E et al. Calcium and potassium are important regulators of barrier homeostasis in murine epidermis. J Clin Invest 1992; 89:530–8.
4. Lee SH, Elias PM, Feingold KR et al. A role for ions in barrier recovery after acute perturbation. J Invest Dermatol 1994; 102:976–9.

34

Comparison of commercial hydrocortisone formulations with regard to their permeation behaviour through excised stratum corneum

I Brinkmann and CC Müller-Goymann

Aims

Dermatologists often prescribe hydrocortisone creams and ointments for the treatment of skin eczema. A variety of formulations, with different hydrocortisone concentrations, and formulation types are obtainable on the pharmaceutical market. However, there is a lack of available data on the permeability of these different formulations through the skin. The aim of this study was to compare different commercially available hydrocortisone formulations with regard to hydrocortisone permeation rates. In addition, the influence of one of these products on stratum corneum (SC) structure was investigated.

Materials and methods

For permeation studies, three hydrocortisone ointments and six creams were tested. The hydrocortisone concentrations ranged from 0.1% to 1.0%. All products were suspension-type formulations, which was demonstrated microscopically. For permeation experiments, a modified Franz diffusion cell was used, whereby the excised human SC was integrated between the hydrocortisone formulation, as the donor compartment, and the receiver, consisting of phosphate buffer pH 7.4. For higher mechanical stability, the SC was placed on a polycarbonate filter, of pore width 5.0 μm. The amount of hydrocortisone in the receiver phase was analysed by high-performance liquid chromatography at 2-hour intervals. In order to investigate the influence of the formulations on the lipid matrix of the SC, differential scanning calorimetry (DSC) was used, at temperatures ranging from –20 to 140°C, with a heating rate of 5°C/min.

Results

All formulations showed similar drug permeation behaviour, regardless of formulation type or hydrocortisone concentration, whereby the permeation curves were typical for formulations with a suspended drug. The permeation coefficients, as well as the fluxes, were in the same range (Table 34.1).

A possible influence of a formulation on the lipid matrix of SC can be registered by DSC, but the data of one of the hydrocortisone formulations (further ones are in progress) show no significant shifts in the transitions of SC (Figure 34.1). This is in accordance with results from Refai and Müller-Goymann,[1] who also demonstrated no significant influence of hydrocortisone within German Pharmacopoeia formulations[2] either on SC DSC transitions or hydrocortisone fluxes and permeability coefficients

Table 34.1 Permeation data of different commercial hydrocortisone formulations.

	Flux J $(g/cm^2.s).\ 10^{-12}$	Permeability-coefficient P (cm/s). 10^{-9}
Dermallerg-ratiopharm 1.0%	30.93 +/− 6.42	2.29 +/− 0.48
Hydrocutan Salbe mild 0.1%	32.25 +/− 8.34	3.38 +/− 0.87
Hydrocutan Salbe 1.0%	34.53 +/− 5.25	3.62 +/− 0.55

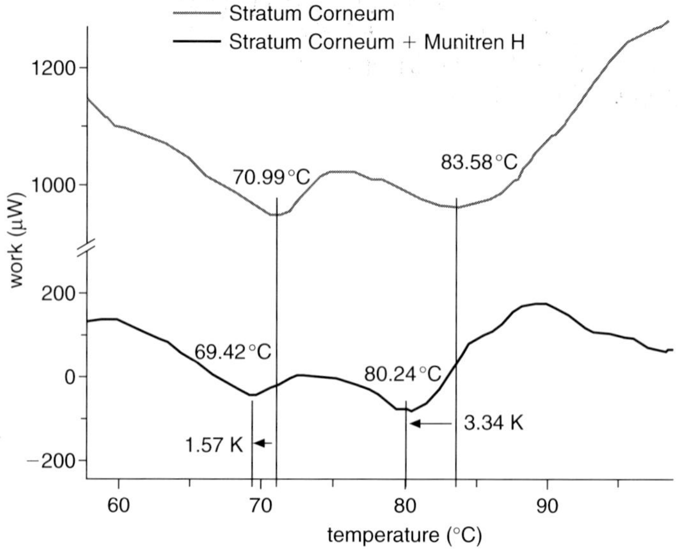

Figure 34.1
DSC thermogram for human SC after pre-treatment with Munitren® H fettarm.

through excised human SC. However, the absolute permeability coefficients of the present and recent studies differ. This can be explained by the inter-individual variation of lipid composition in SC. To prove this, the comparison of one of the commercial formulations and one cream base of water containing hydrophilic ointment[2] was made. In fact, there was no significant difference in permeation between these two formulations.

Conclusion

Permeation of formulations with suspended hydrocortisone is independent of formulation type and concentration. Indeed, the individual composition of the lipid matrix in SC can influence drug permeation. The limiting factor is not the delivery of the drug from the formulation, but the SC permeability itself.

References

1. Refai H, Müller-Goymann CC. Arch Pharm Med Chem 1999; 332.2:37.
2. Deutsches Arzneibuch 1998: Monographien, Deutscher Apotheker Verlag & Govi Verlag: Stuttgart/Frankfurt, 1997.

35
Localization of titanium dioxide microparticles in the horny layer

S Gottbrath and CC Müller-Goymann

Introduction

The present contribution deals with percutaneous penetration of titanium dioxide microparticles as ultraviolet filters in sunscreen formulations. A method developed by Weigmann et al, which combines spectroscopic measurements and tape-stripping to localize microparticles in stratum corneum, was slightly modified. To determine the amount of titanium dioxide on every strip, atomic absorption spectrometry (AAS) was performed. Furthermore, ultraviolet spectroscopy (UVS) was used to find a correlation with AAS.[1]

Methods

Tape-stripping

A concentration of 2 mg/cm^2, according to the COLIPA standard, of Eucerin® Micropigment Creme (Beiersdorf; Hamburg, Germany) was applied on the ventral side of the forearm. After 45 minutes, the formulation was removed. Ten tape-strips (Scotch Transparent tape, 3M; Neuss, Germany) were taken from the pre-treated area and analysed by UVS and AAS.

AAS

Dissolution of titanium dioxide from the strips was performed in sulphuric acid together with ammonium sulphate at boiling temperature. The samples were injected into the graphite oven of an atomic absorption spectrometer (Perkin Elmer 2380; Überlingen, Germany).[2]

Transmission electron microscopy (TEM)

The sample was frozen at –210°C and fractured (Balzers GmbH BAF 400; Wiesbaden, Germany) at –100°C and 5×10^{-6} bar. The fractured surface was shadowed with platinum/carbon and with pure carbon to stabilize the replica. Sulphuric acid was used for cleaning. Replicas were viewed by TEM (Philips EM-300; Kassel, Germany).

UV/VIS spectroscopy (UVS)

Prior to AAS, UVS of every strip was performed with a double-beam spectrometer (Shimadzu UV 210 A; Kyoto, Japan). The maximum absorption at 253 nm was taken as the characteristic absorption.

Results

TEM of Eucerin® Micropigment Creme (Figure 35.1) shows the distribution of titanium dioxide microparticles within the formulation.

The absorptions of every single strip taken from the untreated area were summarized to calculate a percentage of corneocyte aggregates removed.

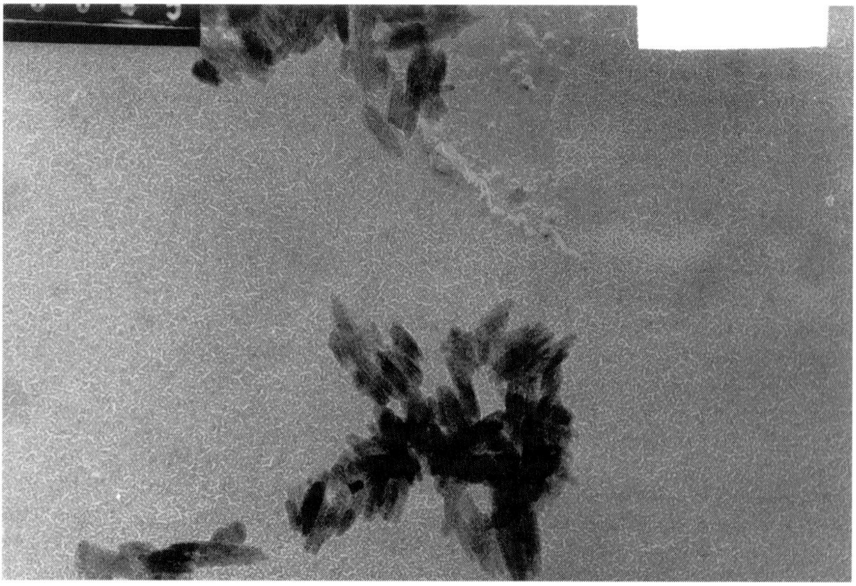

Figure 35.1

TEM micrograph of Eucerin® Micropigment Creme (magnification 140 000×, bar = 229 nm).

Plotting the results (AAS of the strips versus the number of strips) shows an exponential decline. At strip 7, the titanium concentration approaches its lowest value of 0.15 μg/cm^2. The shapes of the curves obtained from UVS are similar to those from AAS. Plotting the UVS results of the specific strips versus the AAS results of the same strips exhibits a linear relationship, of which the correlation coefficient is $R^2 = 0.98$.

Conclusion

According to the results of the spectroscopical measurements, there is a linear relationship between the titanium concentration and the UV/VIS absorption of the strips.

The results of the UV/VIS absorption from the untreated skin area lead to a more precise location of the titanium microparticles. This is because the penetration of the substance is correlated with the number of corneocyte aggregates removed with every single strip, and not with the number of strips, and so the individual differences of the horny layer thickness are eliminated.

References

1. Weigmann H-J, Lademann J, Meffert H et al. Determination of the horny layer profile by tape stripping in combination with optical spectroscopy. Skin Pharmacol 1999; 12:34–45.
2. Müller-Goymann CC, Bennat C. Penetration von partikulären UV-Filtern in die Haut. Parfümerie und Kosmetik 1998; 5:24–6.

Section III
Bioengineering techniques

36

Understanding and measuring the optics that drive visual perception of skin appearance

PJ Matts

Our eyes respond to a narrow bandwidth of the electromagnetic spectrum – visible light, a nominal 400–700 nm. The interaction of these wavelengths with skin, therefore, is of primary importance in our understanding of the way we perceive and are perceived.

Assuming that the stratum corneum has an approximate refractive index of 1.5, Fresnel's Law predicts that incident light at normal to the surface will always have a regular reflectance of between 4% and 8%. In other words, 92–96% of normally incident light will, theoretically, enter the skin surface. Once within the skin medium, two main factors now need to be considered – absorption and scattering. In the visible spectrum, the stratum corneum of an untanned skin behaves much like a neutral density filter, displaying little spectral dependence. The dense concentration of keratinous material at the surface, however, is responsible for a marked absorption of short-wave UV (driven primarily by absorption by peptide bonds (< 240 nm), tyrosine and tryptophan (λ_{max} 275 nm) and urocanic acid (λ_{max} 277 nm)).

In the remainder of the epidermis, the melanins (eumelanin and phaeomelanin) are essentially the only chromophores moderating transmittance of ultraviolet (UV) and visible light. These melanins strongly and selectively absorb UV and shorter wavelength visible light, due to the extensive, conjugated, double bonds within their polymer structures.

In the dermis, the blood-borne pigments haemoglobin and oxyhaemoglobin are the major absorbers of visible light. These strongly-absorbing pigments are highly localized within the vasculature in the dermal matrix. Seen from above, haem-rich capillary bundles appear as discreet dots of pigment, creating a unique optical effect, quite different from that achieved by a homogeneous distribution. This pigment is also unique in that it can influence skin colour dynamically over a few seconds, depending upon the filling and draining of cutaneous vasculature, in response to emotional or environmental influence.

Scattering results from inhomogeneities within the transmitting medium as a consequence of refractive index differences. The shape, size and refractive index of these inhomogeneities drive the extent and intensity of the resulting scatter. For particles or molecules less than one-tenth of the wavelength of incident radiation, scattering is weak, isotropic and inversely proportional to wavelength. When, however, the inhomogeneity is much larger than the wavelength of the incident radiation, scattering is highly forward-directed, with no dependence on wavelength.

Within the epidermis, therefore, the overall effect of the various sub-structures is that of forward-scatter (Table 36.1). The dermis has a profound effect on cutaneous optics and requires special mention. It is a dense, optically-turbid medium, comprising collagen as its major constituent (some 70% of its dry weight). Importantly, collagen exhibits bi-refringence, i.e. the ability to separate unpolarized incident light into two separate, orthogonally-polarized rays. Photons encountering the dermis, therefore, experience intense multiple-scattering; back-scattering is the dominant effect, the dermis reflecting the bulk of light reaching it.

The fate of light impinging upon the skin surface can now be traced. Normally-incident light hits the skin surface. Less than 10% is remitted, the bulk passing into the skin, where it experiences diffusion by the heterogeneous surface and then strong forward-scattering in the stratum corneum and absorption of short-wave UV. In the epidermis, UV and short-wave visible light are absorbed by melanin granules, which also promote forward-scatter. The modified light enters the dermis, where it experiences intense multiple-scattering and absorption by haemoglobin and other blood-borne chromophores. The bulk is back-scattered from

Table 36.1 Light scattering within the skin

Stratum corneum
- Corneocyte gross structure (multiple μm scale) – forward scatter
- Corneocyte internal ultrastructure (angstrom scale) – isotropic scatter
- **Overall, stratum corneum promotes strong forward scattering**

Epidermis
- Melanin particles > 300 nm (melanosomes) – forward scatter
- Melanin dust < 30 nm – isotropic scatter
- Basal, prickle, granular cell gross structure – forward scatter
- Sub-cellular organelles in viable cells – isotropic scatter
- **Overall, epidermis promotes forward scattering**

Dermis
- Collagen fibres in papillary dermis (3 μm) – some forward scatter
- Collagen fibres in reticular dermis (10–40 μm) – forward scatter
- Birefringence and layer thickness promote intense back-scatter
- **Overall, dermis promotes intense back-scattering**

the dermis, experiences a second forward-scatter and absorption in the epidermis and stratum corneum, and is remitted from the skin surface. The integration of reflection and backward scatter from all cutaneous layers reaches our trichromatic retinas, combining the red, green and blue registrations, to form a perceived red-yellow hue within our visual cortex.

To some extent, skin appearance may be modelled and predicted, if certain assumptions are made. For example, if one has reliable data for the optical properties of skin chromophores (spectral absorption, scattering coefficients, molar concentration and viewing path-length), assumes that the system is isotropic in nature, and that remittance from interfaces is ignored, one may use the radiation-transfer equations derived by Kubelka and Munk in 1931. In this type of modelling, it becomes rapidly apparent that three skin components essentially drive the quality of the remittance spectrum of skin – absorption by melanins and haemoglobins, and back-scattering by the dermis.

Any model uses assumptions and application of the Kubelka–Munk equation to skin is no exception. The equation assumes an isotropic system. Recent work, however, has indicated an apparent directional dependence in the propagation of visible light through skin in vivo. Using spatially-resolved, steady-state diffuse reflectometry, Nickell et al found anisotropy in the skin's reduced scattering coefficient across multiple body sites. The orientation of these effects was found to closely match 'Langer's Lines', corresponding to directionality in collagen fibre bundles parallel to the skin surface. It is probable that this subtle directional effect contributes to our perception of skin appearance.

Secondly, most models and, indeed, most methods that are used to measure the remitted light from the skin surface, assume or use sources and detectors at a normal angle. This, however, bears no resemblance to reality. Take the frontal aspect of a human face. Even if we assume a single point source of light, less than 5% of that radiation is normal to the surfaces presented. Firstly, this affects regular reflectance. Using Fresnel's Law again to calculate the amount of light remitted from the skin surface as a function of angle of incidence, it is seen that above incident angles of 45°, there is a dramatic increase in surface reflectance. Secondly, incident angle varies proportionally with path length within the skin, with corresponding changes in relative spectral absorption. Analysis of remittance spectra derived from multiple-angle spectrophotometry, therefore, demonstrates a surprising range of hue and saturation for the same area of skin. Depending on the angle, we may observe any one or any combination of these, which may change in a fraction of a second.

Furthermore, deriving colour measurements does not mean that we can reconstruct a realistic human face. One can take a mannequin head, insert glass eyes, dress it with a wig of real human hair, and then painstakingly apply a map of skin colour derived by remittance spectroscopy. It will still, however, look flat and lifeless. A wax-work, though, can look surprisingly real; in contrast to the solid colour of a mannequin, it is made of layers of coloured translucent wax. In the same way, the chromophores in our skin are not omnipresent, they are located *beneath* an essentially colourless, translucent rind. This natural translucency is derived from the heterogeneity of refractive index within the skin.

Surface texture can also moderate our perception of skin appearance. To separate the internal optics of skin from its surface, we took precise, large replicas of cheek skin taken from female subjects aged 20–70 years. These were recast as positives in optically-opaque silicone rubber, which were then mounted into a goniophotometer (a multiple-angle of incidence/detection photometer). Using white light, the instrument was set to measure angular reflection over a range comprising specular ±45°. Multiple measures across the surface were used to calculate a simple derivative, angular distribution at half maximal reflectance. For this method, the greater the diffuse component of surface reflection, the greater the half-maximal angular distribution. Four replicas (imaged approx. 50×) illustrate the trend of the broad data (Figure 36.1). Replicas A and B were taken from the cheeks of two 25-year-olds; as expected, the surface architecture is in good condition, with an abundance of char-

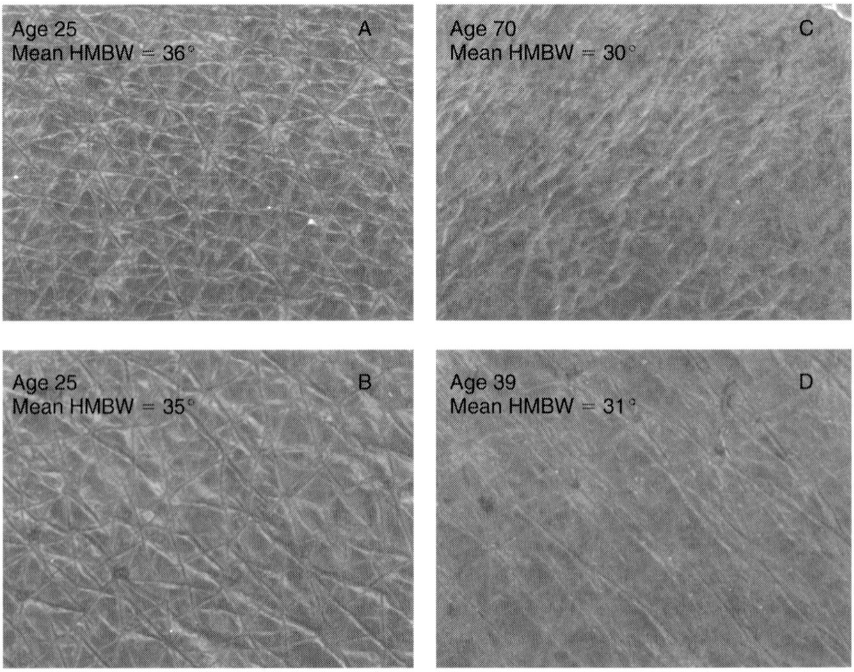

Figure 36.1

Measurement of diffuse reflection from opaque cheek skin replicas (HMBW = half maximal bandwidth).

acteristic fine anisotropic lines and furrows, which we may call 'microtexture'. Replicas C and D were taken from 39- and 70-year-old subjects, respectively. In contrast to A and B, each of these shows a marked absence of the previous fine microtexture, consistent with intrinsic and extrinsic ageing. Importantly, A and B both have higher values of angular distribution than C and D. We have noted consistently that the amount of diffuse reflection detected appears to vary proportionally with abundance of microtexture and not necessarily with age. Intuitively, one would expect 'texture' to increase the diffuse component of surface reflection. It does, but texture must be defined carefully. Somewhat contra-intuitively, there is a lot more texture in young, undamaged skin than in older or photo-damaged skin – it is just on a much smaller scale.

As we age, there is a relentless metamorphosis of texture quality (Figure 36.2). One can define these changes in terms of amplitude and frequency. Young skin contains an abundance of low-amplitude, high-frequency, topographical features. As skin ages, feature amplitude increases and frequency decreases. To the touch, the frequency of features in young skin is so high that they are below the threshold of resolution for human touch – it feels smooth and soft. With age, as feature

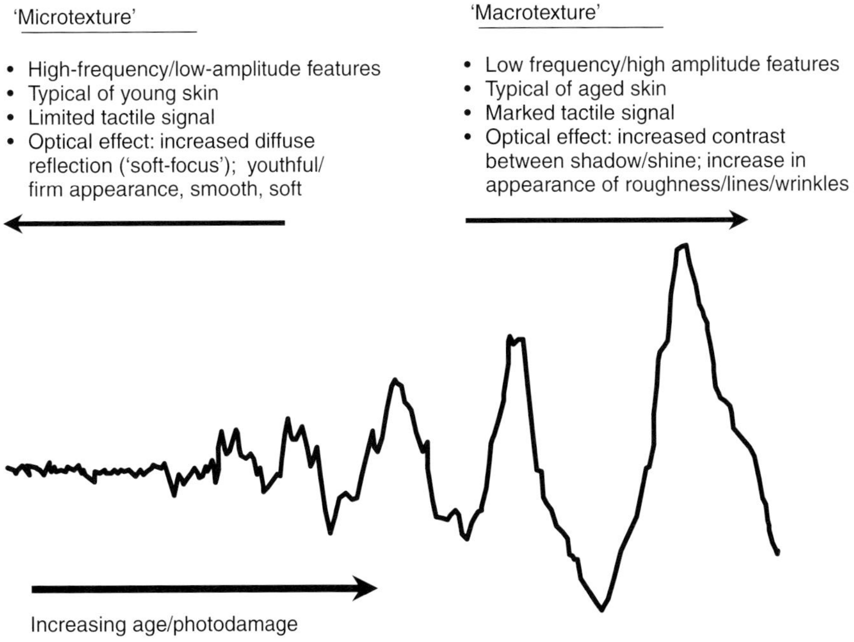

'Microtexture'
• High-frequency/low-amplitude features
• Typical of young skin
• Limited tactile signal
• Optical effect: increased diffuse reflection ('soft-focus'); youthful/ firm appearance, smooth, soft
'Macrotexture'
• Low frequency/high amplitude features
• Typical of aged skin
• Marked tactile signal
• Optical effect: increased contrast between shadow/shine; increase in appearance of roughness/lines/wrinkles
Increasing age/photodamage

Figure 36.2
Texture amplitude and frequency as a function of age and photodamage.

frequency decreases and amplitude increases, we can resolve these features and we perceive roughness. The eye also measures these two components but in a slightly different way. The human eye is a superb contrast meter; in optimal conditions, the human eye can detect contrasts as low as 2%. In Image Analysis terms, our eyes are superlative in identifying *edges*. A skin surface with high-frequency, low-amplitude features promotes diffuse reflectance, or a 'soft-focus' effect, because of the sheer number of reflecting structures per unit area. We tend to perceive the surface as smooth and even. As frequency decreases and amplitude increases, diffuse reflection is increasingly replaced by delineated areas of specular reflection, or edges, which our eyes detect with lightning precision and which our visual cortex interprets as lines, wrinkles and roughness.

The author believes that it is this abundance of microtexture in young skin that is one of the drivers of perception of youth and beauty. Observe the two faces in Figure 36.3 – a woman in her sixties and a girl in her teens. Note how one looks unconsciously for edges and areas of contrast to make one's judgement of age and beauty. Our eyes are drawn not only to edges of light and dark, denoting lines and wrinkles, but also to

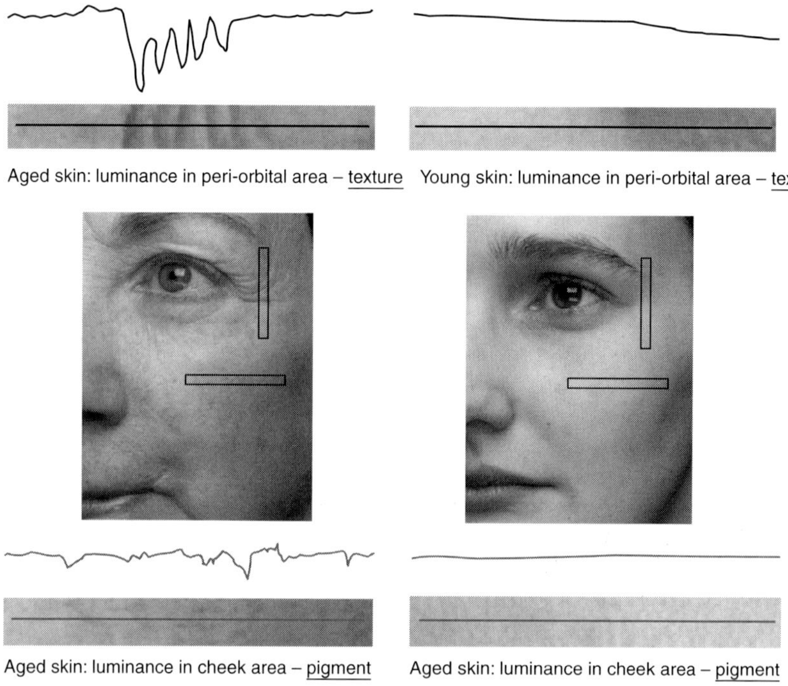

Aged skin: luminance in peri-orbital area – texture
Young skin: luminance in peri-orbital area – texture
Aged skin: luminance in cheek area – pigment
Aged skin: luminance in cheek area – pigment

Figure 36.3

Facial texture and pigment each display changes in frequency and amplitude with age and photodamage.

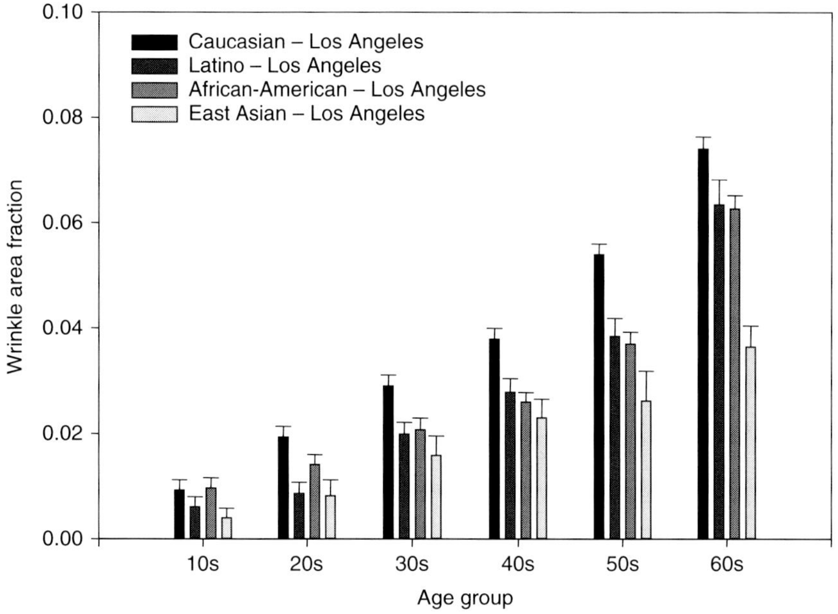

(a) Expression of facial wrinkling by race and age group, Los Angeles subjects

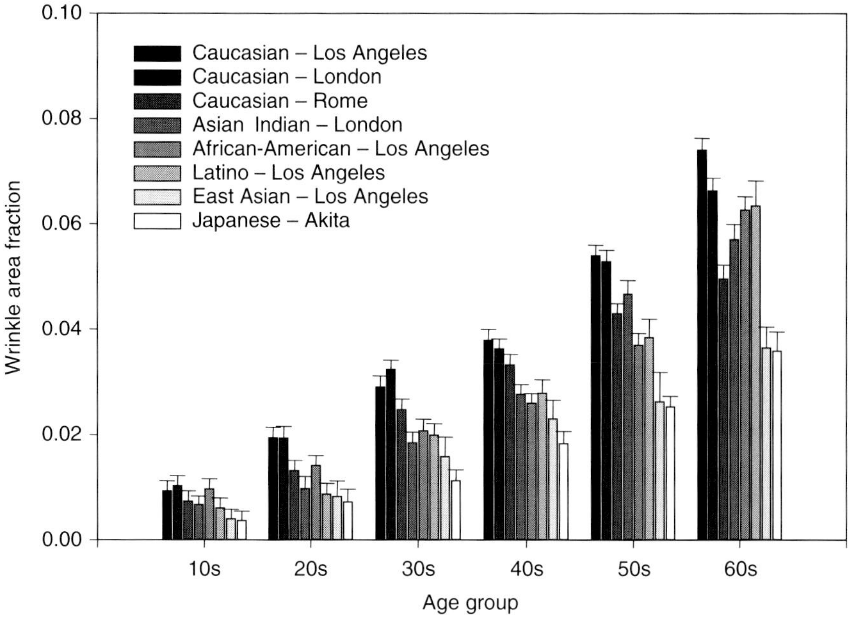

(b) Expression of facial wrinkling by race and age group, all geographies

Figure 36.4

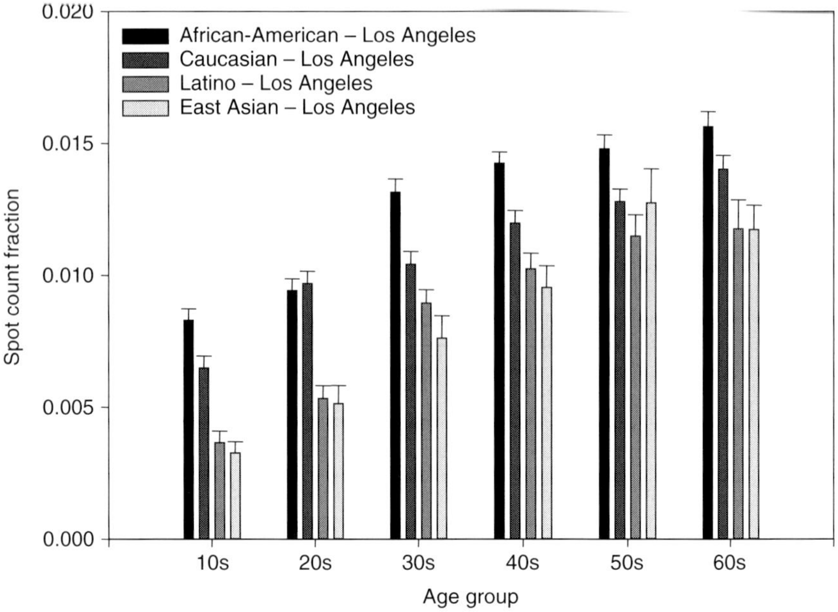

(c) Expression of hyperpigmented spots by race and age group, Los Angeles subjects

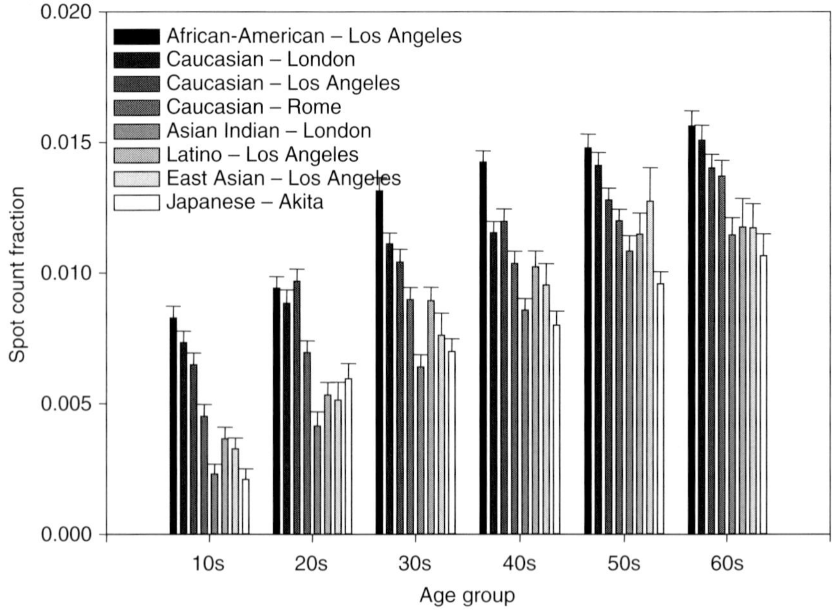

(d) Expression of hyperpigmented spots by race and age group, all geographies

Figure 36.4
Continued

edges between pigmented areas, whether telangiectasia, or hyper-pigmented spots. If regions of interest are selected in both images, and luminance of a mid-line is plotted, a very similar result is obtained for both texture *and* pigment – the frequency/amplitude model appears to hold true for both of these features.

We have led a project to attempt to image and map the visual features of ageing skin. The effort is unique in its inclusion of five different racial groups (i.e. African-American, East Asian, Caucasian, Asian-Indian and Latino), its large base size (some 3160 subjects) and its wide age range (10–70 years). We developed and patented a compact, portable digital imaging system with integrated illumination to obtain facial images. Using this system, we obtained facial images from female subjects aged 10–70 years from five different ethnic groups. Images were then presented to naive judges, who were asked to grade each image for severity of pre-selected markers of skin ageing, including 'lines/wrinkles' and 'hyper-pigmented spots'. Using the significant age/grade relationships observed, a set of image analysis algorithms was developed in-house to evaluate the prominence of the chosen skin markers, which were used to detect features in the images previously graded by naive judges.

In the Los Angeles data (Figure 36.4a), one can see a clear, positive age dependence for wrinkle detection, most prominent in Caucasians and least prominent in East Asians. Considering all ethnic groups and geographies, the trend is confirmed – all Caucasian groups have the most prominent expression of wrinkling, and East Asian groups, the least. African-American and Latino groups lie between the Caucasian and East Asian groups (Figure 36.4b). If one considers hyperpigmentation, in Los Angeles, somewhat surprisingly, African-Americans display the most prominent expression of pigmentation with age, closely followed by Caucasians (Figure 36.4c). In all ethic groupings, the trend is confirmed, with African-Americans and Caucasians from all geographies displaying the most prominent pigment expression by age and, once again, East Asian and Japanese skins, the least (Figure 36.4d). These data offer invaluable insight into the extent and time-tabling of expression visual endpoints that drive perception of age and beauty within ethnic groupings. We have recently adapted the system to also measure hands.

Overall, therefore, an understanding of the physical and biochemical nature of skin optics and the means to measure it allows fundamental insight into the way we consciously and unconsciously perceive our fellow human beings.

Further reading

Anderson RR, Parrish JA. Optical properties of human skin. In: *The Science of Photomedicine.* Plenum Press 1982; 147–94.

Dawson JB, Barker DJ, Ellis DJ et al. A theoretical and experimental study of light absorption and scattering by in vivo skin. Phys Med Biol 1980; 25:695–709.

Hillebrand GG, Levine MJ, Miyamoto K. The age-dependent changes in skin condition in African Americans, Asian Indians, Caucasians, East Asians and Latinos. IFSCC Magazine 2002; in press.

Kollias N, Al Baqer BS. Spectroscopic characteristics of human melanin in vivo. J Invest Dermatol 1985; 85:38–42.

Matts PJ, Hourihan N, Solechnick ND et al. Visual characteristics of ageing hand skin in Northern Europe. Poster presented at American Academy of Dermatology Annual Meeting, Washington, March 2001.

Matts PJ, Solechnick ND. Predicting visual perception of human skin surface texture using multiple-angle reflectance spectroscopy. Poster presented at American Academy of Dermatology Annual Meeting, Washington, March 2001.

Nickell S, Hermann M, Essenpreist M et al. Anisotropy of light propagation in human skin. Phys Med Biol 2000; 45:2873–86.

Young AR. Chromophores in human skin. Phys Med Biol 1997. 42: 789–802.

37

Electrical impedance. A method to evaluate the ability of betaine to reduce the skin-irritating effects of detergents

I Nicander, I Rantanen, E Söderling and S Ollmar

Introduction

We use a non-invasive multifrequency impedance spectrometer (IMP) to measure reactions in the skin. The technique enables measurements of both magnitude and phase at 31 frequencies between 1 kHz and 1 MHz at five depth settings. From the impedance spectra, a set of four indices (MIX = magnitude index, PIX = phase index, RIX = real part index, and IMIX = imaginary part index)[1] has been devised, emphasizing different aspects of the impedance properties of the tissues. These have been found to be valuable for objective analysis in the invisible or barely-visible range[2] and also for discriminating between different types of skin reactions.[1]

Detergents, for example, those widely used in personal-care products and cosmetics, produce a number of side effects of which irritant contact dermatitis is the most common. Therefore, attempts have been made to find both detergents with lower irritating properties as well as products decreasing this side effect. A novel approach is offered by betaine (trimethylglycine), which has recently been found to reduce the skin-irritating properties of ingredients of cosmetics[3] and to have skin-moisturizing effects.[4] For studying the positive ability of betaine to reduce irritation, two detergents were used: sodium lauryl sulphate (SLS) and cocoamino-propylbetaine (CAPB). The latter is considered to be less irritating than SLS.

Methods

Twenty-one healthy test persons with no history of skin diseases or allergy were recruited. The study was performed during one winter month, to eliminate seasonal variation.[5] Seven test sites on both mid-volar forearms were used, and were randomly assigned to the test substances and the controls. The test sites comprised: 4% betaine, 1% SLS, 1% SLS + 4% betaine, 4% CAPB, 4% CAPB + 4% betaine, distilled water and an unoccluded site. The test substances were applied in 12-mm Finn chambers for 24 hours. Distilled water and an unoccluded site were used as controls. For evaluation of the skin reactions, two non-invasive techniques were used.

Readings were taken before application (day 1) of the patches and 24 hours after the removal (day 3) in the following order: transepidermal water loss (TEWL) and IMP. Measurements with IMP must be performed last, as the skin has to be soaked with physiological saline solution before the measurement.

For the statistical analysis, Student's paired t-test and ANOVA were used.

Results and discussion

The TEWL showed a significant increase between day 1 and day 3 for the detergents alone as well as together with betaine, and this increase was more pronounced for SLS. Compared with SLS alone, the reaction decreased significantly after adding betaine. CAPB with betaine had a similar, but not statistically significant, tendency.

The mean values and standard deviations were calculated for the four impedance indices (MIX, PIX, RIX, and IMIX) at all five depth settings at all test sites. Figure 37.1 shows that the reaction pattern differed between the two detergents used. SLS showed a significant decrease for MIX, RIX and IMIX and a significant increase for PIX for both depth settings 1 and 5; CAPB, for depth settings 1 and 5, induced a statistically significant decrease for MIX and IMIX, and for depth setting 5, also a significant increase for RIX.

IMP	Depth 1				Depth 5			
	MIX	PIX	RIX	IMIX	MIX	PIX	RIX	IMIX
SLS	↓	↑	↓	↓	↓	↑	↓	↓
CAPB	↓			↓	↓		↑	↓

Figure 37.1

Statistically significant differences before and after exposure for the detergents SLS and CAPB at depth settings 1 and 5. Arrows indicate the direction of the responses.

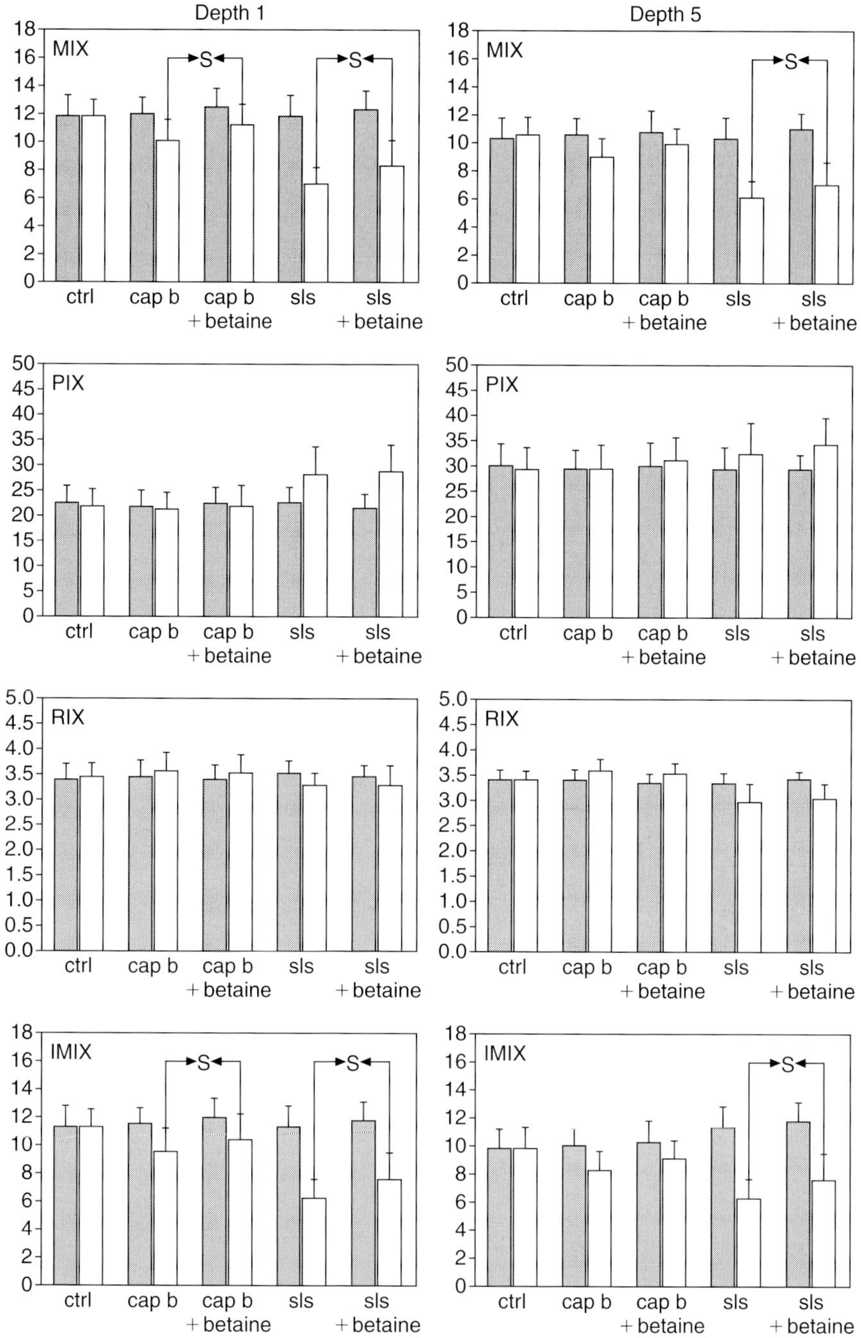

Figure 37.2

Mean values and standard deviations for depth settings 1 and 5 before and after application of SLS and CAPB with and without betaine as reflected in the four impedance indices MIX, PIX, RIX, and IMIX. Filled bars = day 1; empty bars = day 3. S = statistically significant differences.

Furthermore, betaine produced a third impedance pattern group for depth 1, giving a significant increase for IMIX, and a significant reduced response for RIX. For depth setting 5, both MIX and IMIX increased significantly. No significant changes were found for the controls.

The variation in tissue responses reflects the substances' different chemical properties, e.g. how they will attack the skin barrier and interact with the intercellular lipids in different ways. From an earlier study,[1] biopsies were taken from SLS-exposed skin and the most dominant feature was an epidermal oedema. Unpublished data show that biopsies from CAPB-exposed skin differ from those of SLS.

After the addition of betaine, similar changes were found for both SLS and CAPB, with one exception: CAPB showed a significant increase for RIX for both depths 1 and 5.

Compared with the detergents alone, SLS showed a significantly reduced reaction for the indices MIX and IMIX for depth settings 1 and 5 together with betaine, and with CAPB for the same indices but just for depth 1 (Figure 37.2). One reason for the positive effect of betaine might be the fact that this substance acts as a methyl donor, which, to a certain degree, will protect the cells from the attacks of surfactants.

Conclusion

Betaine is a promising ingredient to reduce the side effects of detergents and electrical impedance is a suitable tool to quantify the degree of irritation and also to differentiate various types of reactions.

References

1. Nicander I, Ollmar S, Eek A et al. Correlation of impedance response patterns to histological findings in irritant skin reactions induced by various surfactants. Br J Dermatol 1996; 134:221–8.
2. Nicander I, Ollmar S. Mild and below threshold skin responses to sodium lauryl sulphate assessed by depth controlled electrical impedance. Skin Res Technol 1997; 3:259–63.
3. Jutila K. A method of reducing the irritating properties of a cosmetic composition. EPO Patent 0531387 1996.
4. Söderling E, Bell AL, Kirstilä V et al. Betaine-containing toothpaste relieves subjective symptoms of dry mouth. Acta Odontol Scand 1998; 56:65–9.
5. Nicander I, Ollmar S. Electrical impedance measurements at different skin sites related to seasonal variations. Skin Res Technol 2000; 6:81–6.

38
Electrical capacitance measurement of the stratum corneum hydration: comparison with the dermopharmacokinetics of the active moiety

E Chatelain and B Gabard

Introduction

Urea is an important component of the skin 'natural moisturizing factor' (NMF) and contributes in a significant manner to the hydration of the stratum corneum (SC). It is widely used in dermatology as a humectant in a great number of formulations to treat so-called 'dry skin' conditions or aged skin.[1–4] Patients suffering from diseases such as atopic dermatitis, psoriasis or ichtyosis show a reduced SC urea concentration.[5–8]

Although urea is often reported to influence the skin penetration characteristics of different compounds,[9–11] little data is available on its own skin penetration properties after application of skin-care products. However, penetration characteristics of humectants are important for their moisturizing effects, determined by, for example, measuring the electrical capacitance of the horny layer with the Corneometer or the NOVA DPM.[12,13] The aim of our study was to compare the results of hydration measurements with those of urea SC dermopharmacokinetics, obtained by successive stripping in vivo after topical application of different urea-containing lotions.

Methods

An oil-in-water (O/W) and a water-in-oil lotion (W/O) containing 2% and 4% urea, respectively, (Spirig Pharma Ltd, Egerkingen, Switzerland) were used. Hydration measurements (NOVA DPM) were conducted in a climatized room on the forearms of six volunteers, starting 5 minutes after a 1-hour application of the two moisturizers. Besides hydration (H), the water accumulation capacity (WA) of the SC was assessed by means of the Moisture Accumulation Test (MAT).[12,13]

Release of urea from the lotions was evaluated in vitro using the infinite dose technique and Franz diffusion cells with phosphate-buffered saline as receptor fluid.

The dermopharmacokinetics of urea were investigated using successive stripping of the SC at different time points after product application (reservoir-filling kinetics) and product removal (elimination kinetics). The urea content of the strips was determined with a commercially available enzymatic kit (Roche, Basel, Switzerland). Briefly, the applied product was wiped off at the end of the application time and the skin then stripped 16 times with D-Squames. The content of the first strip was added to urea found on the skin surface, strips 2–8 and 9–16 were pooled and analysed separately. Urea was extracted from the strips using chloroform/water 1:1. The water phase was used for the enzymatic assay.

Results

Urea release in vitro strongly depended on the formulation. An almost linear release was found from the O/W lotion, reaching 25% of the applied dose after 6 hours, but a very slow release was shown for the W/O system (3% of the applied dose after 6 hours), despite higher urea content (Figure 38.1).

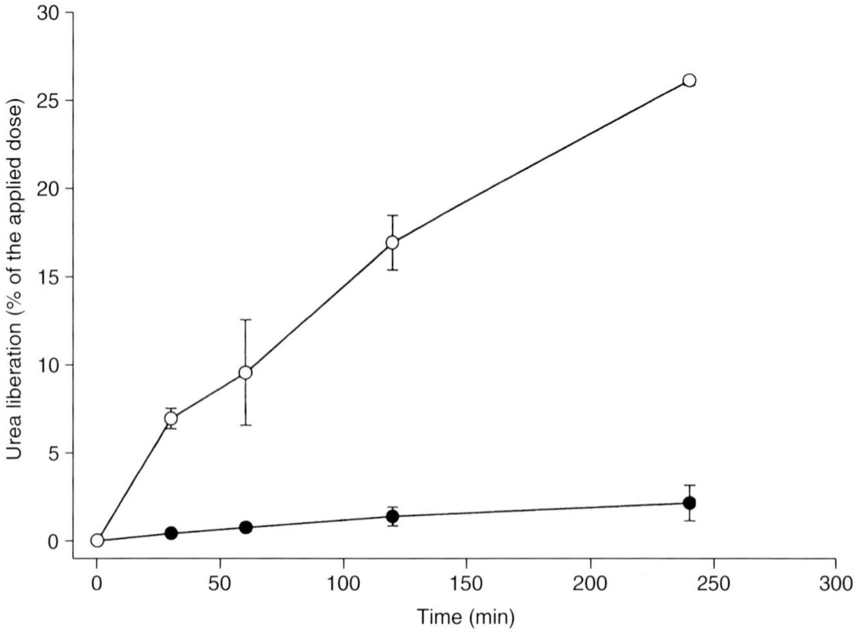

Figure 38.1

In vitro urea release from two different formulations. (•) Water-in-oil lotion containing 4% urea; (o) Oil-in-water lotion containing 2% urea. Results are expressed in % of the applied dose.

In vivo, an average of 150 nmol urea/cm^2 was measured in the SC of untreated control subjects but large interindividual variability was observed. Considering skin penetration kinetics, urea was rapidly taken up by the SC. High concentrations were measured as soon as 5 minutes after application of the formulations. More urea was measured in the strips with the W/O lotion than with the O/W lotion (Figure 38.2), but the percentage of applied dose remained the same for both formulations. SC penetration kinetics may be defined as a rapid uptake from the O/W lotion, with a plateau attained as soon as 5 minutes after application and no changes thereafter. With the W/O lotion, uptake was also rapid and increased steadily until 30 minutes, when a plateau was attained (corresponding to 30% of the applied dose). Differences in the distribution of urea from the two products were measured in the upper layers of the SC – strips 2–8 – but not in the lower layers – strips 9–16 (data not shown).

To investigate the elimination kinetics from the SC, the products were applied for as long as was necessary, to be in the plateau phase (15 minutes for the O/W formulation and 30 minutes for the W/O formulation). Product remnants were then removed and concentrations of urea were measured at different times thereafter. A small increase of the SC urea content was observed during the first 2 hours after product removal. Subsequently, almost linear elimination kinetics were noticed, and urea control values were reached 24 h later (Figure 38.3).

The in vivo SC electrical capacitance measurements are shown, together with the summary of both urea uptake and elimination phases (Figure 38.4). A greater increase in electrical capacitance was measured after application of the W/O lotion compared to the O/W lotion, thus matching found concentration differences. At a first glance, the increase in measured hydration values appears modest compared with the measured increase in urea concentration. Similarly, the differences between hydration values from both formulations also did not really reflect the measured differences in urea concentrations. The WA of the SC was almost maximal as soon as 5 minutes after product removal, but no differences were measured between formulations (data not shown).

Discussion and conclusion

For the first time, SC-dermopharmacokinetics of urea were investigated in vivo and were compared with measurements of SC hydration after application of two different formulations. Penetration results correlate well with published data. Wellner and Wohlrab were the first to investigate the SC penetration of urea after topical application of different formulations using ^{14}C-labelled urea and an in vitro human skin model.[8] They showed that urea penetrated the horny layer rapidly and in high amounts, and also

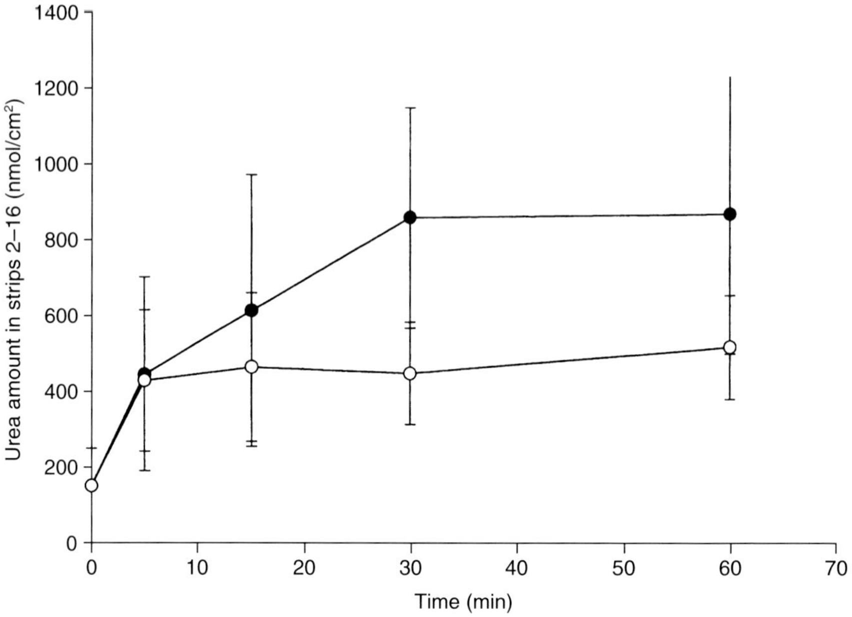

Figure 38.2

Stratum corneum uptake of urea: reservoir-filling kinetic. (•) Water-in-oil lotion containing 4% urea; (o) Oil-in-water lotion containing 2% urea. Results are expressed in nmol urea/cm^2.

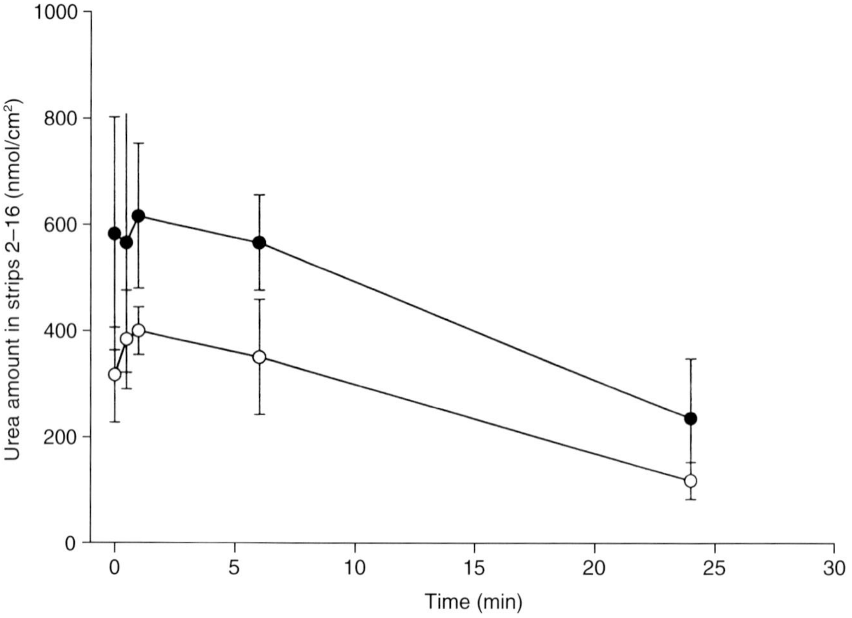

Figure 38.3

Stratum corneum urea content after product removal: elimination kinetic. (•) Water-in-oil lotion containing 4% urea; (o) Oil-in-water lotion containing 2% urea. Results are expressed in nmol urea/cm^2.

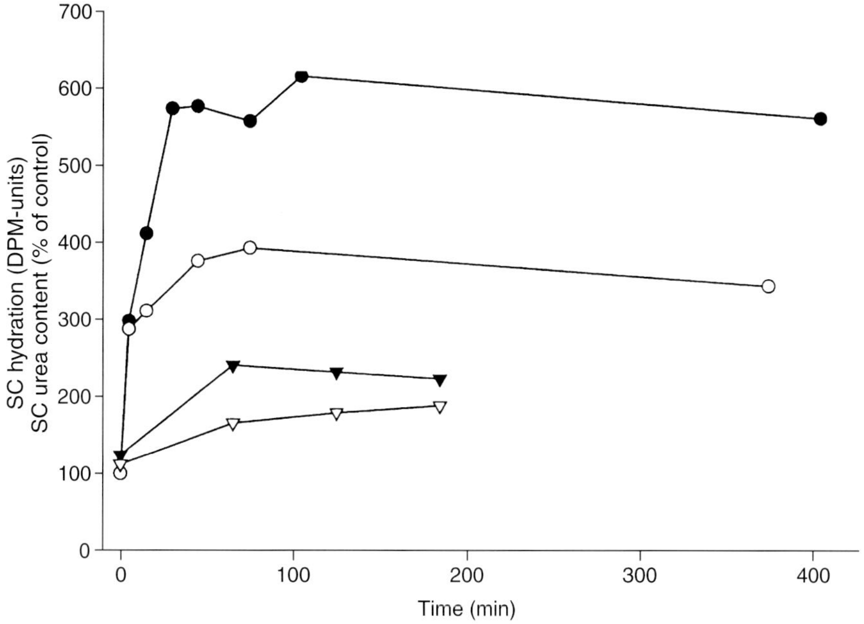

Figure 38.4

In vivo stratum corneum hydration compared with urea uptake and elimination phases following the application of urea-containing lotions. For hydration measurements, the products were removed after 1 hour of application and electrical capacitance measured 5, 60 and 120 minutes thereafter; results are expressed in DPM-units: (▼)Water-in-oil lotion containing 4% urea; (▽) Oil-in-water lotion containing 2% urea. The stratum corneum urea content is expressed as % of untreated control (corresponding to an average of 150 nmol urea/cm^2); (•) Water-in-oil lotion containing 4% urea; (o) Oil-in-water lotion containing 2% urea.

found differences in the amount penetrated, depending on the formulation. Using ^{3}H-labelled water, they showed that the vehicle-dependent rapid uptake of urea directly influenced the water-binding capacity, an effect lasting longer if W/O emulsions were applied compared to O/W formulations.

More recently, Häntschel et al,[14] using a similar enzymatic method, measured urea in the SC of healthy volunteers in vivo. They reported normal values between 3 and 300 nmol urea/cm^2, in good agreement with those that we found (52–274 nmol urea/cm^2). Treatment of skin with water or cleansing products dramatically decreased the extractable urea. On the other hand, they achieved a considerable supply of urea to the SC by treating the skin with a cream containing 5% urea. This increase in extractable urea was accompanied by an increase in electrical capacitance values measured with the Corneometer.

We in turn showed that the SC avidly took up urea. Differences were noticed between O/W and W/O formulations concerning uptake pharmacokinetics. Urea SC penetration in vivo was quicker from the O/W lotion than from the W/O, possibly reflecting different release kinetics from the vehicles. These results in vivo confirm Wellner and Wohlrab's results obtained in vitro.[8] On the other hand, elimination kinetics were almost similar with both formulations. The slight increase in concentration noticed 2 hours after wiping off the products is also apparent if one calculates the percentages of applied dose. This could be due to urea redistribution within the SC (back diffusion of urea from the deeper SC layers towards the surface layers caused by a loss of occlusion after product removal).

Electrical capacitance measurements pointed out differences between the formulations, but these were considered as not reflecting measured SC urea concentration differences. Electrical capacitance may be suitable to reflect the effect of a humectant such as urea on SC hydration and to point out differences between galenical systems (O/W or W/O), but the limits of these measurements are rapidly attained when one faces changes in the distribution of the humectant within the SC, such as back diffusion from the lower toward the upper layers.

Moreover, determination of WA was not useful in our experiments, as apparently, the accumulation of water during the MAT was maximally influenced by urea after rapid penetration into the SC, whereas no differences between the two galenical systems were detected. Thus, one must be very careful in interpreting results from such experiments, as the measurement of SC hydration using electrical capacitance is far from being validated.

Acknowledgments

We thank Ms C Kissling and C Schluep for their excellent technical assistance during this study.

References

1. Müller KH, Pflugshaupt C. Harnstoff in der Dermatologie III. Z Hautkr 1999; 74:732–41.
2. Wohlrab W. The influence of urea in different emulsions on the water-binding capacity of the human horny layer. Z Hautkr 1990; 66:390–5.
3. Schölermann A, Banké-Bochita J, Bohnsack K et al. Efficacy and safety of Eucerin 10% Urea Lotion in the treatment of symptoms of aged skin. J Derm Treat 1998; 9: 175–9.
4. Swanbeck G. Urea in the treatment of dry skin. Acta Derm Venereol 1992; 177:7–8.
5. Küster W, Bohnsack K, Rippke F et al. Efficacy of urea therapy in children with ichtyosis. Dermatol-

ogy 1998; 196:217–22.

6. Wellner K, Fiedler G, Wohlrab W. Investigations in urea content of the horny layer in atopic dermatitis. Z Hautkr 1992; 67:648–50.
7. Wellner K, Fiedler G, Wohlrab W. Investigations in urea content of the horny layer in psoriasis vulgaris. Z Hautkr 1993; 68:102–4.
8. Wellner K, Wohlrab W. Quantitative evaluation of urea in stratum corneum of human skin. Arch Dermatol 1993; 285:239–40.
9. Beastall J, Guy RH, Hadgraft J et al. The influence of urea on percutaneous absorption. Pharm Res 1986; 3:294–7.
10. Wohlrab W, Taube KM, Kuchenbecker I. Penetration and efficiency of vehicles containing low concentrations of hydrocortisone. Z Hautkr 1990; 65:534–7.
11. Wohlrab W. The influence of urea on the penetration kinetics of vitamin-A-acid into human skin. Z Hautkr 1990; 65:803–5.
12. Gabard B. Testing the efficacy of moisturizers. In: Elsner P, Berardesca E, Maibach HI, eds. *Bioengineering of the Skin: Water and the Stratum Corneum.* Boca Raton, USA: CRC Press 1994: 195–201.
13. Treffel P, Gabard B. Stratum corneum dynamic function measurements after moisturizer or irritant application. Arch Dermatol Res 1995; 287:474–9.
14. Häntschel D, Sauermann G, Steinhart H et al. Urea analysis of extracts from stratum corneum and the role of urea-supplemented cosmetics. J Cosmet Sci 1998; 49:155–63.

39
FOITS – corneometry influenced by peripheral experimental conditions

M Rohr and A Schrader

Introduction

Besides a good compatibility, which should be a matter of course for cosmetic products, the skin's physiological effectiveness, in particular moisture and skin-smoothing effects, are of main interest for this kind of product. Techniques such as FOITS (Fast Optical In vivo Topometry of human Skin)[1,2] and corneometry are used to investigate their effectiveness. In order to succeed in reproducible and statistically significant results, experimental side conditions, such as a defined panel, controlled climatic conditions or a test design that includes a positive and a negative standard, are the basic starting tools. As shown before, the outdoor climate is of great influence on any skin physiological investigation.[3] During the summer, it is much more difficult to obtain a very good moisturizing effect, especially if the test design does not include a positive standard product. Keeping these facts in mind, the influence of the indoor climate in the laboratory will be the main focus of this paper. What will happen to the level of skin moisture during the pre-conditioning phase? Will it be influenced by the level of relative room humidity? Will the influence vary for different kinds of products? Will the influence on skin moisture and skin structure be comparable? Will the influence change for different types of volunteers? What is the best time for pre-conditioning?

Materials and methods

In order to answer all these questions on the influence of the indoor laboratory climate on a skin physiological investigation, a kinetic test design was used. The level of skin moisture was monitored by a Corneometer 825 PC. The basic principle, capacitance measurements based on the influence of the high dielectric constant of water, which will change the capacitance of an electric resonant circuit, has been well known for more than 20 years. Skin roughness is measured by FOITS, an optical, touch-free, real-time, three-dimensional analysis of the skin surface by fringe projection. An area of 25 × 35 mm is digitized within 260/500 ms, with a resolution of 28 μm in the X and Y directions and of 4 μm in the Z direction. The analysis was carried out on the basis of Rz and Ra values.[4] Twelve individual values per parameter were calculated along a 20-mm line. All lines were distributed on a circle of 20-mm diameter by a rotation of 30°. Thus, the presented Rz and Ra are the mean values of 12 lines.

The acclimatized laboratory had a relative humidity of 60% or 50% (± 5%) and a temperature of 22°C (± 1°C). Frequent measurements were carried out, commencing immediately after the volunteers' arrival at the institute, and continuing for up to 5 hours. In order to show the basic influence of the indoor climate, no product application was performed for the duration of the investigation. In a second series of measurements, five different brands and five different formulations, with an increasing amount of glycerine (3–25%) as an active ingredient, were investigated in a short time-test design up to 4 hours after product application. In order to quantify the influence of the indoor climate on the product rating, the second test series was carried out twice. In a first run, the relative humidity was set at 60%; in a second run, it was reduced to 50%.

Results and discussion

Figure 39.1a presents the results of the 'no-product Corneometer kinetic'. The kinetic measurements were carried out on four different test areas (lower, middle and upper forearm, and upper arm). Figure 39.1b, shows the summary of the forearm data, based on the first-measured value. The volunteers were divided into three groups: those with starting values below 40 Corneometer Units (cu), those with values between 40 cu and 55 cu, and those with starting values above 55 cu.

Analysing the data of different test areas results in a decrease of about 2 cu for the upper forearm and a little less for the other test areas, independent of the absolute level, which was different for each test site (lower forearm < middle forearm < upper forearm = upper arm). These data were calculated without taking into account the individual skin type of the volunteers. Figure 39.1b picks up this idea, showing the individual starting conditions. As can be seen clearly from the differences to baseline, the 40–55 cu group did not show any changes above ± 1% during 5 hours of investigation. The group below 40 cu showed a constant increase of approximately 2%, whereas, for the group with high starting values, above 55 cu, a decrease of up to 10% was obtained. Independent of the test site, the pre-conditioning phase seems to be most effective for a high skin-moisture level at the beginning of a study. Therefore, a dry skin might be less influenced by the indoor climate. The data to

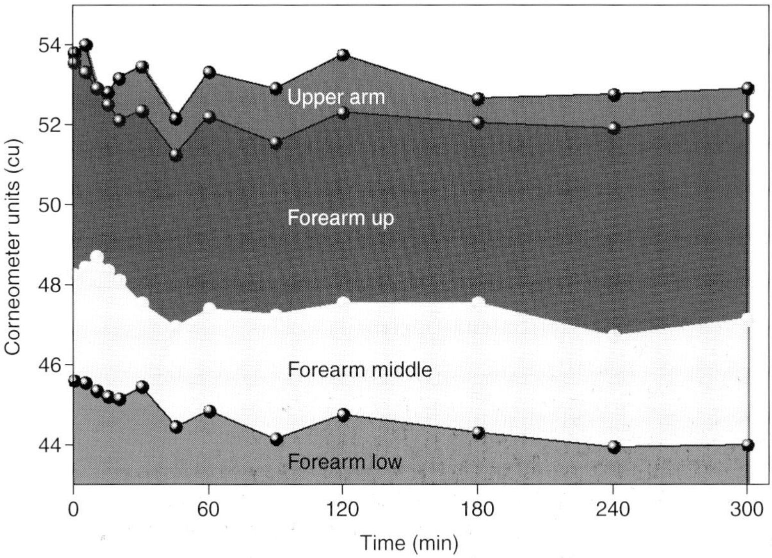

(a)

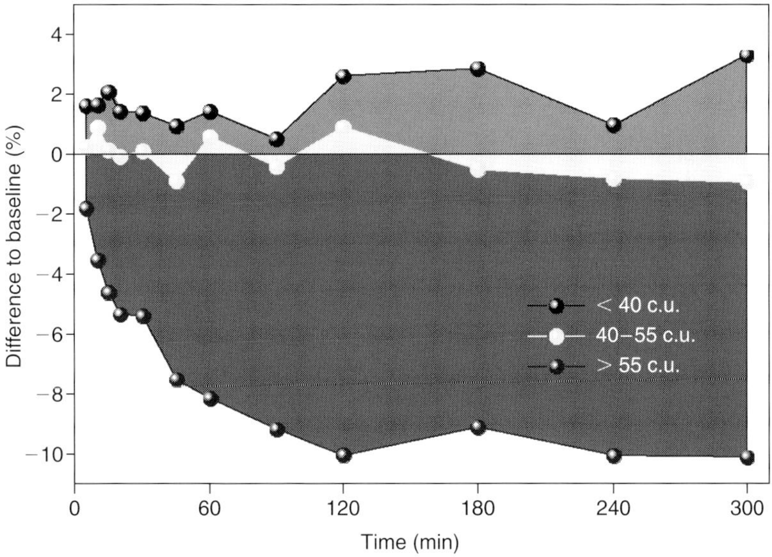

(b)

Figure 39.1

(a) Kinetic Corneometer – data summarized for different test areas, without any product application, n = 120; (b) Kinetic Corneometer – difference to baseline; data summarized for different volunteers, without any product application, n = 120.

determine the optimal time of pre-conditioning in order to generate stable skin conditions are represented in Figure 39.2.

As shown in Figure 39.2a, the difference to baseline (white curve: mean overall) became stabilized at 30 minutes, and remained constant after 60 minutes. Thus, 45 minutes' acclimatization seems to be the best choice – a time not too short for 'moist' skin and not too long to realize a reliable test design.

The data describing the skin surface are given in Figure 39.2b. No significant changes occured during the 4-hour kinetic investigation. Differences between the lower and upper forearm were comparable to the Corneometer measurements. Nevertheless, summing up, for the Rz and Ra values up to 4 hours, no distinguishable trend of change was obtained. Consequently, the influence of the indoor climate seems to be of minor impact if compared to skin moisture. In any case, changes of the skin structure are obviously on a much slower time scale if the producing event is as indirect as the indoor climate.

Changing from the kinetic view to a more static analysis, the data of five different products are summarized in Figure 39.3. Figure 39.3a shows the difference between baseline and end values, 4 hours after unique product application in absolute cu. The dark bars represent the data at an indoor climate of 60% relative humidity, whereas the light bars are obtained at 50% relative humidity.

With the exception of product 1, no difference occurred due to changing the indoor humidity. For product 1, a tendency was calculated for the comparison of both measurements. Taking product 1 as a hint that an influence might be possible, a second run of five formulations, with an increasing amount of glycerine, was carried out under the same conditions. In this case, significant changes occurred for the first two, low-glycerine concentrations (concentration below saturation). At 50% relative humidity, the level of measured absolute units decreased significantly. Thus, the selectivity became better if the relative humidity was reduced and the product contained hygroscopic-active ingredients. The hygroscopic ingredient seems to pick up the air humidity like a sponge, as long as it is in the upper stratum corneum. Nevertheless, the origin of moisture should be irrelevant for the skin, but, in the case of ranking and differentiating products as fast as possible after the product application, it might be helpful to measure at 50% relative humidity.

Summary

As demonstrated by the results obtained, the indoor climate plays an important part in cosmetic efficacy testing. Besides the outdoor climate which might have an effect on a long-term basis, the indoor climate, especially at the time of pre-conditioning, is decisive for short-term and

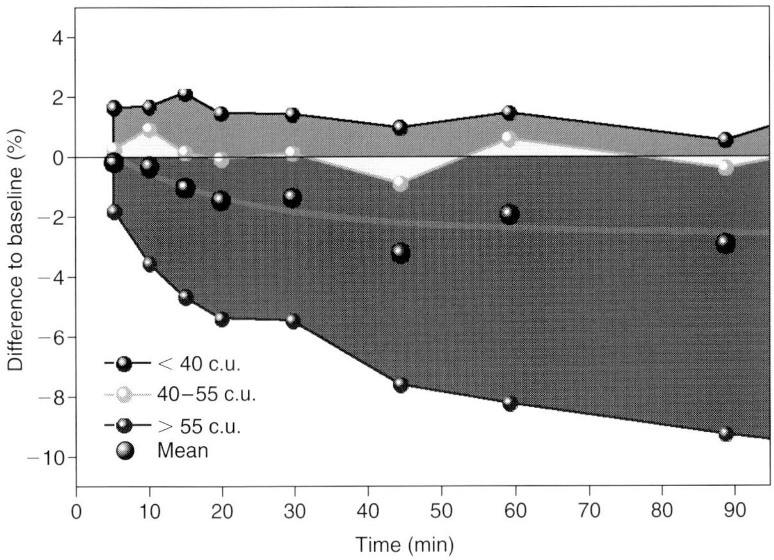

(a)

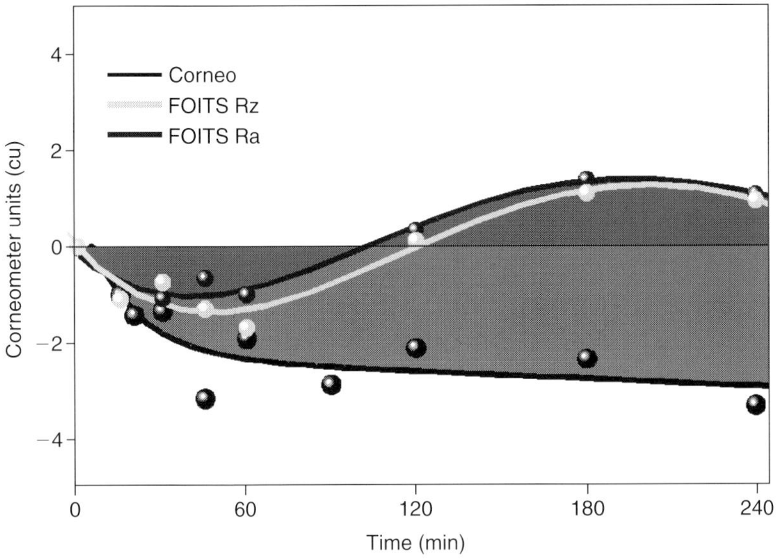

(b)

Figure 39.2

(a) Kinetic Corneometer – difference to baseline; data summarized for different volunteers up to 90 minutes, without any product application, n = 120; (b) Kinetic FOITS and Corneometer – difference to baseline mean overall up to 240 minutes, without any product application, n = 120/40

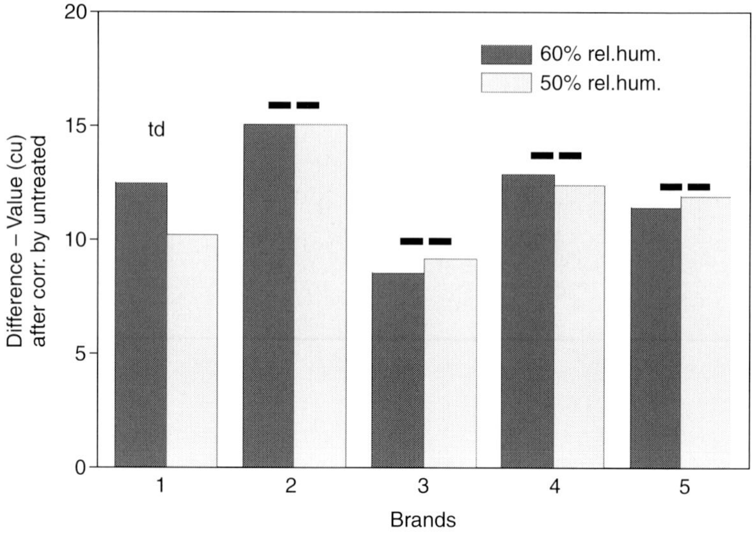

(a)

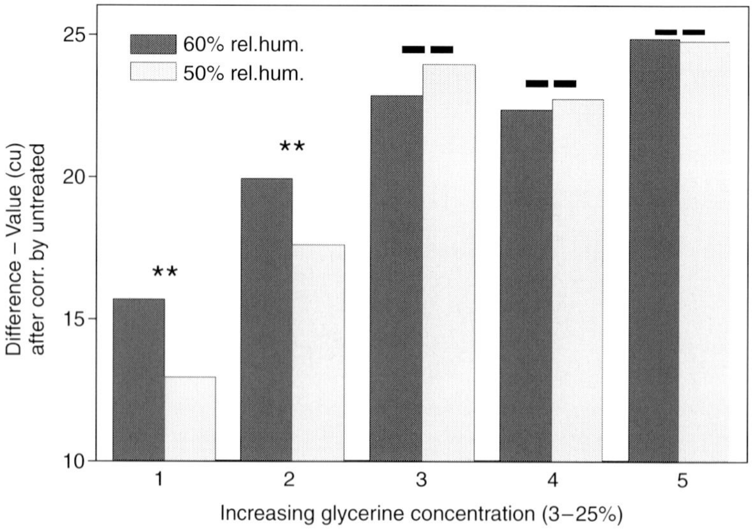

(b)

Figure 39.3

(a) Corneometer, product 1–5 – difference to baseline after correction by untreated, dark bar: 60% relative humidity, light bar: 50% relative humidity; (b) Corneometer, increasing concentration of glycerine (3–25%) – difference to baseline after correction by untreated, dark bar: 60% relative humidity, light bar: 50% relative humidity.

kinetic investigations. While the influence of the moisture level is strongly dependent on the starting value, the changes in skin topometry seem to be less marked. Based on the Corneometer kinetic data shown, 45 minutes of pre-conditioning appears to be an optimal compromise of effect, standardization and costs. The actual laboratory conditions (relative humidity) may be of great influence as well. Depending on the active ingredients (hygroscopic or not), a ranking of products might be of greater selectivity if a lower level of relative humidity is used. All in all, the data presented underline the importance of a standardized procedure in order to investigate cosmetic effects on a statistical and reproducible level.

References

1. Rohr M, Schrader K. Fast Optical In vivo Topometry of Human Skin (FOITS). SÖFW-Journal, 124. Jahrgang 1998; 2:52–9.
2. Rohr M, Brandt M, Schrader A. Skin surface – claim support by FOITS. SÖFW-Journal, 126. Jahrgang 2000, 1: 2–11.
3. Rohr M, Schrader K. Climatic influence on cosmetic skin parameters. In: *Skin Bioengineering – Techniques and Applications in Dermatology and Cosmetology* 1998. Basel: Karger Verlag.
4. DIN 4768. Ermittlung der Rauheitskenngrößen Ra, Rz, Rmax mit elektrischen Tastschnittgeräten, Begriffe, Messbedingungen.

40

The effect of extraction and NMF treatment on the water handling capability of stratum corneum as measured by TEWL and MAT

RR Wickett, G Tolia and M Visscher

Introduction

Electrical properties of the stratum corneum (SC) are intimately related to its water content and water handling capacities. Measurements made at a single point in time are often used to estimate the hydration level of the SC.[1–4] Dynamic measurements can yield additional information about SC function. A dynamic test of SC function that can be made using electrical measurements is the moisture accumulation test (MAT).[5,6] To perform the MAT, the probe of the instrument is held against the skin surface and occlusion by the probe causes the measurement to increase with time. In situations where the skin barrier is compromised, the MAT values are high and often correlate well with the degree of compromise. Thus, MAT has been used as an alternative to transepidermal water loss (TEWL) for assessing SC barrier function in neonatal rats subjected to tape stripping,[7] premature infants,[8] and human skin culture systems before and after transplant to athymic mice.[9,10] However, in situations where dry, flaky skin develops, MAT may go down dramatically while TEWL may either increase slightly or be unaffected. In a study of below-the-knee amputees who wear silicon sleeve suspension systems to hold their prostheses in place, we observed the development of dry flaky skin under the prosthesis, in spite of constant occlusion.[11] In these individuals, MAT was dramatically lower on the site that required the prosthesis compared to the contralateral side, even though TEWL was slightly higher. We hypothesized that MAT was reduced either because of lower levels of natural moisturizing factor (NMF) production at high humidity,[12] or because the patient's own sweat was extracting NMF. To begin to test this hypothesis, we have investigated the effect of water soaking before or after acetone/ether (A/E) extraction on MAT and TEWL. A/E extraction removes lipids but not NMF, and the water soak is expected to remove NMF, especially after the A/E extraction has removed some of the protective lipids.[13]

After the soak procedure, skin was treated with an artificial NMF mixture to test the direct effect of NMF on MAT in both extracted and untreated skin.

Materials and methods

Subjects

Eleven healthy, adult, female subjects were enrolled during June of 2000. Individuals with visually dry forearm skin or dermatological conditions (psoriasis, eczema, irritant dermatitis, etc.), currently on steroid or insulin therapy, were excluded. The Institutional Review Board of the University of Cincinnati Medical Center approved the protocol. All subjects provided informed consent.

Biophysical measurements

TEWL was determined using a DermaLab Evaporimeter. Baseline hydration and rate of moisture accumulation (MAT) were measured with a NOVA Dermal Phase Meter (NOVA DPM; NOVA Technology, Portsmouth, NH, USA). MAT measurements were made using 20 seconds of probe occlusion and determining a linear slope for the DPM units/second curve.

NMF and vehicle formulations

The NMF components (Table 40.1) were added to a vehicle of hydroxy-

Table 40.1 Natural moisturizing factor formulation.

Component	Percent (% by wt)	mg/cm^2 applied to site
Pyrrolidone carboxylic acid	12	0.24
Urea	7	0.14
Sodium chloride	5	0.10
Sodium lactate	5	0.10
Potassium citrate	0.5	0.01
Serine	18.2	0.36
Glycine	9.1	0.18
Arganine	3.2	0.064
Glutamic acid	2.3	0.04
Tyrosine	0.5	0.01
Alanine	6.6	0.13
Hydroxyethyl cellulose*		
Deionized water†		

* Sufficient quantity to provide a viscosity of 300 cps.
† Added as necessary to provide a total of 100% by weight.

ethyl cellulose (Natrosol[T]) in distilled water and the viscosity adjusted to 300 centipoises (cps) to produce a formulation suitable for application to the skin. The formula was based on reported compositions of NMF.[14–16] The levels of pyrrolidone carboxylic acid, urea, citrate, chloride, and total amino acids were taken from the NMF composition reported by Cler and Fourtanier.[15] The relative ratios of neutral, basic, and acidic amino acids were formulated to match the composition of amino acids extracted from the skin after treatment with acetone/ether followed by a water soak.[17] The relative amounts of the neutral amino acids approximated the ratios found in guinea-pig epidermis.[16] The formula pH was 5.6. A vehicle control was prepared in a similar fashion and adjusted to a viscosity of 300 cps and a pH of 5.6.

Treatment protocol

Sites and initial measurements

Six 2 × 2-cm treatment sites areas were marked on each volar forearm. The areas were randomized for left vs right and for position along the arm, and treatments were assigned as shown in Table 40.2. Prior to entry into the study, subjects refrained from using moisturizer on their volar forearms for 72 hours. Measurements were performed after equilibration to environmental conditions (temperature 21 ± 1°C and relative humidity 31 ± 5%) for 30 minutes. Baseline skin measurements of TEWL, skin hydration and MAT were made for each of the 12 treatment sites (time = 0 minutes).

Acetone/ether extraction

Three sites on each forearm (six in total) were treated with a 1:1 mixture of A/E to remove surface lipids and intercellular lipids from the outer SC layers. The A/E extraction procedure was expected to remove only very small quantities of water-soluble materials from the skin.[17] The sites were exposed to A/E for 5 minutes, using a glass extraction cup to hold the solvent. The areas were then wiped repeatedly with cotton pads dipped in the A/E mixture. This process was continued until the TEWL reading increased to approximately twice the baseline value. Following extraction, the biophysical measurements were repeated for each of the six sites.

Soaking

Once the A/E extraction was complete, one forearm was soaked in fresh water (temperature 104 ± 2.5°F) for 10 minutes and blotted dry. The sites on the other (unsoaked) forearms served as control sites. Fifteen minutes after soaking, the biophysical measurements were repeated for all 12 sites.

NMF and vehicle treatment

The NMF formulation was applied (2 mg/cm^2) to four sites: untreated (no extraction, no soak), A/E treated, soaked, and A/E plus soak). The vehicle control (2 mg/cm^2) was applied to another set of sites (untreated, A/E treated, soaked, A/E plus soak). The biophysical measurements were made 30 minutes after application for all 12 sites (Table 40.2). The test areas were left undisturbed for 3.5 hours. The subjects returned to the test facility and the measurements were made following the 30-minute equilibration.

Analysis of data

Analysis of variance was used to compare treatment groups. Repeated measures statistics were used to evaluate the changes in the treatment sites over time. The paired comparison t-test was used to evaluate the effects of treatment variables. To normalize the data for variations in skin condition along the forearm, the change from baseline was used in the paired comparison procedures (SigmaStat, Jandel Scientific). Additional analyses were conducted using PROC MIXED SAS version 6.09.

Results

Soak/NMF study

The effect of extraction on TEWL is shown in Figure 40.1. The effect of extraction and soaking on MAT is shown in Figure 40.2.

The error bars in the figures represent standard errors of the mean. Extraction with A/E increased both TEWL and MAT compared to the baseline averages for the sites before treatment. Water soak decreased MAT significantly and the A/E followed by the 10-minute water soak had a very dramatic effect on MAT. Figure 40.3 shows the effect of the NMF treatment on MAT values 30 minutes after NMF treatment for skin that had been given the various extraction and soaking treatments.

NMF treatment increased the MAT values for all of the sites and

Table 40.2 Experimental treatments.

Site	Arm A	Site	Arm B
1	Untreated	7	Soak
2	Untreated + vehicle	8	Soak + vehicle
3	Untreated + NMF	9	Soak + NMF
4	A/E extraction	10	A/E + soak
5	A/E + vehicle	11	A/E + soak + vehicle
6	A/E + NMF	12	A/E + soak + NMF

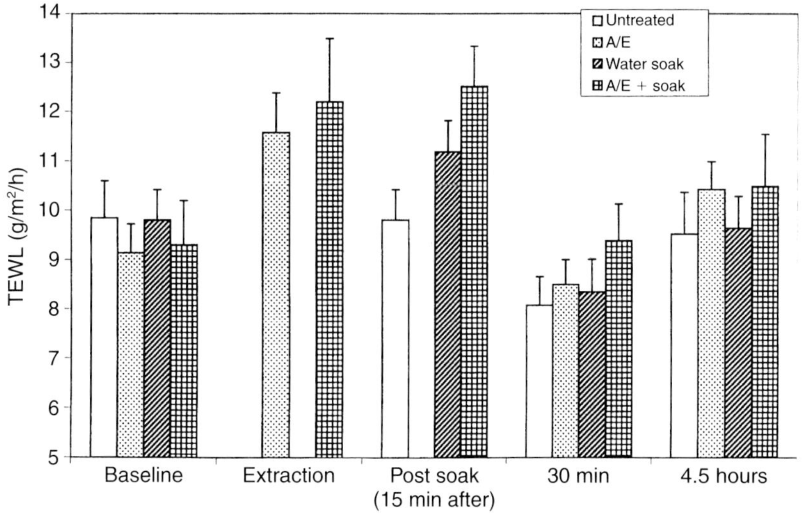

Figure 40.1

Effect of extraction and soaking on TEWL.

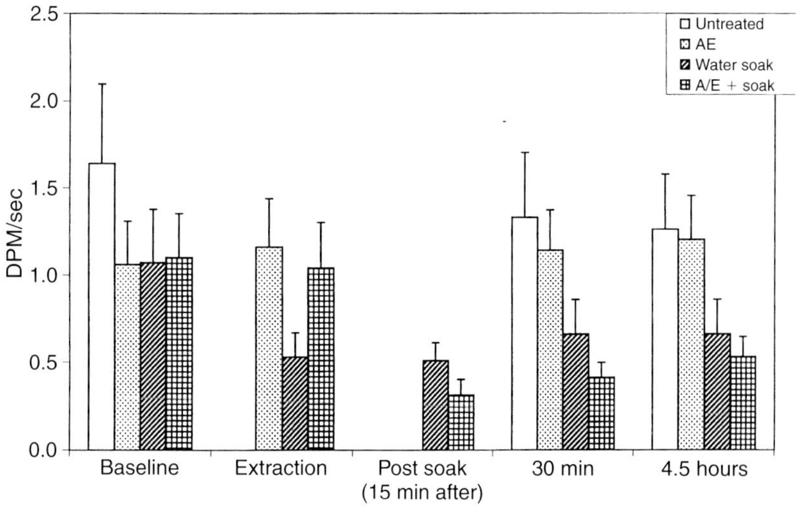

Figure 40.2

Effect of extraction and soaking on MAT.

brought the values for even the A/E + soak-treated skin back to approximately the initial baseline values. The NMF treatment also reduced TEWL for the extracted sites (data not shown).

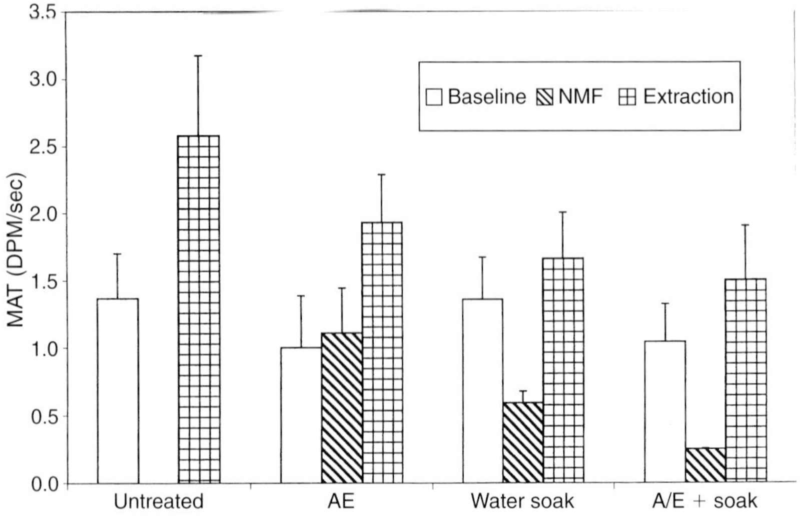

Figure 40.3
Effect of NMF on MAT.

Discussion

We had previously observed that patients wearing silicone sleeve prosthetic limbs suffer from a number of skin problems on the residual limb due to occlusion by the silicone.[11] Dry, scaly skin is often one of the manifestations of amputee dermatitis. We reported that TEWL was elevated, but NOVA DPM instantaneous measurements and MAT were reduced compared to the normal limb, with MAT being dramatically lower. We hypothesized that this reduction in MAT and NOVA are due to reduced NMF production in skin that is occluded for long periods of time each day, based on the work of Scott and Harding,[12] who reported that NMF production in rat skin is reduced at high humidity or possibly due to extraction of NMF by the patient's own sweat.

In the work reported here we tested the effects of treatments designed to first deplete, and then replace, NMF. Extraction of the skin with A/E led to increased TEWL but had little effect on MAT (Figure 40.1). Soaking in water for 10 minutes reduced MAT dramatically, even on sites that not been subjected to A/E treatment but the effect was most dramatic on A/E-treated sites (Figure 40.2). Treatment with an artificial NMF formulation led to recovery of the MAT to approximately baseline levels on soaked or soaked-and-extracted skin, and elevated the MAT of untreated skin above baseline (Figure 40.3). The data reported here are consistent with the hypothesis that MAT is reduced in dry, scaly skin, due to reduced levels of NMF. In order to substantiate this hypothesis more directly, it will be necessary to determine the actual NMF levels in the skin after treatments that reduce MAT.

References

1. Li F, Conroy E, Visscher M et al. The ability of electrical measurements to predict skin moisturization. I. Effects of NaCl and glycerin on short-term measurements. J Cosmet Sci 2001; 52:13–22.
2. Tagami H, Ohi M, Iwatsuki K et al. Evaluation of the skin surface hydration in vivo by electrical measurement. J Invest Dermatol 1980; 75:500–7.
3. Loden M, Lindberg M. The influence of a single application of different moisturizers on the skin capacitance. Acta Derm Venereol 1991;71:79–82.
4. Serup J. A three-hour test for rapid comparison of effects of moisturizers and active constituents (urea). Measurement of hydration, scaling and skin surface lipidization by noninvasive techniques. Acta Derm Venereol Suppl (Stockh) 1992; 177:29–33.
5. Van Neste D. In vivo evaluation of unbound water accumlation in stratum corneum. Dermatologica 1990; 181:197–201.
6. Treffel P, Gabard B. Stratum corneum dynamic function measurements after moisturizer or irritant application. Arch Dermatol Res 1995; 287:474–9.
7. Wickett RR, Nath V, Tanaka R et al. Use of continuous electrical capacitance and transepidermal water loss measurements for assessing barrier function in neonatal rat skin. Skin Pharmacol 1995; 8:179–85.
8. Okah FA, Wickett RR, Pickens WL et al. Surface electrical capacitance as a noninvasive bedside measure of epidermal barrier maturation in the newborn infant. Pediatrics 1995; 96:688–92.
9. Boyce ST, Supp AP, Harriger MD et al. Surface electrical capacitance as a noninvasive index of epidermal barrier in cultured skin substitutes in athymic mice. J Invest Dermatol 1996; 107:82–7.
10. Supp AP, Wickett RR, Swope VB et al. Incubation of cultured skin substitutes in reduced humidity promotes cornification in vitro and stable engraftment in athymic mice. Wound Repair Regen 1999; 7:226–37.
11. Wickett RR, Tolia G, Visscher M et al. Bioengineering evaluation of the water handling capabilities of stratum corneum in vivo. In: *Creation and Hope, Proceedings of the 2001 IFSCC International Conference, Taipei, Taiwan.* Taipei Taiwan: International Federation of Societies of Cosmetic Chemists; 2001; 37–46.
12. Scott IR, Harding CR. Filaggrin breakdown to water binding compounds during development of the rat stratum corneum is controlled by the water activity of the environment. Dev Biol 1986; 115: 84–92.
13. Imokawa G, Kuno H, Kawai M. Stratum corneum lipids serve as a bound-water modulator. J Invest Dermatol 1991; 96:845–51.
14. Jacobi OK. About the mechanism of moisture regulation in horny layer of skin. Proc Sci Sec Toilet Goods Assoc 1959; 31:22–4.
15. Cler EJ, Fourtanier A. L'acide purrolidone caboxylique (PCA) et la peau. Int J Cosmet Sci 1981; 3:101.

16. Tabachnick J, LaBadie JH. Studies on the biochemistry of epidermis. IV. The free amino acids, ammonia, urea, and pyrrolidone carboxylic acid content of conventional and germ-free albino guina pig epidermia. J Invest Dermatol 1970; 54:24–31.

17. Jokura Y, Ishikawa S, Tokuda H et al. Molecular analysis of elastic properties of the stratum corneum by solid-state 13C-nuclear magnetic resonance spectroscopy. J Invest Dermatol 1995; 104: 806–12.

41

Evaluation of surfactant effects on stratum corneum using squamometry, transepidermal water loss measurements and the sorption–desorption test

D Black, A Del Pozo and Y Gall

Introduction

Overexposure to certain cleansers will result in skin damage, manifested by impaired barrier function, leading to irritant reactions with prolonged use. Evaluation of barrier function deterioration is thus a useful indicator of early stratum corneum (SC) damage, and may help to predict potential skin irritancy for these products. The squamometry technique has been used for assessing cleansers in terms of their degree of 'mildness', and appears useful as a complementary method for screening their irritant potential.[1,2] The aim of this study was to use squamometry on SC, treated in two ways: ex vivo post-sampling, and in vivo by washing, and to compare this with measurements of SC barrier function and dynamic hydration tests.

Methods

Subjects

Fourteen women volunteers, who had given their written, informed consent, were included in the study (mean age 25 ± 4.6 years). All subjects had clinically normal-appearing skin, lying within the normal hydration index range when measured using an electrical capacitance technique (Corneometer 825, Courage & Khazaka; Germany). The right volar forearm was used for all measurements.

Protocol

On day 1, the forearm was marked with six circular areas, 20 mm in diameter. From adjacent sites, six samples of SC were taken, using 23-mm diameter D-squame® discs, and treated with the surfactants for subsequent squamometric evaluation, which we shall call the 'ex-vivo' method. The marked sites were then treated with the surfactant solutions by washing, this being repeated on days 2 and 3. On day 4, transepidermal water loss (TEWL) was measured on the 6 marked sites followed by dynamic hydration measurements with the water sorption-desorption test (WSDT). Finally, also on day 4, D-squame® samples of the same sites were taken for squamometry evaluation, this being called the ex vivo method. The marked sites were then treated with the surfactant solutions by washing, this being repeated on days 2 and 3.

On day 4 transepidermal water loss (TEWL) was measured on the six marked sites, followed by dynamic hydration measurements with the water sorption–desorption test (WSDT). Finally, also on day 4, Dsquame® samples of the same sites were taken for squamometry evaluation, this being called the in vivo method.

Treatments

Solutions (5%) of the following surfactants were used: anionic surfactants sodium lauryl sulphate (SLS) and disodium laureth-2 sulphosuccinate (DSLS); non-ionic surfactants polysorbate 20 (PS20) and decylpolyglucoside (DPG). Controls included distilled water (DW) and untreated (U) sites. For the in vivo method, treatments were randomly allocated and applied by 1-minute washes, then rinsed and patted dry. For the ex vivo method, SC samples were immersed for 5 minutes in the same solutions, and then rinsed for 1 minute.

Assessments

Squamometry

The technique of Piérard et al was used, with some modifications.[1,2] D-squame® (CuDerm Corp; USA) samples of SC were completely immersed in a toluidine blue/basic fuschin stain for 1 minute, then rinsed in distilled water for 1 minute. On drying, stained D-squame® samples were placed on a white calibration tile and measured colorimetrically (Chromameter CR300, Minolta, Japan). CIE values of L^* and C^* were used to calculate the colorimetric index of mildness (CIM), where $CIM = L^* - C^*$. SC samples treated ex vivo and in vivo were evaluated in this way.

Transepidermal water loss

SC barrier function was assessed, using an evaporimeter (EP1 Servo-Med; Sweden) for measuring TEWL. Stable readings over 3 minutes were averaged.

Water sorption–desorption test

Dynamic hydration measurements were made using a WSDT.[3] The sorption phase used soaked cotton wool inside rubber washers, held on the skin for 20 seconds. Afterwards, excess water was patted dry for 10 seconds, and the hydration index immediately measured (HI_0). Measurements were repeated every 30 seconds for 3 minutes during the desoprtion phase ($HI_{0.5-3}$). Before the sorption phase, a baseline reading was taken (HI_b).

Data were processed by subtracting baseline for all desorption values (HI_{0-3}–HI_b). The HI_0–HI_b value indicates maximal water sorption, often referred to as hygroscopicity value. From plotted HI_{0-3}–HI_b values, the area under the curve was calculated, and is called the water-holding capacity (WHC) of the SC.

Unpublished data from our group has shown that dry, flaky skin of the calf has high hygroscopicity and WHC values, and these decrease with emollient use and increase with SLS application. The WSDT detects changes in SC porosity, whereby intact SC is less permeable to brief water contact than a drier, flakier SC. In the latter case, applied water remains longer in the more porous SC, due to a brief reservoir effect, giving higher corneometer values.

Results

Combined squamometry CIM values for ex vivo and in vivo treatment variants are expressed graphically (Figure 41.1). The ex vivo method showed more significant differences between treatments, with SLS having the lowest CIM value, and, thus, the harshest surfactant effect. DSLS- and PS20-treated samples had significantly higher CIM values compared to SLS and were similar in effect, while DPG, water-treated and untreated sites had the highest values, with no significant differences between these three treatments and that of PS20. With regard to the in vivo method, the same general pattern was observed; however, only SLS had a significantly lower CIM compared to the other treatments.

TEWL was significantly increased with SLS-treated skin only. All other treatments were similar, showing no real change from untreated sites (Figure 41.2). With regard to WSDT results, these are summarized as desorption curves with HI_b values subtracted (Figure 41.3). Hygroscopicity was greatest for SLS-treated skin, being significantly different from that of water-treated and untreated sites. All other treatments were the same. The WHC was significantly higher for SLS compared to the other treatments, with no significant differences between the latter, although DSLS and PS20 were higher than the rest.

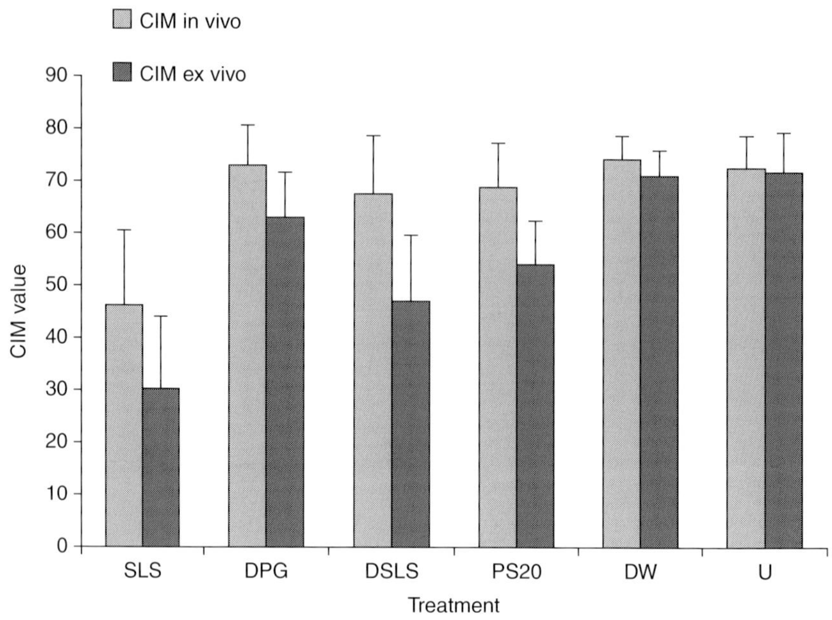

Figure 41.1

CIM values for the surfactants used for ex vivo and in vivo squamometry variants (means + 1 sd). Significant treatment differences ($p < 0.05$) for ex vivo CIM values: SLS < DSLS/PS20 < DPG/PS20/DW/U, and for in vivo CIM values: SLS < all other treatments.

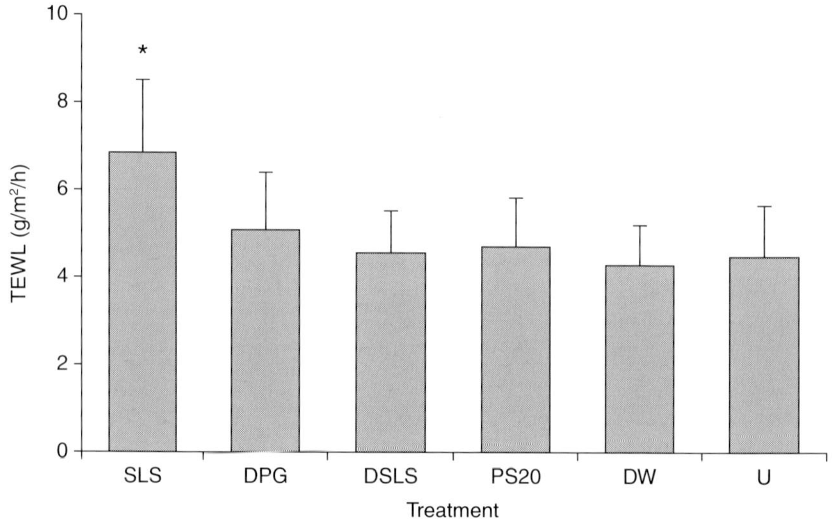

Figure 41.2

TEWL values for the surfactant used (means + 1 sd). Significant treatment differences ($p < 0.05$), with SLS > all other treatments.

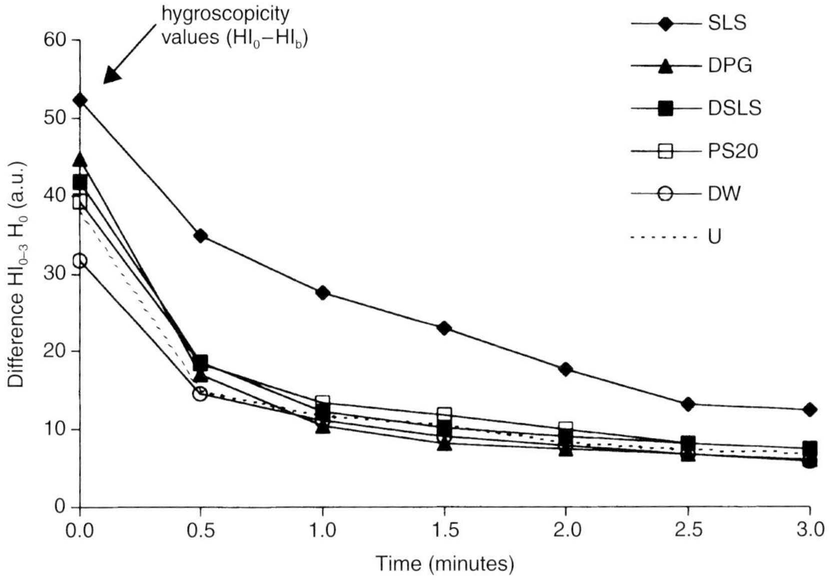

Figure 41.3

WSDT results as mean desorption/time curves, with baseline hydration indices subtracted (HI_{0-3}–HI_b). Significant treatment differences ($p < 0.05$) between hygroscopicity values: SLS > DW/U, and between WHC values: SLS > all other treatments.

Discussion

The two squamometry variants showed essentially the same pattern of results. The ex vivo method showed more significant product differences than the in vivo method, and, thus, could be considered as more discriminatory. However, this conclusion is misleading, since the main reason for this method difference may be due to the way the product is applied to the SC. With the ex vivo approach, the product and subsequent stain are both applied to the same under-surface of the Dsquame®-sampled SC in the space of 6 minutes. The in vivo approach applies the product to the top surface for 3 days, followed by staining of the under-surface. Thus, with the latter method, the test-product effect is less, since it is more diluted after permeating two to three corneocyte layers before reaching the surface to be stained. Also, it is assumed with squamometry that the test products have the same, but variable, mode of action on the SC. This is debatable, since, along with lipid interaction, there are also protein effects with stronger anionic surfactants. Furthermore, the structural components of the SC, which are specifically stained by toluidine blue and basic fuschin, remain unclear.

When these results are compared with barrier-function tests using

TEWL and WSDT, the in vivo version compares better than the ex vivo one. Here, significant differences were seen only between SLS and the other treatments. This is not surprising, since the reasons behind the choice of surfactant were to test those frequently used in current formulations, which are well tolerated by the skin, with the exception of SLS, which was included as a positive control due to its known irritant effects.

Conclusion

Surfactant effects have been assessed using squamometry on SC, treated both ex vivo and in vivo.

Greater treatment differences were observed ex vivo than in vivo, although both approaches showed similar treatment ranking. The in vivo results are corroborated by TEWL and WSDT data, where only 5% SLS gave significant changes. The ex vivo approach is less time-consuming than the in vivo one, and may be more sensitive, due to better product discrimination. However, the ex vivo approach may overestimate product harshness, since test conditions are unrealistic. If correlated with the in vivo method, it may be useful for rapid initial screening. Nonetheless, caution is required when extrapolating the squamometry technique to the general in vivo situation, with regard to potential product irritancy.

References

1. Piérard GE, Piérard-Franchimont C, Saint Léger D et al. Squamometry: the assessment of xerosis by colorimetry of D-squame adhesive discs. J Soc Cosmet Chem 1992; 40:297–305.
2. Piérard GE, Goffin V, Piérard-Franchimont C. Squamometry and corneosurfametry for rating interactions of cleansing products with stratum corneum. J Soc Cosmet Chem 1994; 45:269–77.
3. Tagami H, Kanamaru Y, Inoue K et al. Water sorption–desorption test of the skin in vivo for functional assessment of the stratum corneum. J Invest Dermatol 1982; 78:425–8.

42

Epidermal in vivo and in vitro studies by attenuated total reflection spectroscopy using a novel mid-infrared fibre probe

HM Heise, L Küpper, W Pittermann and M Kietzmann

For studies of the upper horny skin layer, attenuated total reflection (ATR) infrared spectroscopy has often been used, allowing a shallow micrometer probing depth for the surface measurement. The range of applications is increased by the development of a fibre-optic probe made from a polycrystalline infrared-transparent silver halide material with ductile and non-toxic characteristics,[1] which provides more flexibility for the epidermal surface characterization than that available with conventional accessories. Largest transmittance of the fibres is observed particularly within the information-rich infrared fingerprint region (about 1500–600 cm^{-1}).[2] Our aim was to study the chemistry of the human horny layer and that of the upper bovine udder skin, and a comparison was made possible on the grounds of their ATR-spectra. Further potential of the measurement technique in combination with adhesive tape-stripping for penetration studies of topically applied active substances is illustrated.

The in vitro model of isolated perfused bovine udder skin (BUS model) has been proposed as a substitute for human in vivo tests.[3] Due to the continuous perfusion, the horny layer demonstrates active barrier and reservoir functions. The in vitro BUS model is widely used in dermatological and cosmetic research as well, and exhibits hair follicles and sebaceous glands, providing the corneal compartment with sebum similar to the human in vivo situation. Histological studies also prove the similarity of the BUS-model to human skin.

In Figure 42.1, the measurement instrument, including the attachment of the fibre-probe, is shown. The spectrometer was a Fourier-transform infrared (FTIR)-spectrometer (model Vector 22 from Bruker Optik GmbH; Ettlingen, Germany). The set-up, with mirror optics, fibre-probe and fibre-detector coupling, was a development from the Institute of Spectrochemistry and Applied Spectroscopy and Infrared Fiber Sensors, which includes a semiconductive mercury-cadmium-telluride (MCT)-detector (liquid-nitrogen cooled, from Infrared Associates, Inc.; Stuart, FL, USA).

The silver halide fibre-optic probe consisted of a shaft with one fibre for transmitting and a second one for receiving infrared radiation from the ATR-measuring head. The measurement principle, with the evanescent electrical radiation field outside the optically dense fibre, which is either air or the sample in contact with the fibre for the respective background or sample measurement, is illustrated in Figure 42.1a. The transmitting and receiving fibres were 2 m in length (either of square cross-section of 750 μm × 750 μm or of circular cross-section with a diameter of 700 μm; optical numerical aperture of 0.5).

The shaft length was 20 cm (12 mm in diameter), and one prototype also had the means for attaching detachable short U-shaped silver halide fibre pieces for ATR measurements (see Figure 42.1c).

An example of the spectral measurements of bovine udder and human forearm skin using the fibre-optic ATR-probe is provided in Figure 42.2. Skin areas of less than 1 mm^2 were measured with a probe made from a

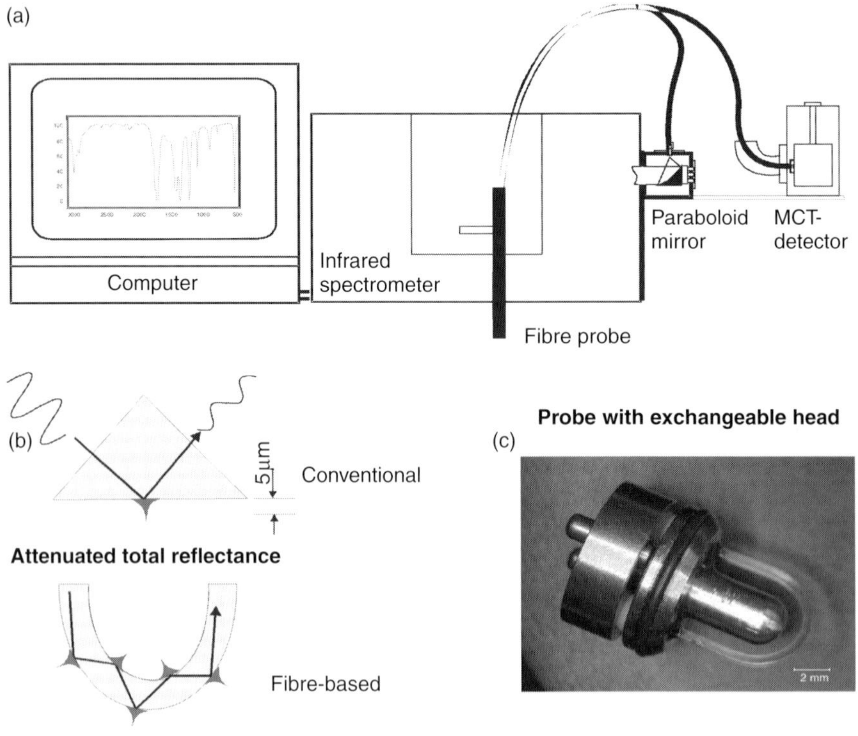

Figure 42.1

(a) Set-up of the FTIR spectrometer with a fibre-based accessory; (b) measurement principle of an ATR experiment with a conventional ATR-crystal and an U-shaped fibre configuration, respectively (the penetration of the evanescent field is wavelength dependent and estimated for an interface of ZnSe as crystal material and skin at around 1000 cm^{-1}); (c) exchangeable fibre-probe head.

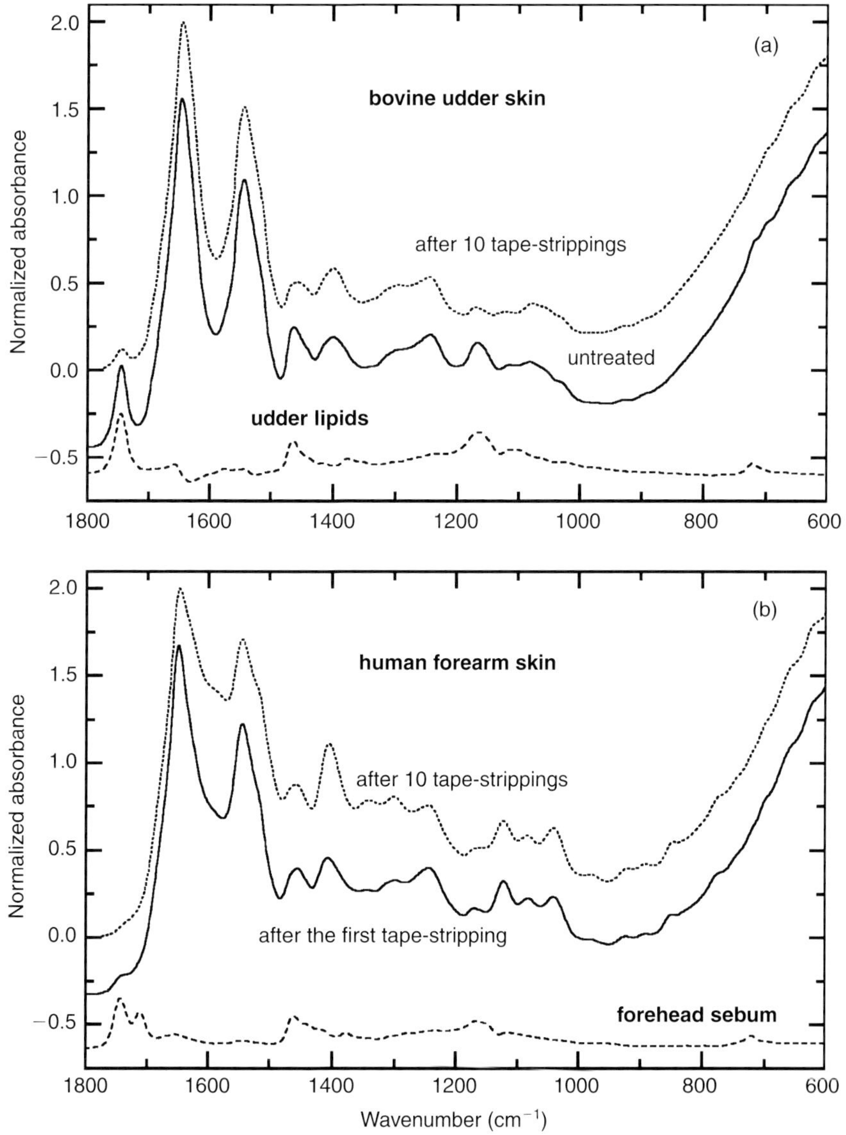

Figure 42.2

Surface spectra of bovine udder skin (a), and of human forearm skin (b), including a spectrum of the pure skin lipid components.

silver halide fibre of square cross-section. Repeat skin stripping by application of adhesive tape was also performed, similar to the technique described recently.[4] Besides spectra measured from the skin surface, a spectrum of the lipids within the udder skin and of sebum from a human, male forehead are also shown (Figure 42.2a and b, respectively). Differences in the spectra are due to keratin differences (see the strong amide I bands at 1650 cm^{-1}, mainly C=O stretching vibration, and the most striking features in the C–O and C–C-stretching region between 1150 and 1000 cm^{-1}) and the amount of lipids observed. For the latter, the absorption band of the ester C=O stretching at 1740 cm^{-1} and an overlapped band at about 1460 cm^{-1} from CH_2-deformation vibrations are characteristic. There is an astonishing similarity in both lipid spectra, giving evidence of a similar chemistry, apart from the absorption band at 1710 cm^{-1}, which is found in the human sebum spectrum and can be assigned to a free fatty acid component.

In Figure 42.3, the exemplary results from experiments with the application of a lamellar cream applied to udder skin are shown. In Figure 42.3a, the ATR-spectrum of a dry film of the cosmetic cream is also given, which eases the interpretation of the in situ measurements that were carried out after subsequent tape-stripping. The disappearance of cream constituents is obvious after 10 tape-strippings. Complementary information is obtained from the measurements on the adhesive tapes used (Figure 42.3b), which can be exploited also for a quantitative determination of the stripped corneal material and cream constituents.

Conclusion

The non-invasive infrared spectroscopic measurement technique can be applied to human studies as well as in vitro studies using skin models with fully functional horny layers and natural sebum excretion. The technique, based on probes made from fibres, in particular of square cross-section, is very promising, since it opens the field for new medical and cosmetic applications that were not possible with conventional ATR-crystals and bulky sampling compartment-based accessories.

Acknowledgements

HMM and LK from the Institute of Spectrochemistry and Applied Spectroscopy acknowledge gratefully the financial support by the Ministerium für Schule, Wissenschaft und Forschung des Landes Nordrhein-Westfalen and the Bundesministerium für Bildung und Forschung.

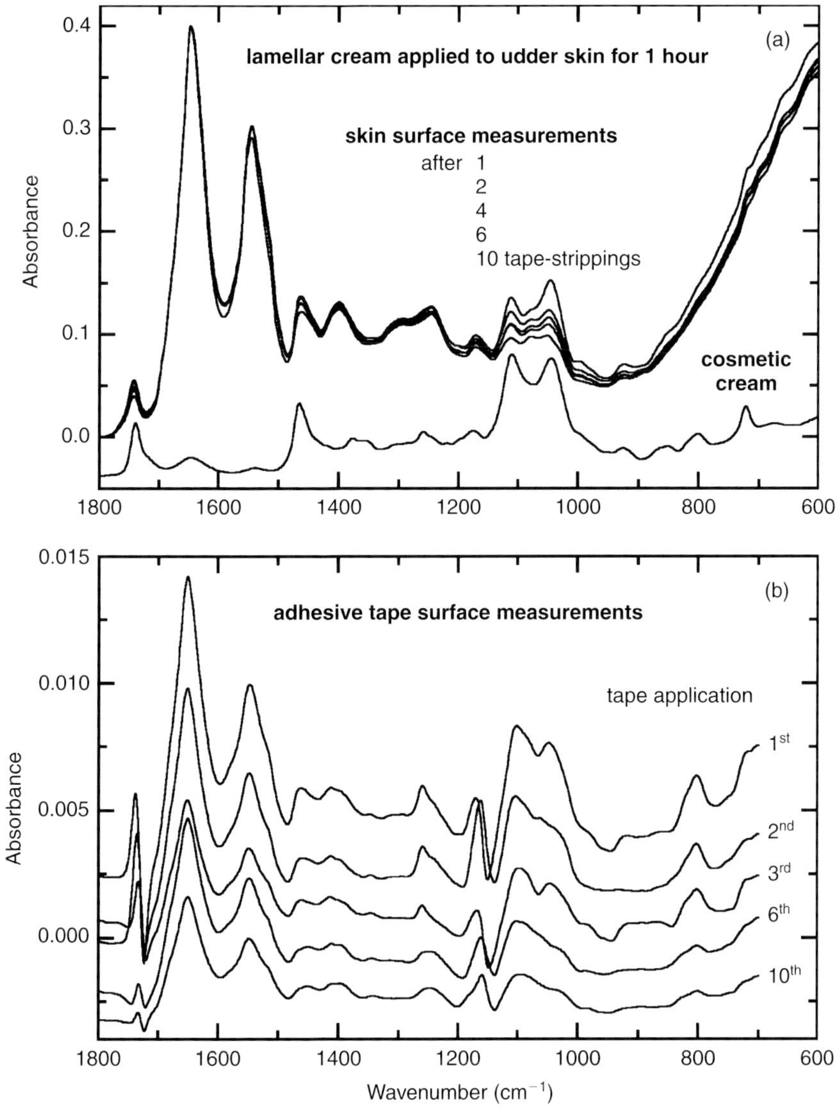

Figure 42.3

Skin surface measurements after topical cream application and repeat tape-stripping, including a spectrum of a pure dry cream film (a), and complementary measurements on the tape surfaces after topical application (b).

References

1. Küpper L, Heise HM, Butvina LN. Novel developments in mid-IR fiber optic spectroscopy for analytical applications. J Mol Struct 2001; 563/564:173–81.
2. Küpper L, Heise HM, Pittermann W et al. New tool for epidermal and cosmetic formulation studies by attenuated total reflection spectroscopy using a flexible mid-infrared fiber probe. Fresenius J Anal Chem 2001; 371:753–7.
3. Förster Th, Pittermann W, Schmitt M et al. Skin penetration properties of cosmetic formulations using a perfused bovine udder model. J Cosmet Sci 1999; 50:147–57.
4. Laugel C, Do Nascimento C, Ferrier D et al. Contribution of ATR/FT-IR spectroscopy for studying the in vivo behavior of octylmethoxycinnamate (OMC) after topical application. Appl Spectrosc 2001; 55:1173–80.

43

TEWL and stratum corneum hydration changes caused by prolonged contact with a new TEWL measurement head

LI Ciortea, E Fonseca, J Sarramagnan and RE Imhof

Introduction

The aim of this research was to investigate the effect on transepidermal water loss (TEWL) and stratum corneum (SC) hydration of prolonged contact with the measurement head of a patented new instrument for measuring water vapour flux (Cool-TEWL[1]). It uses a closed measurement chamber, to eliminate fluctuations due to ambient air movements, whilst removing trapped water vapour with an electronically cooled condensing surface opposite the measurement orifice. In consequence, the skin surface is exposed to a precisely controlled and highly reproducible microclimate of ~10% relative humidity and it was thought worthwhile to investigate and quantify any consequential changes in skin properties.[2]

Experimental details

Volar forearm skin was exposed to repeated cycles of prolonged contact with the Cool-TEWL measurement head in two measurement series, as summarized in Table 43.1.

At baseline, and immediately after each period of contact (within 30 seconds), the mean hydration of the top ~10 μm of the SC under study

Table 43.1 Main experimental parameters.

Parameter	Series (1)	Series (2)
No. of volunteers	4	3
No. of contact cycles	6	5
Duration of contact (minutes)	5	30

was measured using the OTTFR technique.[3] The measurements were normalized to the first measurement from each volunteer and fitted to a linear relationship of the form $y = A + B^*t$, where B is the gradient characterizing the mean change with time of exposure.

Results

Measurement Series (1) did not reveal any underlying trend above the noise. Measurement Series (2) revealed a trend of decreasing TEWL (–0.10 ± 0.03% per minute, see Figure 43.1a) and increasing SC hydration (+0.05 ± 0.05% per minute, see Figure 43.1b).

Discussion and conclusions

The most surprising aspect of these experiments is how small the observed changes of SC properties were, given the long exposure times to which the test sites were subjected. The weak increase in SC hydration with contact time is clearly not the result of exposure to the microclimate, where the opposite effect would be expected. Metabolic changes occurred in the volunteers during these experiments. For example, a decrease in skin-surface temperature in measurement Series (2) was

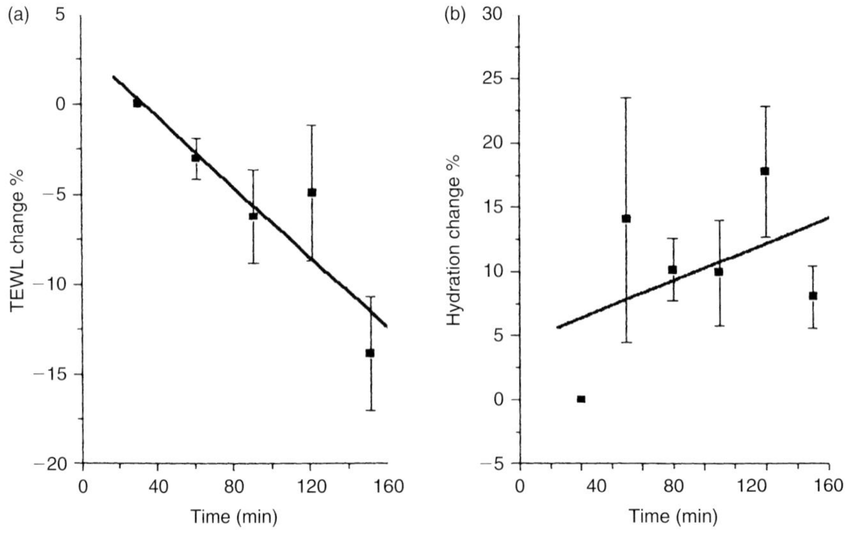

Figure 43.1
Time Series (2) results for (a) TEWL, and (b) SC hydration with fitted trend lines.

observed. We attribute the relatively large error bars in the TEWL data to (a) instrument imperfection in the crude prototype used, and (b) bio-noise.

In conclusion, the results show that prolonged exposure of skin to the low relative humidity microclimate within the Cool-TEWL[T] measurement head has little discernible effect on TEWL and SC hydration.

References

1. Imhof RE, O'Driscoll D, Xiao P, Berg E. New sensor for water vapour flux. In: *Sensors and their Applications X*. Bristol: IoP Publishing, 1999:173–7.
2. Pinnagoda J. Transepidermal water loss – hardware and measuring principles: evaporimeter. In: Elsner P, Berardesca E, Maibach HI, eds. *Bioengineering of the Skin: Water and the Stratum Corneum*. CRC Press Inc, 1994:51–65.
3. Bindra RMS, Imhof RE, Mochan A, Eccleston GM. Opto-thermal technique for in-vivo stratum corneum hydration measurement. Journal de Physique 1994; C7:465–8.

44
Basal TEWL rates and skin permeability

RP Chilcott, CH Dalton, AJ Emanuel, A Patel, Z Ashley, CE Allen and ST Bradley

Introduction

Transepidermal water loss (TEWL) is the normal, constitutive loss of water vapour from the skin in the absence of sweat-gland activity.[1] The development of robust instrumentation for measuring TEWL rates has provided an invaluable tool for the non-invasive evaluation of skin function in diseased and damaged skin.[2–4] As such, TEWL has become a ubiquitous parameter of in vivo skin studies.

TEWL is commonly ascribed to be a measure of skin barrier function, either at baseline,[5,6] or following topical treatments.[7,8] More precisely, TEWL is thought to represent the water-barrier function of the skin.[9]

The purpose of this study was to investigate the relationship between TEWL and skin permeability in vitro, to validate the assumption that TEWL is an appropriate measure of skin barrier function. Excised skin is free of many factors that may potentially affect TEWL and/or skin absorption rates, such as variations in blood perfusion,[10] temperature fluctuations,[11] sweat-gland activity,[12] metabolism,[13] and other diurnal variations.[14,15] In addition, the permeability of excised skin can be measured directly using validated, standard techniques.[16] Thus, an in vitro investigation of the relationship between TEWL and skin permeability may arguably be considered superior to in vivo studies. In this study, sulphur mustard (bis-[2-chloroethyl]sulphide, SM) was used as a model lipophilic penetrant[17,18] to complement the use of tritiated water.

Materials and methods

Chemicals

Dulbecco's phosphate-buffered saline (DPBS), gentamycin and ethanol (100%) were purchased from the Sigma-Aldrich Chemical Company (Poole, UK). Liquid scintillation (LS) counting fluid (Emulsifier-safe) was purchased from the Canberra-Packard Chemical Co (Michigan, USA).

Tritiated water (^3H_2O) was purchased from NEN Life Science Products (Hounslow, UK). Radiolabelled sulphur mustard (^{35}SM) was synthesized at CBD Porton Down (purity >98%). The majority of experiments were conducted in an environmentally controlled chamber (40 ± 2% relative humidity (RH), 20 ± 0.5°C). Skin absorption of ^{35}SM was measured in a normal laboratory fume cupboard (35–55% RH, 20 ± 3°C).

Skin

Full-thickness, pig-back skin was obtained from Large White pigs (*Sus scrofa domestica*) bred at CBD Porton Down (six animals in total, weight range 30–40 kg). Subcutaneous fat was dissected from each piece of skin and the (epidermal) surface was carefully clipped to remove excess hair prior to storage at –25°C for a maximum of 14 days. Human epidermal membranes were prepared and stored as previously described[17] by heat separation of full-thickness breast skin.[19]

Diffusion cells

Full-thickness pig skin or human epidermal membranes were placed into Franz-type[20] glass diffusion cells, with an available skin surface area of 2.54 cm^2, and a 5-ml receptor chamber containing DPBS (containing 86.6 $\mu g.ml^{-1}$ gentamycin) or 50% aqueous ethanol (for SM penetration study). Groups of six diffusion cells were mounted on purpose-built aluminium heating blocks (CBD Porton Down), heated to 35°C to attain a skin-surface temperature of 31 ± 1.5°C. Each heating block was placed on a six-place magnetic stirrer bed (Whatman; Kent, UK) that stirred the receptor fluid of each diffusion cell via a magnetic follower.

Measurement of transepidermal water loss

TEWL was measured using a calibrated, ServoMed EP-3 Evaporimeter (ServoMed; Varberg, Sweden) in accordance with current guidelines.[12] A 1.5-cm stainless steel collar was attached to the TEWL probe in order to ensure contact with the pig skin or human epidermal membranes in each diffusion cell. The probe collar was placed on the skin surface for 60 seconds prior to an average rate being taken over a 15-second measurement period. The probe was immediately serviced after the experiments, using 50% ethanol water receptor chamber fluid, as ethanol has been reported to have adverse effects on the TEWL probe.[21]

Measurement of skin permeability

Skin water-barrier function was measured directly using ^3H_2O (1 ml, 10 $\mu Ci.ml^{-1}$) placed into the donor chamber of cells containing full-thickness pig skin or human epidermal membranes. Samples (20 μl) of receptor chamber fluid were removed at 0-, 1-, 2-, 4- and 6-hour intervals, placed into 5 ml LS counting fluid and analysed using a Wallac 1409DSA LS counter. The amount of radioactivity in each sample was related to the amount of ^3H_2O, by reference to standards prepared and measured simultaneously. Skin absorption rates were calculated by linear regression analysis of the amount of ^3H_2O penetrated against time between 2 and 6 hours (steady state, where the amount penetrating per unit time was constant). Skin absorption of ^{35}SM through human epidermal membranes was measured under unoccluded conditions, as previously described.[17]

Protocol

Diffusion cells (containing heat-separated human epidermal membranes or full-thickness pig skin) were assembled in an environmentally controlled chamber on day 1. On day 2, baseline measurements of TEWL were taken, prior to measurement of ^3H_2O skin permeability (conducted in situ) or ^{35}SM (conducted within a fume cupboard in a laboratory that was not equipped with a rigorous environmental-control system).

Statistical analysis

Rates of TEWL were analysed using a multivariate analysis of variation, followed by Dunnet's adjustment for multiple comparisons post test (one-sided). Correlation coefficient (r^2) values were used to evaluate the linear regression analysis of skin absorption rates. If r^2 was <0.90, the data was deemed to be non-linear (i.e. steady-state conditions were not attained).

Results

Penetration of ^3H_2O through human epidermal membranes

A total of 48 epidermal membranes were placed into diffusion cells and subject to ^3H_2O-permeability measurements. Following linear regression analysis (of the amount of ^3H_2O penetrated against time), six of these membranes were rejected on the basis of the correlation coefficient (r^2) being <0.90. A further two were subsequently rejected, as nearly all ($>93\%$) the applied dose had penetrated within 1 hour and, whilst the linear correlation coefficients were high ($r^2>0.94$), the apparently low calculated fluxes (measured between 2 and 6 hours) were meaningless. The remaining flux values were plotted against initial TEWL rates (Figure 44.1a), which indicated that there was no correlation between TEWL rates and ^3H_2O permeability ($r^2=0.26$). Similarly, a plot of the total amount

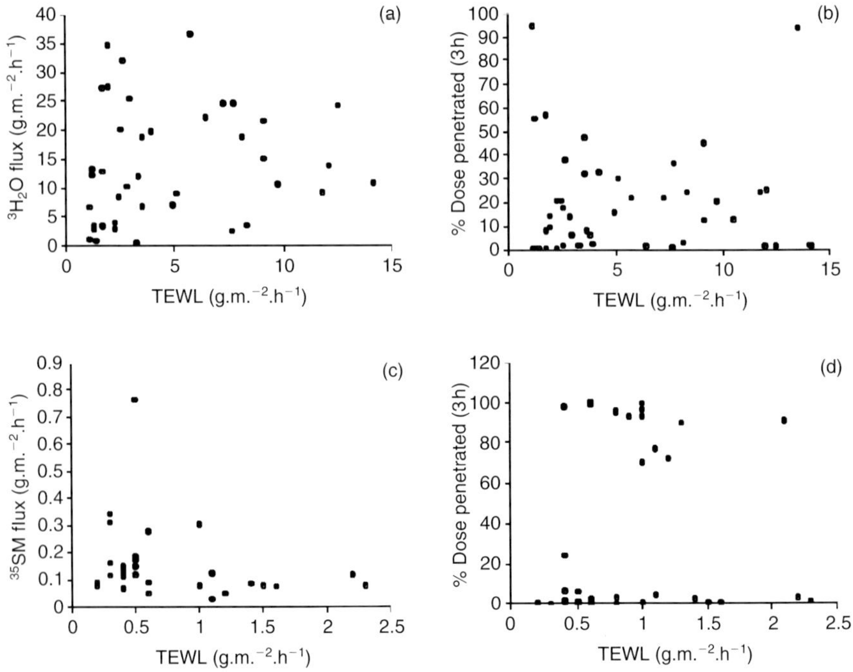

Figure 44.1

(a–d) Skin absorption rates of ^3H_2O (a; n = 40) and ^{35}SM (c; n = 32) and percentage of applied dose of ^3H_2O (b; n = 48) and ^{35}SM (d; n = 48) penetrated at 3 hours, through heat-separated human epidermal membranes, plotted as a function of TEWL rate, measured under controlled environmental conditions (40% RH, 20°C). Diffusion cells contained skin derived from up to seven individuals.

of ^3H_2O penetrated (at 3 hours) against TEWL rates for all 48 epidermal membranes did not indicate any correlation (Figure 44.1b).

Penetration of ^{35}SM through human epidermal membranes

Skin absorption rates of ^{35}SM were subject to the same criteria as above, and resulted in 15 membranes being rejected from 48, on the basis of allowing a high percentage of applied dose to penetrate (>70%); one additional membrane was rejected on the basis of a poor linear correlation coefficient ($r^2 < 0.90$). A plot of ^{35}SM skin absorption rates against TEWL (n = 32) indicated no apparent correlation ($r^2 = 0.24$; Figure 44.1c), as did a plot of percentage of applied dose penetrated at 3 hours against TEWL for all epidermal membranes (n = 48, Figure 44.1d).

Penetration of ^3H_2O through full-thickness pig skin

Fluxes of ^3H_2O and TEWL rates were measured using a total of 144 pieces of skin (obtained from six separate animals). When plotted as ^3H_2O flux against TEWL, there was no correlation between the two parameters (Figure 44.2).

A summary of the linear regression analysis for all data is presented in Table 44.1.

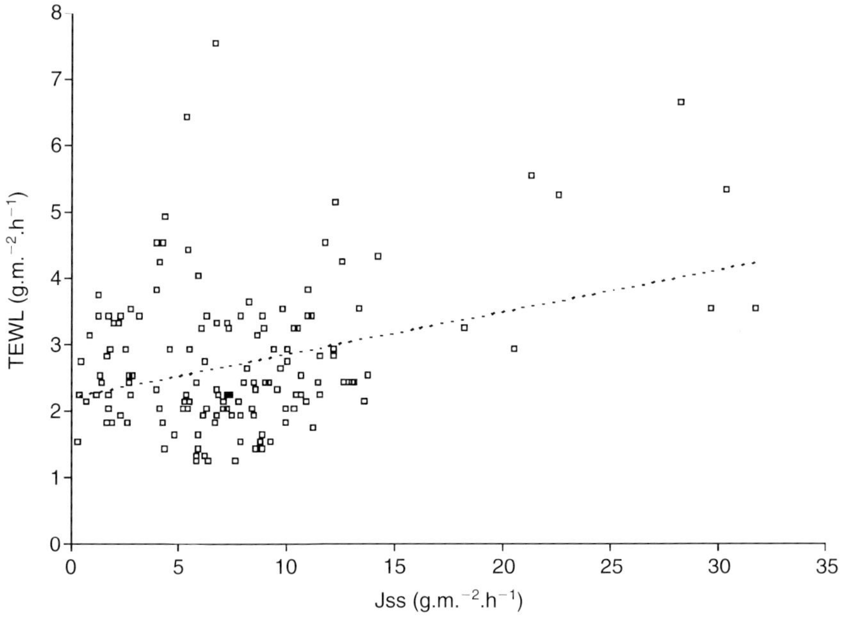

Figure 44.2

Baseline ^3H_2O-permeation and baseline TEWL-rate data from all experiments, using full-thickness pig skin, conducted during this study (using n = 144 pieces of skin from n = 6 animals). Dotted line indicates result of linear regression analysis ($r^2 = 0.1075$).

Table 44.1 Summary of the statistical relationship between TEWL and skin permeability to tritiated water (^3H_2O) or sulphur mustard (^{35}SM), measured in this in vitro study.

Species	Penetrant	TEWL:^3H_2O Flux	p
Human epidermal membranes	^{35}SM	No correlation	0.74
	^3H_2O	No correlation	0.72
Full-thickness pig skin	^3H_2O	No correlation	0.68

Discussion

It is logical to assume that changes in TEWL represent alterations to the skin's 'barrier function' (permeability), as it is consistent with the fact that the stratum corneum is the main barrier to the egress of water and ingress of most xenobiotics.[22] Thus, TEWL rates are frequently interpreted as damage to skin barrier function following exposure to various chemical or physical insults. Indeed, studies by Lotte et al[5] and Nangia et al[6] have indicated a linear correlation between TEWL rates and skin permeability in vivo and in vitro. The results of this in vitro study clearly do not concur with the supposition that baseline TEWL rates are a reflection of intrinsic skin barrier function.

The environment under which measurements of TEWL and skin permeability were conducted during this study was subject to rigorous control. In addition, each group of six diffusion cells contained human skin matched from the same individual, where possible. These measures were introduced to reduce variation due to temperature, humidity or inter-individual variation, etc., factors which are known to influence TEWL and skin permeability.[23] In addition, a post-study analysis was used to identify both structurally viable and damaged skin membranes. The results of this study clearly indicate that there was no correlation between TEWL and skin permeability to $^{3}H_2O$ or ^{35}SM in structurally viable human skin. Furthermore, TEWL failed to identify damaged epidermal membranes. This was particularly evident for ^{35}SM skin absorption, where there was a distinct difference in the percentage dose penetrated between viable and compromised skin membranes. In addition, the full-thickness pig skin data for baseline $^{3}H_2O$ fluxes measured in this study also showed a lack of correlation ($r^2 = 0.11$) with baseline TEWL values (Figure 44.2). Therefore, these data strongly imply that baseline TEWL rates cannot be used as a tool to evaluate epidermal membrane integrity prior to in vitro percutaneous absorption experiments using epidermal membranes or full-thickness pig skin.

The results of this study clearly demonstrate that basal TEWL rates do not correlate with baseline skin permeability to water or SM. These data infer that TEWL rates should not be unconditionally ascribed to be a measure of skin barrier function. It is evident that further work is required to elucidate the meaning of TEWL rates, given their increasing utility in clinical studies. With regard to measuring skin barrier function by evaporimetry, perhaps the fundamental principle, that the gradient of water vapour on the skin surface represents skin barrier function, should be questioned.

Acknowledgements

The authors would like to thank Mr Ben Stubbs for his technical assistance. This work was funded by the UK Ministry of Defence (MoD), at facilities operated by the Defence science technology laboratory (Dstl).

References

1. Pinson EA. Evaporation from human skin with sweat glands inactivated. Am J Physiol 1942; 187:492–503.
2. Lamke L-O, Nilsson GE, Reithner HL. Insensible perspiration from the skin under standardized environmental conditions. Scand J Clin Lab Invest 1977; 37:325–31.
3. Nilsson GE. Measurement of water exchange through skin. Med Biol Eng Comput 1977; 15: 209–18.
4. Idson B. In vivo measurement of transepidermal water loss. J Soc Cosmet Chem 1978; 29:573–80.
5. Lotte C, Rougier A, Wilson DR et al. In vivo relationship between transepidermal water loss and percutaneous penetration of some organic compounds in man: effect of anatomic site. Dermatol Res 1987; 279:351–6.
6. Nangia A, Berner B, Maibach HI. Transepidermal water loss measurements for assessing absorption experiments. In: RL Bronaugh RL, Maibach HI, eds. *Percutaneous Absorption: Drugs – Cosmetics – Skin Barrier Function During In Vitro Percutaneous Mechanisms – Methodology.* Third edn. New York: Marcel Dekker Inc, 1999:chap 34.
7. Nicander I, Ollmar S, Eek A et al. Correlation of impedance response patterns to histological findings in irritant skin reactions induced by various surfactants. Br J Dermatol 1996; 134:221–8.
8. Freeman S, Maibach HI. Study of irritant contact dermatitis produced by repeat patch test with sodium lauryl sulfate and assessed by visual methods, transepidermal water loss, and laser Doppler velocimetry. J Am Acad Dermatol 1988; 19:496–502.
9. Pinnagoda J, Tupker RA. Measurement of transepidermal water loss. In: Serup J, Jemec GBE, eds. *Handbook of Non-invasive Methods and the Skin.* London: CRC Press, 1995:chap 9.
10. Benowitz NL, Jacob III, Olsson P et al. Intravenous nicotine retards transdermal absorption of nicotine: evidence of blood-flow limited percutaneous absorption. Clin Pharmacol Ther 1992; 52:223–30.
11. Blank IH, Scheuplein RJ. Transport into and within the skin. Br J Dermatol 1969; 81:4–10.
12. Pinnagoda J, Tupker RA, Agner T et al. Guidelines for transepidermal water loss (TEWL) measurement. Contact Dermatitis 1990; 22:164–78.
13. Kao J, Hall J, Shugert LR et al. An in vitro approach to studying cutaneous metabolism and disposition of topically applied xenobiotics. Toxicol Appl Pharmacol 1984; 75:289–98.
14. Yosipovitch G, Xiong GL, Haus E et al. Time dependant variations of the skin barrier function in humans: transepidermal water loss, stratum corneum hydration, skin surface skin temperature. J Invest Dermatol 1998; 110:20–3.

15. Chilcott RP, Farrar R. Biophysical measurements of human forearm skin in vivo: effects of site, gender, chirality and time. Skin Res Technol 2000; 6:64–9.
16. Howes D, Guy R, Hadgraft J et al. Methods for assessing percutaneous absorption. ATLA 1996; 24:81–106.
17. Chilcott RP, Jenner J, Carrick W et al. Human skin absorption of bis-2-(chloroethyl)sulphide (sulphur mustard) in vitro. J Appl Toxicol 2000; 20:349–55.
18. Chilcott RP, Jenner J, Hotchkiss SAM et al. In vitro skin absorption and decontamination of sulphur mustard: comparison of human and pig ear skin. J Appl Toxicol 2001; 21:279–83.
19. Kligman AM, Christophers E. Preparation of isolated sheets of human stratum corneum. Arch Dermatol 1963; 88:70–3.
20. Franz TJ. Percutaneous absorption. On the relevance of in vitro data. J Invest Dermatol 1975; 64:190–5.
21. Abrams K, Harvell JD, Shriner S et al. Effect of organic solvents on in vitro human skin water barrier. J Invest Dermatol 1993; 101: 609–13.
22. Scheuplein RJ, Blank IH. Permeability of the skin. Physiol Rev 1971; 51:702–45.
23. Schaefer H, Redelmeier TE. Factors affecting percutaneous absorption. In: Schaefer H, Redelmeier TE, eds. *Skin Barrier: Principles of Percutaneous Absorption*. London: Karger 1996:153–212.

45
The effects of chemical damage on TEWL

RP Chilcott, A Patel, Z Ashley, JN Hughes and JA Parkes

Introduction

The gradient of water vapour immediately above the skin surface can be accurately measured by evaporimetry.[1–3] This gradient can be equated to the rate at which water is lost from the skin, and is termed transepidermal water loss (TEWL). As a semipermeable membrane, there is a constant level of TEWL in normal skin,[4–6] and exposure to certain skin-damaging agents can elevate in vivo TEWL rates.[7–11] An obvious interpretation of increased TEWL is that damage has occurred to the barrier layer of the skin, resulting in increased permeability to water.

Whilst it is logical to assume that TEWL is a reflection of skin water-barrier function,[12] it is difficult to investigate this relationship in vivo without making direct measurements of skin permeability. In contrast, the use of excised skin in vitro is free of many factors that may potentially affect TEWL and/or skin absorption rates, such as variations in blood perfusion,[13] temperature fluctuations,[14] sweat-gland activity,[15] metabolism,[16] and other diurnal variations.[17,18] In addition, the permeability of excised skin can be measured directly using validated, standard techniques.[19] Thus, an in vitro investigation of the relationship between TEWL and skin permeability may arguably be considered superior to in vivo studies.

The purpose of this study was to investigate the relationship between TEWL and skin permeability in vitro (measured directly using tritiated water), following exposure to the model skin irritant sodium lauryl sulphate (SLS), to validate the assumption that TEWL is an appropriate measure of skin barrier function.

Materials and methods

Chemicals

Dulbecco's phosphate-buffered saline (DPBS), gentamycin and SLS

(>99.9%) were purchased from the Sigma-Aldrich Chemical Company (Poole, UK). Liquid scintillation (LS) counting fluid (Emulsifier-safe) and Soluene-350 were purchased from the Canberra-Packard Chemical Co (Michigan, USA). Tritiated water (^3H_2O) was purchased from NEN Life Science Products (Hounslow, UK). Radiolabelled SLS (^{14}C-SLS, >99%) was obtained from Tocris Cookson (Bristol, UK). All experiments were conducted in an environmentally controlled chamber (40 ± 2% relative humidity (RH), 20 ± 0.5°C).

Skin

Full-thickness pig-back skin was freshly obtained from Large White pigs (*Sus scrofa domestica*), bred at CBD Porton Down (two animals in total, weight range 30–40 kg). Subcutaneous fat was dissected from each piece of skin and the (epidermal) surface was carefully clipped to remove excess hair prior to storage at –25°C for a maximum of 14 days.

Diffusion cells

Full-thickness pig skin was placed into a Franz-type[20] glass diffusion cell, with an available skin surface area of 2.54 cm^2 and a 5-ml receptor chamber containing DPBS (containing 86.6 $\mu g.ml^{-1}$ gentamycin). Groups of six diffusion cells were mounted on purpose-built aluminium heating blocks (CBD Porton Down), heated to 35°C to attain a skin-surface temperature of 31 ± 1.5°C. Each heating block was placed on a six-place magnetic stirrer bed (Whatman; Kent, UK) that stirred the receptor fluid of each diffusion cell via a magnetic follower. All diffusion cells were left to equilibrate in the environmental chamber for at least 24 hours prior to measurements of TEWL or skin permeability.

Measurement of TEWL

TEWL was measured using a calibrated, ServoMed EP-3 Evaporimeter (ServoMed; Varberg, Sweden) in accordance with current guidelines.[15] A 1.5-cm stainless steel collar was attached to the TEWL probe in order to ensure contact with the pig skin or human epidermal membranes in each diffusion cell. The probe collar was placed on the skin surface for 60 seconds prior to an average rate being taken over a 15-second measurement period.

Measurement of skin permeability

Skin water-barrier function was measured directly using ^3H_2O (1 ml, 10 $\mu Ci.ml^{-1}$) placed into the donor chamber of cells containing full-thickness pig skin. Samples (20 µl) of receptor-chamber fluid were removed at

0-, 1-, 2-, 4- and 6-hour intervals, placed into 5 ml LS counting fluid and analysed using a Wallac 1409DSA LS counter. The amount of radioactivity in each sample was related to the amount of $^{3}H_2O$ by reference to standards prepared and measured simultaneously. Skin absorption rates were calculated by linear regression analysis of the amount of $^{3}H_2O$ penetrated against time between 2 and 6 hours (steady state, where the amount penetrating per unit time was constant).

SLS skin damage

Five concentrations (0.25%, 0.5%, 1.0%, 2.0% and 5.0% w/v) of SLS were investigated. Aliquots (1 ml) were placed into donor chambers that were subsequently sealed using parafilm (American National Can Corp; Greenwich, USA). After 2 hours, the solution remaining on the skin surface was removed by continuous swabbing with cotton until the surface was visually dry.

Skin absorption of SLS

Skin absorption of ^{14}C-SLS (1 ml, 10 μCi.ml^{-1}) was measured following 2 hours' exposure to various SLS solutions (0.25–5.0% w/v) by removal of 20-μl samples of receptor chamber fluid. The donor chambers were rinsed with 5 × 2 ml DPBS and the skin removed and placed into 20 ml Soluene-350. Samples (20 μl) of donor rinses and solublized skin were analysed by LS counting, as above, with appropriate standards prepared and measured simultaneously.

Skin-damage protocol

Diffusion cells were assembled within the environmentally controlled chamber on day 1. On day 2, baseline (–24 h) TEWL and $^{3}H_2O$ measurements were taken. Skin damage (by SLS) was conducted on the third day. Day 4 comprised a 24-hour post-damage measure of TEWL and $^{3}H_2O$ permeability, which was followed on subsequent days (relating to 48, 72 and 96 hours post-damage) with TEWL measurements only.

Electron microscopy

Following removal from the diffusion cells, the SLS-treated skin samples were fixed with 3% (v/v) glutaraldehyde solution in 0.1 mol.l^{-1} sodium cacodylate buffer (pH 7.4) for a minimum of 24 hours. Four transverse strips (1 × 2 mm) of fixed skin were cut from random areas of each sample, dehydrated in graded ethanol and dried in a Polaron CPD7501 critical point drier (Agar Scientific; Essex, UK) using carbon dioxide as the transitional fluid. Skin strips were orientated for cross-sectional imaging, sputter-coated with gold under vacuum, and examined using a Hitachi S800 field emission scanning electron microscope (Hitachi Scientific Instruments; Wokingham, UK). Skin morphology was observed and, in a blind study, electron micrographs were taken of the upper skin layers from central and end regions of each of the sample strips, and digitally recorded using a Printerface image-capturing system (KE Developments Ltd; Cambridge, UK). Using a pre-determined template, measurements of the number of coherent layers of corneocytes within the stratum corneum (SC) (layer number) and total SC thickness were made directly from the calibrated micrographs.

Statistical analysis

Comparison of ^3H_2O flux pre- and post-damage were analysed using a paired, non-parametric test (Wilcoxon signed rank) subject to adequate pairing, as indicated by the Spearman correlation coefficient. Ineffectively paired data were analysed using the Mann–Whitney test. Rates of TEWL were analysed using a multivariate analysis of variation, followed by Dunnet's adjustment for multiple comparisons post-test (one-sided). Correlation coefficient (r^2) values were used to evaluate the linear regression analysis of skin absorption rates. If r^2 was <0.90, the data was deemed to be non-linear (i.e. steady-state conditions were not attained).

Results

Effects of SLS exposure on full-thickness pig skin

Rates of TEWL significantly increased ($p<0.05$) after 2 hours of exposure to 1%, 2% and 5% solutions of SLS (Figure 45.1). This increase was dose dependent ($r^2=0.94$), with the highest increase in TEWL being attained following exposure to the 5% solution (2.5-fold at 48 hours) and the lowest increase for the 1% solution (1.2-fold at 48 hours). There was no significant change in TEWL rates for skin exposed to 0% (control), 0.25% or 0.5% solutions.

A similar change was measured in ^3H_2O fluxes, in that 2-hour exposure to 1%, 2% and 5% solutions resulted in a significant increase in permeability at 24 hours (Figure 45.2) relating to a 1.5-fold, 1.9-fold and 2.2-fold increase, respectively ($r^2=0.97$). Concentrations of SLS up to 0.5% caused a corresponding decrease in both SC thickness and layer number (Table 45.1). Above a concentration of 1%, there was no further decrease in thickness or layer number. The concentration-dependent effects of SLS on SC morphology are illustrated in Figure 45.3.

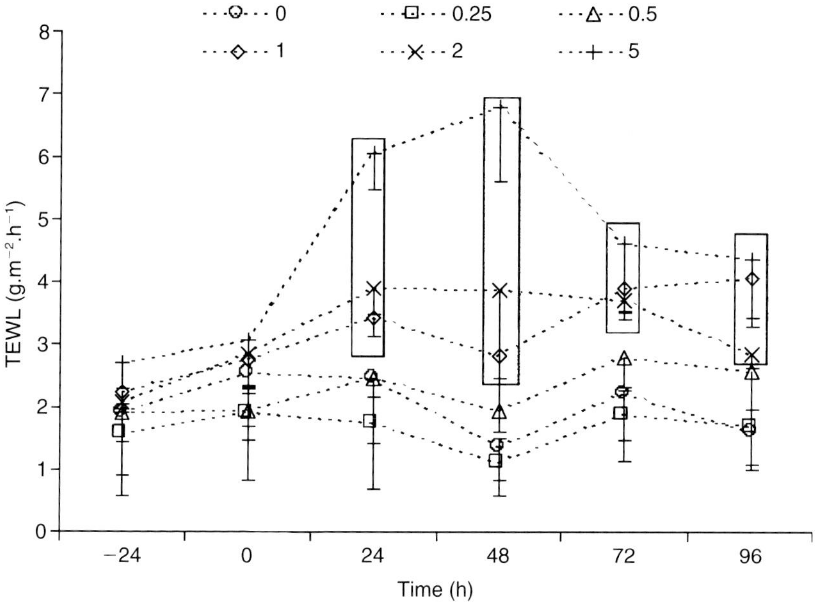

Figure 45.1

Variation in TEWL measured from full-thickness pig-back skin before (–24 hours) and up to 96 hours after exposure (2 hours) to SLS (dose expressed in legend as % w/v). Study was conducted under controlled environmental conditions (40% RH, 20°C). All values are mean ± SD of n = 6 diffusion cells, containing skin from up to two animals. Boxed TEWL values indicate values that are significantly different ($p < 0.05$) from those of controls.

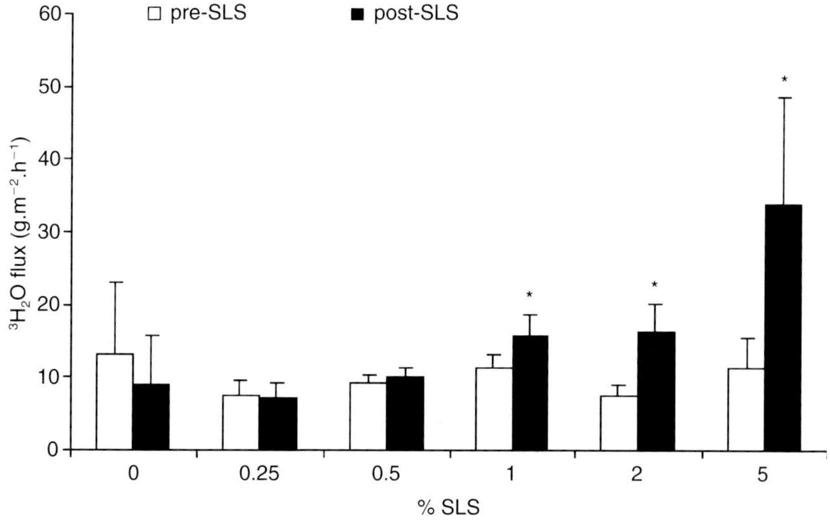

Figure 45.2

Variation in ^3H_2O flux measured from full-thickness pig-back skin pre (–24 hours) and post (24 hours) exposure (2 hours) to SLS (dose expressed in legend as % w/v). Study was conducted under controlled environmental conditions (40% RH, 20°C). All values are mean ± SD of n = 6 diffusion cells, containing skin from up to two animals. ^3H_2O fluxes with an asterisk are significantly different ($p < 0.05$) from those of controls at that time point.

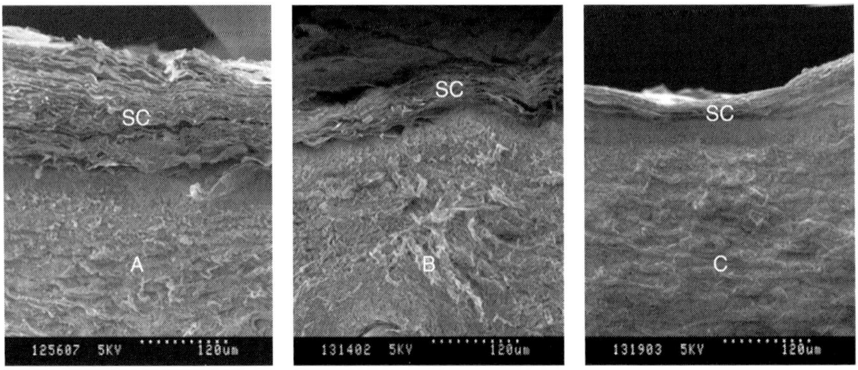

Figure 45.3

Representative scanning electron micrographs of upper region of full-thickness pig skin, demonstrating changes in the thickness of SC exposed to (A) 0% (control), (B) 1%, and (C) 5% solutions of SLS for 2 hours.

Table 45.1 Number of layers comprising the SC (layer number), SC thickness (thickness) and ^3H_2O skin permeability, 24 hours after a 2-hour exposure to varying concentrations of SLS. All values are mean ± SD of n=6 measurements. Asterisks indicate significant difference between exposed and control skin.

% SLS (w/v)	Layer number	Thickness (μm)	Permeability ($g.m^{-2}.h^{-1}$)
0	31 ± 14	94 ± 35	9.0 ± 6.8
0.25	18 ± 3*	58 ± 7*	7.2 ± 1.9
0.50	11 ± 2*	70 ± 12	10.0 ± 1.2
1.0	12 ± 1*	50 ± 4*	15.8 ± 2.8*
2.0	14 ± 2*	55 ± 7*	16.3 ± 3.8*
5.0	12 ± 1*	54 ± 11*	33.8 ± 14.9*

Skin absorption and dose distribution of ^{14}C-SLS

Baseline skin absorption rates of ^3H_2O (conducted 24 hours prior to the addition of ^{14}C-SLS) averaged 9.14 ± 3.06 $g.m^{-2}.h^{-1}$. The amount of ^{14}C-SLS recovered from the donor chambers was dose dependent ($p < 0.05$), as was the quantity of ^{14}C-SLS recovered from within the skin after the 2-hour exposure (Table 45.2). There was no significant difference in the amount of ^{14}C-SLS recovered from the receptor chambers after 2 hours.

Table 45.2 Quantities of ^{14}C-SLS (delivered from five concentrations) recovered from the donor, skin and receptor-chamber compartments of diffusion cells, 2 hours post-exposure. All values are mean ± SD of n = 6 diffusion cells, containing skin from two animals. Superscript letters indicate a significant difference ($p < 0.05$) between different concentrations of the same-labelled parameter within each compartment.

	Compartment				
Concentration SLS (%w/v)	Donor (mg)	Skin (μg)	Receptor (mg)	Total (mg)	Recovery (%)
0.25	1.8 ± 0.1[a]	3.9 ± 0.3[d]	1.2 ± 0.2	2.9 ± 0.2	117
0.50	4.0 ± 0.3[b,c]	5.0 ± 0.6[e,f]	1.0 ± 0.2	5.0 ± 0.5	99
1.00	8.6 ± 0.3	8.8 ± 2.0	1.4 ± 0.2	9.9 ± 0.5	99
2.00	14.9 ± 0.4[c]	15.1 ± 8.0[f]	1.3 ± 0.1	16.2 ± 0.5	80
5.00	42.9 ± 5.0[a,b]	24.6 ± 8.0[d,e]	1.4 ± 0.3	44.4 ± 5.2	88

Discussion

This study has confirmed that SLS causes a dose-dependant increase in TEWL and ^3H_2O permeability. There was a good correlation between the change in TEWL rates and ^3H_2O flux ($p = 0.02$). However, the increases in TEWL rates were substantially lower than in previous in vivo studies, indicating that, in vivo, the increase in TEWL following exposure to SLS may be mediated by other factors in addition to a compromised barrier.

Pig skin has been utilized previously as a model for measuring both skin permeability[21,22] and changes in TEWL following exposure to dermatotoxic chemicals,[23,24] and is generally accepted to be a good model for human skin.[19,25] In this study, skin disposition of SLS measured in pig skin in vitro was similar to that previously measured in vitro using human skin,[26,27] indicating good inter-species correlation. However, few studies have investigated the effect of irritants such as SLS on pig skin, in vitro or in vivo. In one relevant study, 24 hours of exposure to 2.5–10% SLS caused a dose-independent, transient increase in TEWL that was attributable to occlusion of the test site rather than an irritant reaction.[23] In this present study, 2 hours of exposure to 1%, 2% or 5% SLS led to a small, but significant, dose-dependent elevation in TEWL with a concomitant increase in skin permeability to ^3H_2O. Thus, the dose-dependent results of this in vitro study with pig skin are not in accordance with in vivo studies using hairless micropigs, but are in agreement with previous studies using other animal models[28] and human skin, both in vivo[29,30] and in vitro.[9]

The increase in TEWL following SLS exposure measured in this in vitro study was notably less than in comparable studies using human skin in vivo. Whilst this may have been due to the relatively short exposure time (2 hours), a similar disparity in the order of magnitude of change of TEWL between in vitro and in vivo conditions has previously been reported with human skin.[9] Together, these data indicate that only a limited proportion of the change in TEWL rates is due to altered water-barrier function and, thus, it is conceivable that other factors are mainly responsible for the elevation of TEWL in vivo, such as blood perfusion, temperature, sweat-gland activity and diurnal variation.[13–15,17,18]

The dose-dependent increases in TEWL and ^3H_2O permeability measured in this study indicate that SLS impairs the water-barrier function of the SC by altering one or more of the parameters affecting water diffusion, such as diffusional path length, partitioning and/or diffusivity. The actual mechanism of barrier impairment by SLS is of some debate. For example, the assumption of SC delipidization[31] has been questioned.[9,32,33] Alternatively, it has been suggested that SLS may hyperhydrate the SC through the creation of water-binding sites on denatured proteins.[9,32,34,35] Additionally, there may also be changes in the morphology of the SC and lower epidermal layers.[7,33,36–38] The results of this study indicate that removal of the upper layers of the SC may be involved in the increase in TEWL and skin permeability (Figure 45.3). This would be in agreement with previous work demonstrating desmosomal damage that may loosen cohesion between adjacent corneocytes.[38] This process could reasonably be expected to be irreversible in this in vitro study, as the skin had been frozen and subject to nutrient-free media for at least 24 hours prior to tape-stripping. Previous studies have demonstrated that skin tissue, placed in diffusion cells under optimum conditions, is viable for less than 24 hours and may also contain necrotic tissue.[39,40] Consequently, any energy-requiring repair processes would almost certainly be absent in our in vitro model and the skin tissue could be considered to be 'dead'. However, the maximum increase in TEWL (at 48 hours) following exposure to 5% SLS was followed by a notable decrease after 72 hours. It is possible that this was due to subsequent dehydration of the skin,[35] conceivably a direct consequence of increased water loss from the SC or subsequent penetration of the SLS into the receptor chamber fluid,[27,32] i.e. removal of the causative agent from the SC. Alternatively, SLS may cause enhanced TEWL and permeability by increasing the thermodynamic activity of water within the SC. This could be caused by hyperhydration (as already mentioned), its surfactant activity allowing more water to 'dissolve' within the lipid matrix, or through releasing water from previously irreversible binding sites within the SC (which would explain subsequent skin dehydration). Whilst this study suggests an additional mechanism for SLS-induced skin barrier damage through premature sloughing of the SC, it is clear that the effects of SLS are complex and further investigation is warranted.

In summary, there is a correlation between TEWL and skin permeability to ^3H_2O in vitro following exposure to SLS, but the magnitude of change in TEWL rates is lower than that generally observed in vivo.

Acknowledgements

The authors would like to thank Mr B Stubbs and Mrs J Platt for their technical help. This work was funded by the UK Ministry of Defence (MoD), at facilities operated by the Defence science and technology laboratory (Dstl).

References

1. Lamke L-O, Nilsson GE, Reithner HL. Insensible perspiration from the skin under standardized environmental conditions. Scand J Clin Lab Invest 1977; 37:325–31.
2. Nilsson GE. Measurement of water exchange through skin. Med Biol Eng Comput 1977; 15: 209–18.
3. Idson B. In vivo measurement of transepidermal water loss. J Soc Cosmet Chem 1978; 29:573–80.
4. Pinson EA. Evaporation from human skin with sweat glands inactivated. Am J Physiol 1942; 187:492–503.
5. Lotte C, Rougier A, Wilson DR et al. In vivo relationship between transepidermal water loss and percutaneous penetration of some organic compounds in man: effect of anatomic site. Dermatol Res 1987; 279:351–6.
6. Nangia A, Berner B, Maibach HI. Transepidermal water loss measurements for assessing skin barrier function during in vitro percutaneous absorption experiments. In: Bronaugh RL, Maibach HI, eds. *Percutaneous Absorption: Drugs – Cosmetics – Mechanisms – Methodology*. Third edn. New York: Marcel Dekker Inc, 1999: chap 34.
7. Nicander I, Ollmar S, Eek A et al. Correlation of impedance response patterns to histological findings in irritant skin reactions induced by various surfactants. Br J Dermatol 1996; 134:221–8.
8. Freeman S, Maibach HI. Study of irritant contact dermatitis produced by repeat patch test with sodium lauryl sulfate and assessed by visual methods, transepidermal water loss, and laser Doppler velocimetry. J Am Acad Dermatol 1988; 19:496–502.
9. Lévêque JL, de Rigal J, Saint-Léger D et al. How does sodium lauryl sulfate alter the skin barrier function in man? A multiparametric approach. Skin Pharmacol 1993; 6:111–15.
10. Van der Valk PGM, Maibach HI. A functional study of the skin barrier to evaporative water loss by means of repeated cellophane-tape stripping. Clin Exp Dermatol 1990; 15:180–2.
11. Lamaud E, Schalla W. Influence of UV irradiation on penetration of hydrocortisone. In vivo study in hairless rat skin. Br J Dermatol 1984; 111:152–7.
12. Pinnagoda J, Tupker RA. Measurement of transepidermal water loss. In: Serup J, Jemec GBE, eds. *Handbook of Non-invasive*

Methods and the Skin. London: CRC Press, 1995:chap 9.

13. Benowitz NL, Jacob III, Olsson P et al. Intravenous nicotine retards transdermal absorption of nicotine: evidence of blood-flow limited percutaneous absorption. Clin Pharmacol Ther 1992; 52:223–30.
14. Blank IH, Scheuplein RJ. Transport into and within the skin. Br J Dermatol 196; 81:4–10.
15. Pinnagoda J, Tupker RA, Agner T et al. Guidelines for transepidermal water loss (TEWL) measurement. Contact Dermatitis 1990; 22:164–78.
16. Kao J, Hall J, Shugert LR et al. An in vitro approach to studying cutaneous metabolism and disposition of topically applied xenobiotics. Toxicol Appl Pharmacol 1984; 75:289–98.
17. Yosipovitch G, Xiong GL, Haus E et al. Time dependant variations of the skin barrier function in humans: transepidermal water loss, stratum corneum hydration, skin surface skin temperature. J Invest Dermatol 1998; 110:20–3.
18. Chilcott RP, Farrar R. Biophysical measurements of human forearm skin in vivo: effects of site, gender, chirality and time. Skin Res Technol 2000; 6:64–9.
19. Howes D, Guy R, Hadgraft J et al. Methods for assessing percutaneous absorption. ATLA 1996; 24: 81–106.
20. Franz TJ. Percutaneous absorption. On the relevance of in vitro data. J Invest Dermatol 1975; 64: 190–5.
21. Bartek MJ, LaBudde JA, Maibach HI. Skin permeability in vivo: comparison in rat, rabbit, pig and man. J Invest Dermatol 1972; 58: 114–23.
22. Dick IP, Scott RC. Pig ear skin as an in vitro model for human skin permeability. J Pharm Pharmacol 1992; 44:640–5.
23. Gabard B, Treffel P, Charton-Pickard F et al. Irritant reactions on hairless micropig skin: a model for testing barrier creams? In: Elsner P, Maibach HI, eds. Irritant Dermatitis. *New Clinical and Experimental Aspects. Current Problems in Dermatology.* Basel: Kerger, 1995; 23:271–87.
24. Chilcott RP, Brown RFR, Rice P. Noninvasive quantification of skin injury following exposure to sulphur mustard and Lewisite vapours. Burns 2000; 26:245–50.
25. Montagna W, Yun Y. The skin of the domestic pig. J Invest Dermatol 1964; 43:11–21.
26. Blank IH, Gould E. Penetration of anionic surfactants (surface active agents) into skin. J Invest Dermatol 1959; 33:327–35.
27. Fullerton A, Broby-Johansen U, Agner T. Sodium lauryl sulphate penetration in an in vitro model using human skin. Contact Dermatitis 1994; 30:222–5.
28. Frosch PJ, Schulze-Dirks A, Hoffman M et al. Efficacy of skin barrier creams. (II) Ineffectiveness of a popular 'skin protector' against various irritants in the repetitive irritation test in the guinea pig. Contact Dermatitis 1993; 29:74–7.
29. Tupker RA, Willis C, Berardesca E et al. Guidelines on sodium lauryl sulfate (SLS) exposure tests. Contact Dermatitis 1997; 37:53–69.
30. Welzel J, Metker C, Wolff HH et al. SLS-irritated human skin shows no correlation between degree of proliferation and TEWL increase. Arch Dermatol Res 1998; 29: 615–20.
31. Froebe TCL, Simon TFA, Rhein TLD et al. Stratum corneum lipid removal by surfactants: relation to in vivo irritation. Dermatologica 1990; 181:277–83.
32. Abrams K, Harvell JD, Shriner S et al. Effect of organic solvents on in vitro human skin water barrier. J

Invest Dermatol 1993; 101: 609–13.

33. Fartasch M, Schnetz E, Diepgen TL. Characterisation of detergent-induced barrier alterations – effect of barrier cream on irritation. J Invest Dermatol Symp Proc 1998; 3:121–7.
34. Wilhelm KP, Cua AB, Wolff HH et al. Surfactant-induced stratum coreum hydration in vivo: prediction of the irritation potential of anionic surfactants. J Invest Dermatol 1993; 101:310–15.
35. Wilhelm KP, Freitag G, Wolff HH. Surfactant-induced skin irritation and skin repair. Evaluation of the acute human irritation model by non-invasive techniques. J Am Acad Dermatol 1994; 30:944–9.
36. Willis CM, Stephens CJM, Wilkinson JD. Epidermal damage induced by irritants in man: a light and electron microscopic study. J Invest Dermatol 1989; 93:696–9.
37. Denda M, Koyama J, Namba R et al. Stratum corneum lipid morphology and transepidermal water loss in normal skin and surfactant-induced scaly skin. Arch Dermatol Res 1994; 286:41–6.
38. Warner RR, Boissy YL, Lilly NA et al. Water disrupts stratum corneum lipid lamellae: damage is similar to surfactants. J Invest Dermatol 1999; 113:960–6.
39. Holland JM, Kao JY, Whitaker MJ. A multisample apparatus for kinetic evaluation of skin penetration in vitro: the influence of viability and metabolic status of the skin. Toxicol Appl Pharmacol 1984; 72:272–80.
40. Collier SW, Sheikh NM, Sakr A et al. Maintenance of skin viability during in vitro percutaneous absorption/metabolism studies. Toxicol Appl Pharmacol 1989; 99:522–33.

46
The effects of physical damage on TEWL

RP Chilcott, CH Dalton, AJ Emanuel, CE Allen and ST Bradley

Introduction

Transepidermal water loss (TEWL) is commonly ascribed to be a measure of skin 'barrier function'.[1–3] Therefore, an obvious application of TEWL measurements is for the evaluation of skin damage following topical insult or drug therapy.[4,5] As the measurements are non-invasive, TEWL is an ideal research tool for investigating barrier function of normal and diseased skin in vivo, on both human and animal models.[6–8]

The purpose of this study was to investigate the relationship between TEWL and skin permeability to tritiated water in vitro, following physical damage (by tape-stripping, ultraviolet (UV) irradiation and skin punctures) in order to validate the assumption that TEWL is an appropriate measure of skin barrier function. Excised skin is free of many factors that may potentially affect TEWL and/or skin absorption rates, such as variations in blood perfusion,[9] temperature fluctuations,[10] sweat-gland activity,[11] metabolism,[12] and other diurnal variations.[13,14] In addition, the permeability of excised skin can be measured directly using validated, standard techniques.[15] Thus, an in vitro investigation of the relationship between TEWL and skin permeability may arguably be considered superior to in vivo studies.

Materials and methods

Chemicals

Dulbecco's phosphate buffered saline (DPBS) and gentamycin were purchased from the Sigma-Aldrich Chemical Company (Poole, UK). Liquid scintillation (LS) counting fluid (Emulsifier-safe) and Soluene-350 were purchased from the Canberra-Packard Chemical Co (Michigan, USA). Tritiated water (^3H_2O) was purchased from NEN Life Science Products (Hounslow, UK). Tape-stripping was performed with 14-mm diameter D-Squame® stripping discs (CuDerm; Texas, USA). All experiments were conducted in an environmentally controlled chamber (40 ± 2% relative humidity (RH), 20 ± 0.5°C).

Skin

Full-thickness pig-back skin was freshly obtained from Large White pigs (*Sus scrofa domestica*), bred at CBD Porton Down (six animals total, weight range 30–40 kg). Subcutaneous fat was dissected from each piece of skin and the (epidermal) surface was carefully clipped to remove excess hair prior to storage at –25°C for a maximum of 14 days.

Diffusion cells

Full-thickness pig skin was placed into Franz-type[16] glass diffusion cells, with an available skin surface area of 2.54 cm^2 and a 5-ml receptor chamber containing DPBS (containing 86.6 $\mu g.ml^{-1}$ gentamycin). Groups of six diffusion cells were mounted on purpose-built aluminium heating blocks (CBD Porton Down), heated to 35°C to attain a skin-surface temperature of 31 ± 1.5°C. Each heating block was placed on a six-place magnetic stirrer bed (Whatman; Kent, UK) that stirred the receptor fluid of each diffusion cell via a magnetic follower. All diffusion cells were left to equilibrate in the environmental chamber for at least 24 hours prior to measurements of TEWL or ^3H_2O permeability.

Measurement of transepidermal water loss

TEWL was measured using a calibrated, ServoMed EP-3 Evaporimeter (ServoMed; Varberg, Sweden) in accordance with current guidelines.[11] A 1.5-cm stainless steel collar was attached to the TEWL probe, in order to ensure contact with the pig skin or human epidermal membranes in each diffusion cell. The probe collar was placed on the skin surface for 60 seconds, prior to an average rate being taken over a 15-second measurement period.

Measurement of skin permeability

Skin water-barrier function was measured directly, using ^3H_2O (1 ml, 10 $\mu Ci.ml^{-1}$) placed into the donor chamber of cells containing pig skin. Samples (20 µl) of receptor chamber fluid were removed at 0-, 1-, 2-, 4- and 6-hour intervals, placed into 5 ml LS counting fluid and analysed using a Wallac 1409DSA LS counter. The amount of radioactivity in each sample was related to the amount of ^3H_2O, by reference to standards prepared and measured simultaneously. Skin absorption rates were calculated by linear regression analysis of the amount of ^3H_2O penetrated against time between 2 and 6 hours (steady state, where the amount penetrating per unit time was constant).

UV irradiation skin damage

Ultraviolet-B (UVB) irradiation of pig skin was achieved using ten 100-W tubes (Philips TL-100W/01) that emitted radiation between 305 and 320 nm (λ_{max} = 315 nm, > 95%). Ultraviolet-A (UVA) irradiation was achieved using ten standard 100-W sunbed lamps (Philips 'Cleo Professional' 100WR) that emitted radiation between 300 and 410 nm (λ_{max} = 355 nm, 52%). The lamps were housed in a canopy (Leisure Time Sunbeds Ltd; Doncaster, UK) suspended on a purpose-built stereotactic frame with integral wave-guide system (CBD Porton Down) to ensure uniform irradiance[17] over each group of diffusion cells, and were allowed to 'burn in' for 5 hours before use. Irradiance was measured at the skin level of each diffusion cell position using a hand-held UV Meter (model TKA-ABC, TKA Scientific Instruments; St Petersburg, Russia), in accordance with prescribed guidelines.[18] The skin surface in each diffusion cell was 0.59 m from the UV tube array. The dose of UVB or UVA was controlled by exposing skin over a pre-determined period, calculated from irradiance measurements (Table 46.1). No UVC was detectable 0.59 m from the UVA or UVB tube arrays.

Tape-stripping damage

Stripping discs were applied to pig skin for 10 seconds, using a purpose-built applicator that applied a constant pressure of approximately

Table 46.1 Summary of UV dose required, actual irradiance (average ± SD) and exposure times for each group comprising six diffusion cells. Coefficient of variance of irradiation was 5.2% (UVA) and 7.5% (UVB) within each experiment, and 5.2% (UVA) and 3.3% (UVB) between experiments.

Source	Average irradiance ($mJ.s^{-1}.cm^{-2}$)	Dose ($mJ.cm^{-2}$)	Exposure time (min)
UVA	0	0	0
	3.36 ± 0.15	7086	35.2
	3.61 ± 0.17	15234	70.4
	3.63 ± 0.25	23010	105.6
	3.65 ± 0.17	30905	140.8
	3.51 ± 0.19	37012	176.0
UVB	0	0	0
	0.558 ± 0.052	660	19.7
	0.603 ± 0.050	1320	39.5
	0.598 ± 0.049	2640	73.6
	0.606 ± 0.041	5280	145.2
	0.597 ± 0.031	10560	294.7

0.5 N.m^{-2}.[19] The number of tape-strips ranged from 1 to 20. For comparison, epidermis-free 'full-thickness' skin was obtained by heat separation, as previously described.[20]

Skin puncture damage

Skin in each diffusion cell was punctured (one to four times) using a lancet needle delivered from an auto-injector (Monojector Lancet Device), set to a maximum penetration depth of 2 mm. A new needle was used for each puncture.

Skin damage protocol

Diffusion cells were assembled within the environmentally controlled chamber on day 1. On day 2, baseline (–24 hours) TEWL and ^3H_2O measurements were taken. Skin damage (by UVB, tape-stripping or punctures) was conducted on the third day and was accompanied, where appropriate, with TEWL measurements. Day 4 comprised a 24-hour post-damage measure of TEWL and ^3H_2O permeability, which was followed on subsequent days (relating to 48, 72 and 96 hours post-damage) with TEWL measurements only.

Statistical analysis

Comparison of ^3H_2O flux pre- and post-damage were analysed using a paired, non-parametric test (Wilcoxon signed rank), subject to adequate pairing, as indicated by the Spearman correlation coefficient. Ineffectively paired data were analysed using the Mann–Whitney test. Rates of TEWL were analysed using a multivariate analysis of variation, followed by Dunnet's adjustment for multiple comparisons post test (one-sided). Correlation coefficient (r^2) values were used to evaluate the linear regression analysis of skin absorption rates. If r^2 was < 0.90, the data was deemed to be non-linear (i.e. steady-state conditions were not attained).

Results

Effects of UV radiation exposure on full-thickness pig skin

Rates of TEWL did not significantly change for the duration of the experiment following exposure to UVA (Figure 46.1). There was a small, but significant, decrease in ^3H_2O fluxes at the highest UVA dose (37 012 mJ.cm^{-2}; Figure 46.2).

After exposure to UVB, rates of TEWL did not significantly change for the duration of the experiment (Figure 47.3). Similarly, there was no sig-

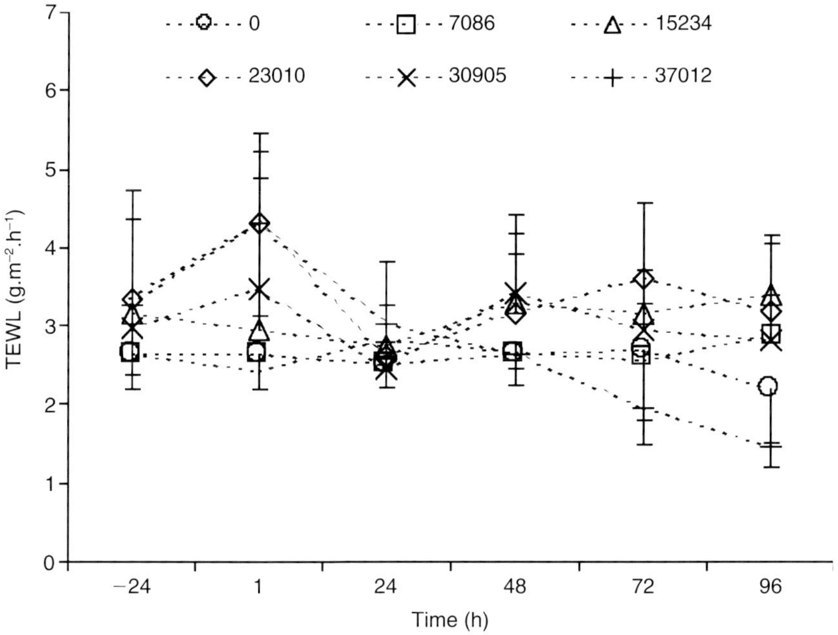

Figure 46.1

Variation in TEWL from full-thickness pig-back skin before (−24 hours) and up to 96 hours after exposure (2 hours) to UVA radiation (dose expressed as $mJ.cm^{-2}$). The study was conducted under controlled environmental conditions (40% RH, 20°C). All values are mean ± SD of n = 6 diffusion cells, containing skin from up to two animals.

nificant change in ^3H_2O skin permeability 24 hours post-exposure (Figure 46.4).

Effects of tape-stripping on full-thickness pig skin

Changes in TEWL rates were dependent on exceeding a certain number of tape-strips (Figure 46.5). Up to six strips had no significant effect. After 10 strips, there was a small (1.9-fold), but significant ($p < 0.05$) increase in TEWL, 1 hour after stripping. Following 15 tape strips, there was a significant (3.4-fold) increase in TEWL for up to 3 hours, whereas 20 strips significantly increased (2–6-fold) TEWL for the duration of the experiment.

Skin permeability to ^3H_2O, 24 hours post-stripping, did not significantly alter until 15 or 20 tape-strips, which resulted in a 6- or 7-fold increase in ^3H_2O permeability, respectively (Figure 46.6), relating to skin absorption rates of 3.18 ± 2.89 and 6.98 ± 2.73 $g.m^{-2}.h^{-1}$, respectively, in comparison to controls (0.36 ± 0.25 $g.m^{-2}.h^{-1}$). The skin absorption rate of ^3H_2O through epidermis-free (heat-separated) skin was 13.43 ± 5.25 $g.m^{-2}.h^{-1}$.

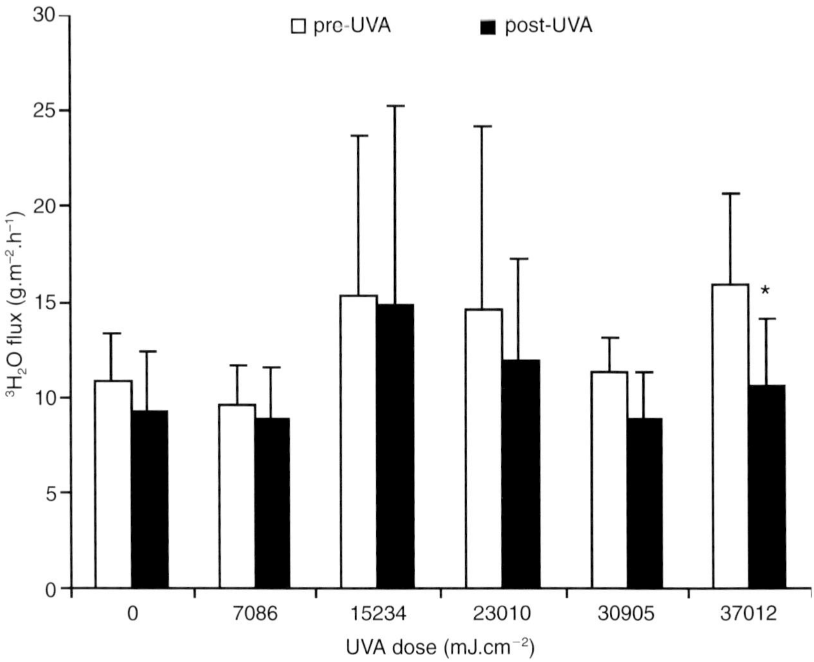

Figure 46.2

Variation in ^3H_2O penetration rates, measured from full-thickness pig-back skin before (–24 hours) and up to 96 hours after exposure (2 hours) to UVA radiation (dose expressed as mJ.cm^{-2}). The study was conducted under controlled environmental conditions (40% RH, 20°C). All values are mean ± SD of $n = 6$ diffusion cells, containing skin from up to two animals. Fluxes of ^3H_2O marked with an asterisk are significantly different ($p < 0.05$) from those of controls at that time point.

Effects of single or multiple skin punctures on full-thickness pig skin

There was a significant ($p < 0.05$) increase in TEWL rates 1 hour after puncturing the skin, the magnitude of which was proportional to the number of punctures (Figure 46.7). After 24 hours, TEWL rates were not significantly different from those of controls (non-punctured). Two or more punctures caused a significant increase in ^3H_2O permeability at 24 hours (Figure 46.8).

Discussion

This study has demonstrated that there is, at best, a poor correlation between TEWL and skin permeability following a physical insult. Moreover, the magnitude of the change in TEWL following skin damage in vitro is less than that measured in previous in vivo studies.

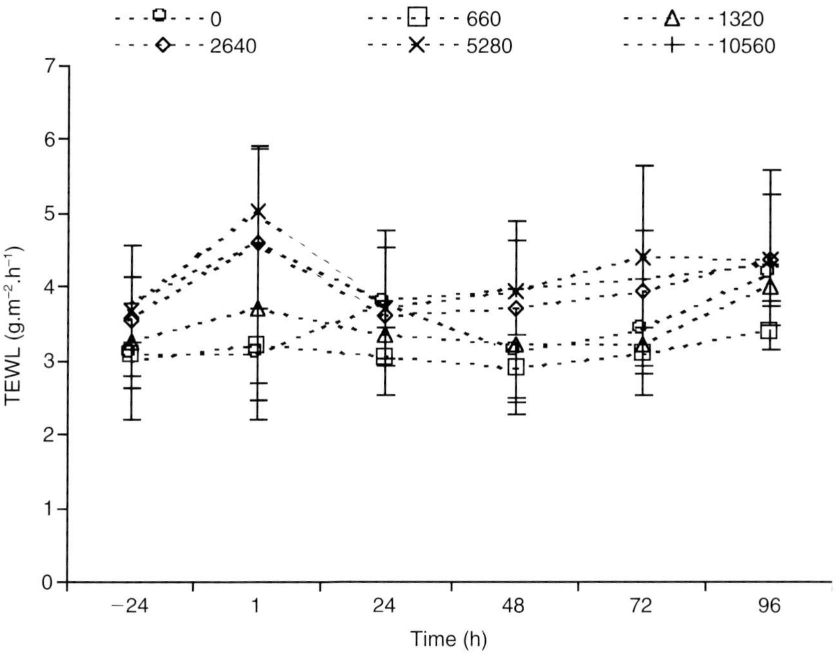

Figure 46.3

Variation in TEWL, measured from full-thickness pig-back skin before (−24 hours) and up to 96 hours after exposure (2 hours) to UVB radiation (dose expressed as mJ.cm^{-2}). The study was conducted under controlled environmental conditions (40% RH, 20°C). All values are mean ± SD of n = 6 diffusion cells, containing skin from up to two animals.

Effects of UV radiation

Arbitrarily, UV radiation can be classified[21] as UVA (315–400 nm), UVB (280–315 nm) and UVC (100–280 nm). The difference in wavelength between the classes of UV dictate their different biological effects. It should be noted that, in this study, the majority (> 95%) of the UVB source was emitting at 315 nm, but it also emitted small (< 5%) quantities of UVA, whereas radiation from the UVA source was normally distributed between 300 and 410 nm, and, thus, contained a small (2%) component of UVB.

The doses of UVA and UVB used in this study were selected so that the lowest doses were equivalent to the highest of those previously studied in vivo. Relatively high doses were employed to augment any possible changes in permeability. Previous in vitro studies have demonstrated that a high-dose exposure (20 000 mJ cm^{-2}) to UVA may increase permeability to certain chemicals, such as methanol and ethanol.[22] Irradiation with UVC may also affect barrier function.[23] An increase in skin permeability and TEWL rates has been well documented in vivo (Table 46.2).

Table 46.2 Summary of several studies investigating the effects of UVA and UVB radiation on TEWL of human or animal skin.

Dose range ($mJ.cm^{-2}$)	Source	Species	Comments	Reference
165–1320	UVB	Rat	72-h delay before ↑ TEWL	Lamaud and Schalla[37]
140–540	UVB	Human	↑ TEWL at 7 d	Abe and Mayuzumi[38]
510–2040	UVA/UVB	Rat	↑ TEWL at 3 d	Bronaugh and Stewart[24]
2500–7500	UVA	Mouse	No effect on TEWL	Bissett et al[39]
20–60	UVB	Mouse	↑ TEWL	Bissett et al[39]
150	UVB	Mouse	↑ TEWL after 72–96 h	Haratake et al[40]
40*	UVB	Rat	↑ TEWL	Meguro et al[41]

*Dose was given daily for 15 days.

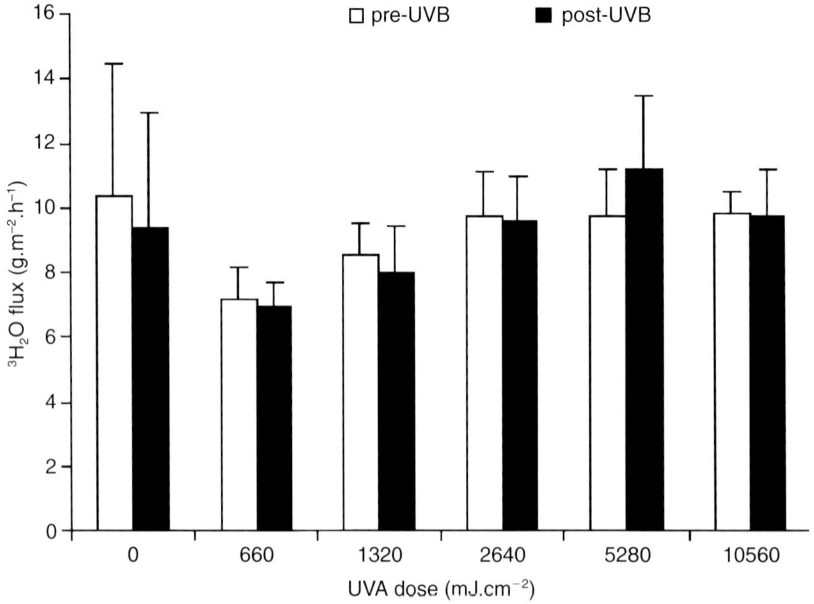

Figure 46.4

Variation in ^3H_2O penetration rates, measured from full-thickness pig-back skin before (–24 hours) and up to 96 hours after exposure (2 hours) to UVB radiation (dose expressed as $mJ.cm^{-2}$). The study was conducted under controlled environmental conditions (40% RH, 20°C). All values are mean ± SD of n = 6 diffusion cells, containing skin from up to two animals.

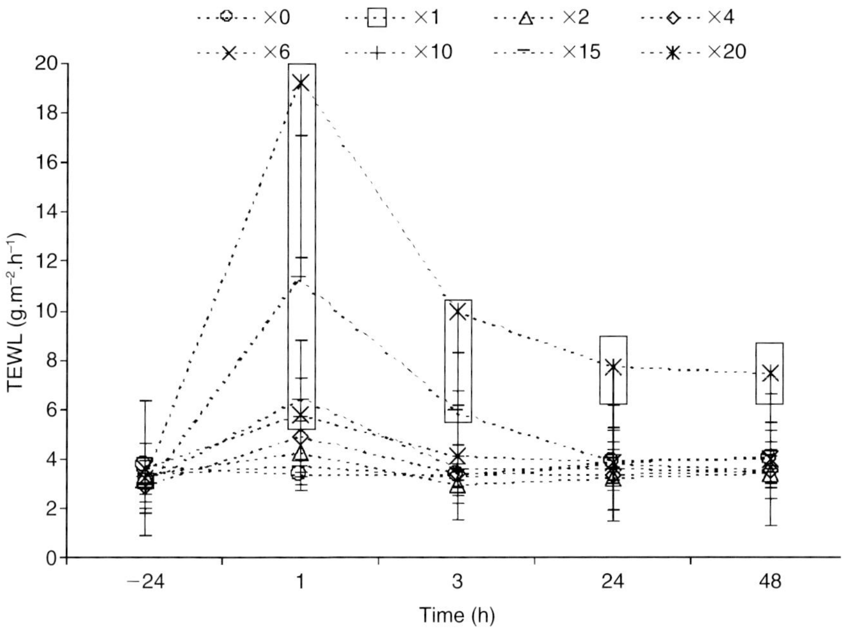

Figure 46.5

Variation in TEWL, measured from full-thickness pig-back skin before (–24 hours) and up to 96 hours after tape-stripping (numbers in legend refer to number of serial tape-strips). The study was conducted under controlled environmental conditions (40% RH, 20°C). All values are mean ± SD of n = 6 diffusion cells, containing skin from up to two animals. Boxed TEWL values are significantly different ($p < 0.05$) from those of controls at that time point.

In this study, using relatively high doses of UVA (≤37 012 mJ.cm^{-2}) and UVB (≤10 560 mJ.cm^{-2}), no increases in skin permeability to ^3H_2O or TEWL rates were measured. Given that the delayed response in vivo may be a consequence of physiological processes,[24] and that these responses may be absent in our in vitro system, this is not surprising. Therefore, these data confirm that UVA and UVB do not have direct effects on skin water-barrier function, in contradiction to previous in vitro studies using short-chain alcohol penetrants.[22] This disparity may be due to differences in relative humidity under which skin permeability was measured, or the time at which permeability measurements were conducted after UV exposure.[25]

There was a small, but significant, decrease in skin permeability following the highest UVA exposure (37 012 mJ.cm^{-2}). It is conceivable that the exposure time (176 minutes) was sufficient to cause drying of the skin. If this represents an actual effect, it has little practical relevance. The difference in water permeability between pre- and post-exposure skin was less than 50% – the fact that this was significant indicates that the

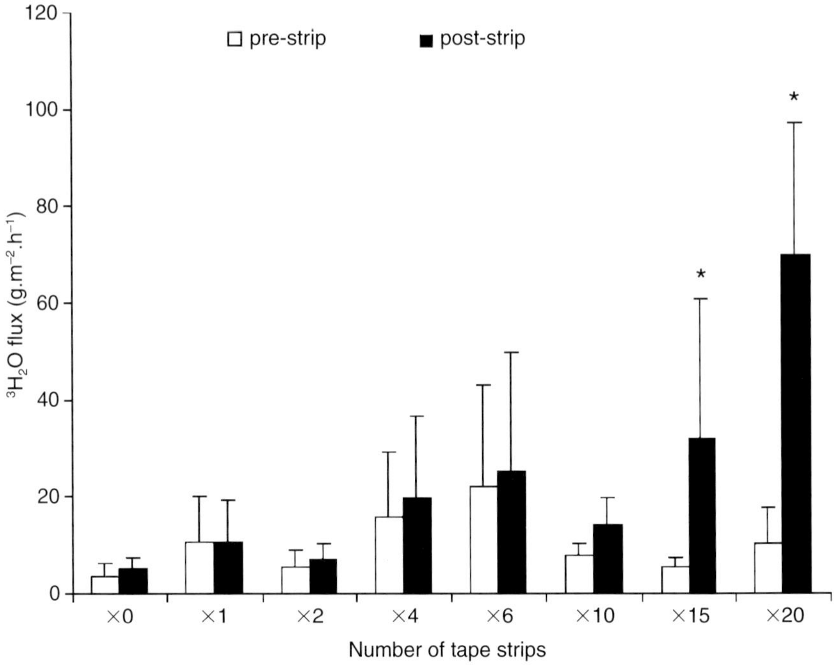

Figure 46.6

Variation in ^3H_2O penetration rates, measured from full-thickness pig-back skin before (–24 hours) and up to 96 hours after tape-stripping (numbers in legend refer to number of serial tape-strips). The study was conducted under controlled environmental conditions (40% RH, 20°C). All values are mean ± SD of $n = 6$ diffusion cells, containing skin from up to two animals. Fluxes of ^3H_2O marked with an asterisk are significantly different ($p < 0.05$) from those of controls at that time point.

measures introduced to limit skin variability in this study were effective. Under standard laboratory conditions, such small variations in skin permeability would probably not be statistically different.[26]

Effects of tape-stripping

Previous studies have demonstrated that sequential removal of the stratum corneum (SC) by tape-stripping results in an increase in TEWL rates, particularly when the lowest cornified layers are removed.[27] This has been interpreted as evidence that the bulk water-barrier of skin resides in the lower (20%) portion of the SC.[28] In vivo, restitution of the barrier following tape-stripping is said to comprise a biphasic mechanism.[29] The primary ('early-repair') stage ($t_{1/2} \approx 0.7$–2.3 days) involves the development of parakeratotic cells, which are thought to be responsible for the large, but incomplete, restoration of barrier function. Parakeratosis may be the result of a pertubation in ion gradients within the SC, such as cal-

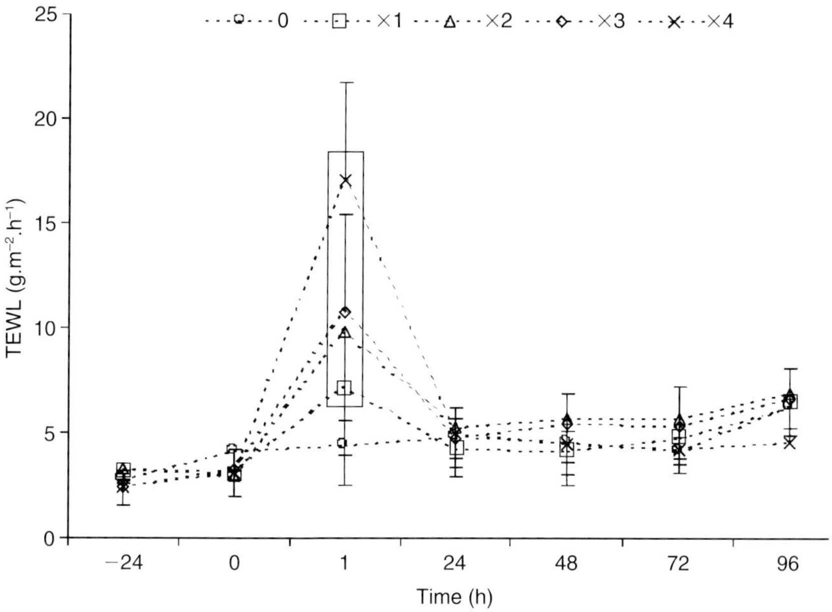

Figure 46.7

Variation in TEWL measured from full thickness pig-back skin before (−24 h) and up to 96 h after administration of skin punctures (numbers in legend refer to number of punctures made). The study was conducted under controlled environmental conditions (40% RH, 20°C). All values are mean ± SD of n = 6 diffusion cells containing skin from up to two animals. Boxed TEWL values are significantly different ($p < 0.05$) to controls at that time

cium.[30] The second phase of repair is slower ($t_{1/2} \approx 1.4$–6.2 days), and possibly seasonally-dependent,[31] but results in the complete restoration of barrier function. The whole process takes about 14 days in normal skin.[32]

Mechanisms of barrier restoration observed in vivo would not be expected to be reproducible in our in vitro system, as the skin had been frozen and subject to nutrient-free media for at least 24 hours prior to tape-stripping. Therefore, any 'healing' processes could reasonably be expected to be absent in this in vitro study, as the skin had been frozen and subject to nutrient-free media for at least 24 hours prior to tape-stripping. Previous studies have demonstrated that skin tissue, placed in diffusion cells under optimum conditions, is viable for less than 24 hours and may also contain necrotic tissue.[33,34] Consequently, any energy-requiring repair processes, such as parakeratosis, would almost certainly be absent in our in vitro model. Therefore, the introduction of barrier damage caused by tape-stripping in this in vitro study would be expected to be irreversible if repair was primarily due to energy-requiring mechanisms. However, the results of this study were similar to the early-repair

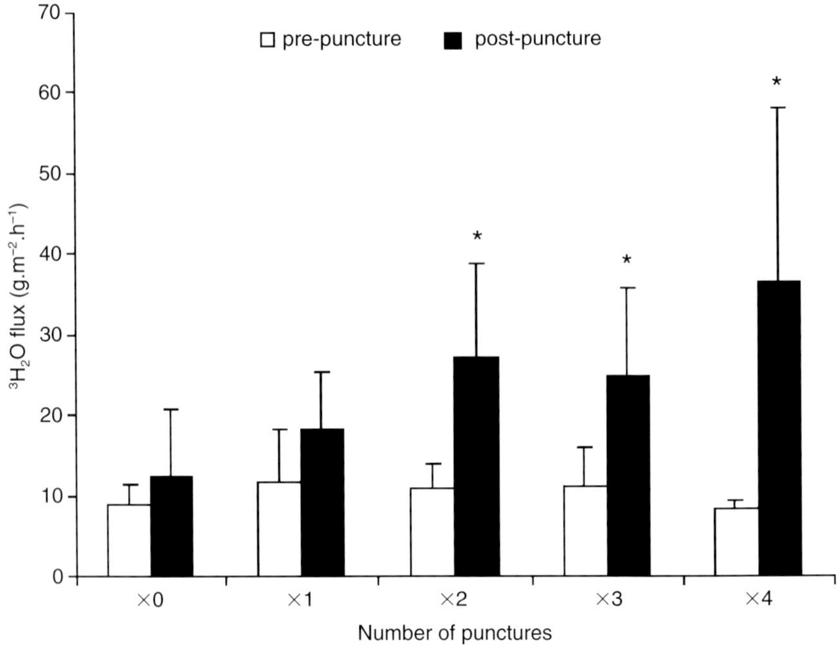

Figure 47.8

Variation in ^3H_2O penetration rates measured from full thickness pig-back skin before (−24 h) and up to 96 h after administration of skin punctures (numbers in legend refer to number of punctures made). The study was conducted under controlled environmental conditions (40% RH, 20°C). All values are mean ± SD of n = 6 diffusion cells containing skin from up to two animals. Fluxes of ^3H_2O marked with an asterisk are significantly different ($p < 0.05$) to controls at that time point.

phase observed in vivo. That is, an immediate increase in TEWL followed by a rapid decrease, to basal (up to 15 strips) or suprabasal TEWL rates (20 strips). There are three obvious interpretations of these data: (1) either the apparent restoration of barrier function (as indicated by a decrease in TEWL) is a non-energy-dependent mechanism; (2) the transient increase in TEWL is due to the temporary exposure of deeper, hydrated tissue, which subsequently re-equilibrates (with a consequent decrease in TEWL); or (3) TEWL rates are not indicative of 'barrier function'. It is possible that the transient increase in TEWL for moderate (up to ×10) strippings is due to the exposure of more hydrated tissue that subsequently undergoes a re-establishment of the water gradient, leading to an apparently normal TEWL value.[19] The rate of re-establishment of the water gradient may be proportional to the diffusivity of water within the remaining SC. This may explain why some individuals appear to be resistant to an increase in TEWL following tape-stripping,[35] as an individual with a high water diffusivity will more rapidly re-establish the gradient, leading to apparently normal TEWL values. This may also explain why certain pathologic skin appears to have a faster early-repair phase after stripping,[36] as water within the SC is more mobile and may equilibrate faster with the surrounding air.

Irrespective of the actual mechanism controlling the transient increase in TEWL, the fact that skin permeability to $^{3}H_2O$ was elevated 6-fold 24 hours after 15 strips, yet without any significant elevation of TEWL at that time, would imply that TEWL is, at best, a poor indicator of skin (water) barrier function. The 2-fold increase in TEWL (24 hours) after 20 strips was also an insensitive measure of the actual 7-fold increase in $^{3}H_2O$ permeability. The permeability of heat-separated (epidermis-free) skin was approximately 2-fold higher than skin stripped $\times 20$, 4-fold higher than skin stripped $\times 15$, and 37-fold higher than controls, confirming that substantial damage was inflicted by tape-stripping.

Effects of needlestick injury

The results of this study are in agreement with previous work, which demonstrated that damage caused by scratching the skin surface with a needle results in a significant increase in permeability to $^{3}H_2O$ and also to a range of other compounds.[24] Whilst there was a transient increase in TEWL that was related to the number of punctures administered, TEWL rates at 24 hours were not significantly different from those of controls, despite a 2–5-fold increase in $^{3}H_2O$ permeability. Thus, TEWL did not identify frank, physical damage to the water-barrier layer. It is possible that the transient alteration in TEWL may be attributable to exposure of deeper, hydrated tissue, as discussed above.

General conclusions

The results of this study indicate that elevated TEWL rates should not be unconditionally ascribed to an alteration of skin barrier function following physical damage, as other factors may be largely responsible for variation in TEWL rates in vivo. Perhaps most importantly, there are occasions when TEWL does not indicate significant skin damage.

Acknowledgements

The authors would like to thank Mr B Stubbs and Mrs J Platt for their technical help. This work was funded by the UK Ministry of Defence (MoD), at facilities operated by the Defence science and technology laboratory (Dstl).

References

1. Pinnagoda J, Tupker RA. Measurement of transepidermal water loss. In: Serup J, Jemec GBE, eds. *Handbook of Non-invasive Methods and the Skin*. London: CRC Press, 1995:chap 9.
2. Lotte C, Rougier A, Wilson DR et al. In vivo relationship between transepidermal water loss and percutaneous penetration of some organic compounds in man: effect of anatomic site. Dermatol Res 1987; 279:351–6.
3. Nangia A, Berner B, Maibach HI. Transepidermal water loss measurements for assessing skin barrier function during in vitro percutaneous absorption experiments. In: Bronaugh RL, Maibach HI, eds. *Percutaneous Absorption: Drugs – Cosmetics – Mechanisms – Methodology*. Third edn. New York: Marcel Dekker Inc, 1999:chap 34.
4. Nicander I, Ollmar S, Eek A et al. Correlation of impedance response patterns to histological findings in irritant skin reactions induced by various surfactants. Br J Dermatol 1996; 134:221-8.
5. Freeman S, Maibach HI. Study of irritant contact dermatitis produced by repeat patch test with sodium lauryl sulfate and assessed by visual methods, transepidermal water loss, and laser Doppler velocimetry. J Am Acad Dermatol 1988; 19:496–502.
6. Lamke L-O, Nilsson GE, Reithner HL. Insensible perspiration from the skin under standardized environmental conditions. Scand J Clin Lab Invest 1977; 37:325–31.
7. Nilsson GE. Measurement of water exchange through skin. Med and Biol Eng Comput 1977; 15: 209–18.
8. Idson B. In vivo measurement of transepidermal water loss. J Soc Cosmet Chem 1978; 29:573–80.
9. Benowitz NL, Jacob III, Olsson P et al. Intravenous nicotine retards transdermal absorption of nicotine: evidence of blood-flow limited percutaneous absorption. Clin Pharmacol Ther 1992; 52:223–30.
10. Blank IH, Scheuplein RJ. Transport into and within the skin. Br J Dermatol 1969; 81:4–10.
11. Pinnagoda J, Tupker RA, Agner T et al. Guidelines for transepidermal water loss (TEWL) measurement. Contact Dermatitis 1990; 22: 164–78.
12. Kao J, Hall J, Shugert LR et al. An in vitro approach to studying cutaneous metabolism and disposition of topically applied xenobiotics. Toxicol Appl Pharmacol 1984; 75:289–98.
13. Yosipovitch G, Xiong GL, Haus E et al. Time dependant variations of the skin barrier function in humans: transepidermal water loss, stratum corneum hydration, skin surface skin temperature. J Invest Dermatol 1998; 110:20–3.
14. Chilcott RP, Farrar R. Biophysical measurements of human forearm skin in vivo: effects of site, gender, chirality and time. Skin Res Technol 2000; 6:64–9.
15. Howes D, Guy R, Hadgraft J et al. Methods for assessing percutaneous absorption. ATLA 1996; 24: 81–106.
16. Franz TJ. Percutaneous absorption. On the relevance of in vitro data. J Invest Dermatol 1975; 64: 190–5.
17. Dalton CH. Effects of ultraviolet radiation on skin barrier function and transepidermal water loss in vitro. MSc Thesis, University of Birmingham, UK 2000.
18. Gasparro FP, Brown DB. Photobiology 102: UV sources and dosimetry – the proper use and measurement of photons as a

reagent. J Invest Dermatol 2000; 114:613–15.

19. Emanuel A. Effects of controlled physical damage on transepidermal water loss and permeability of human and pig skin. MSc Thesis, University of Birmingham, UK 1999.
20. Kligman AM, Christophers E. Preparation of isolated sheets of human stratum corneum. Arch Dermatol 1963; 88:70–3.
21. Commision Internationale de l'Eclairage (International Commission on Illumination). International Lighting Vocabulary, Publication CIE 1970:No. 17.
22. McAuliffe DJ, Blank IH. Effects of UVA (320–400nm) on the barrier characteristics of the skin. J Invest Dermatol 1991; 96:758–62.
23. Solomon AE, Lowe NJ. Percutaneous absorption in experimental epidermal disease. Br J Dermatol 1979; 100:717–22.
24. Bronaugh RL, Stewart RF. Methods for in vitro percutaneous absorption studies. V: permeation through damaged skin. J Pharm Sci 1985; 74:1062–6.
25. Jacques SL, McAuliffe DJ, Blank IH et al. Low dose ultraviolet radiation alters human stratum corneum. Photochem Photobiol (Abstract) 1987; 45S:94.
26. Williams AC, Cornwell PA, Barry BW. On the non-Gaussian distribution of human skin permeabilities. Int J Pharm 1992; 86:69–77.
27. Blank IH. Further investigations on factors which influence the water content of the stratum corneum. J Invest Dermatol 1953; 12:259–71.
28. Van der Valk PGM, Maibach HI. A functional study of the skin barrier to evaporative water loss by means of repeated cellophane-tape stripping. Clin Exp Dermatol 1990; 15:180–2.
29. Matoltsy AG, Schragger A, Matoltsy MN. Observation on regeneration of the skin barrier. J Invest Dermatol 1962; 38:251–3.
30. Ahn SK, Hwang SM, Jiang SJ et al. The changes of epidermal calcium gradient and transitional cells after prolonged occlusion following tape stripping in the murine epidermis. J Invest Dermatol 1999; 113:189–95.
31. Spruit D, Malten KE. Epidermal water-barrier function after stripping of normal skin. J Invest Dermatol 1965; 45:6–14.
32. Frödin T, Skogh M. Measurement of transepidermal water loss using an evaporimeter to follow the restitution of the barrier layer of human epidermis after stripping the stratum corneum. Acta Derm Venereol 1984; 64:537–40.
33. Holland JM, Kao JY, Whitaker MJ. A multisample apparatus for kinetic evaluation of skin penetration in vitro: the influence of viability and metabolic status of the skin. Toxicol Appl Pharmacol 1984; 72:272–80.
34. Collier SW, Sheikh NM, Sakr A et al. Maintenance of skin viability during in vitro percutaneous absorption/metabolism studies. Toxicol Appl Pharmacol 1989; 99:522–33.
35. Bashir SJ, Chew A-L, Anigbogu A et al. Physical and physiological effects of stratum corneum tape stripping. Skin Res Technol 2001; 7:40–8.
36. Tanaka M, Zhen YX, Tagami H. Normal recovery of the stratum corneum barrier function following damage induced by tape stripping in patients with atopic dermatitis. Br J Dermatol 1997; 136: 966–7.
37. Lamaud E, Schalla W. Influence of UV irradiation on penetration of hydrocortisone. In vivo study in hairless rat skin. Br J Dermatol 1984; 111:152–7.

38. Abe T, Mayuzumi J. The change and recovery of human skin barrier function after ultraviolet light irradiation. Chem Pharm Bull 1979; 27:458–62.

39. Bisset DL, Hannon DP, Orr TV. An animal model of solar aged skin: histological, physical and visible changes in UV-irradiated hairless mouse skin. Photochem Photobiol 1987; 46:367–78.

40. Haratake A, Uchida Y, Mimura K et al. Intrinsically aged epidermis displays diminished UVB-induced alterations in barrier function associated with decreased proliferation. J Invest Dermatol 1997; 108:319–23.

41. Meguro S, Aral Y, Masukawa K et al. Stratum corneum lipid abnormalities in UVB-irradiated skin. Photochem Photobiol 1999; 69: 317–21.

47
Reverse electroporation of glucose: a preliminary study

RP Chilcott and CA Rowland

Introduction

Electrically-assisted transdermal drug delivery systems use iontophoresis or electroporation to deliver molecules through the skin.[1] Iontophoresis involves application of a small, constant electric current to the skin, which causes molecules to move across the stratum corneum (SC), mainly through appendageal routes by electrorepulsion or electroosmosis.[2] In contrast, electroporation causes transdermal drug delivery by forming transient 'pores' using short, high-voltage pulses.[3,4]

Reverse iontophoresis has previously been used to extract biologically relevant molecules from the interstitial fluid of the skin.[5,6]

Analysis of chemicals dissolved in the extracted fluid can be related to the systemic circulation, as both are in equilibrium.[7] It is also conceivable that reverse electroporation may enable extraction of molecules from within the body. Theoretically, reverse electroporation would cause increased amounts of glucose to be extracted across the skin, as electroporation is generally accepted to be more efficient than iontophoresis.[8] Electroporation also has a very short lag time for drug delivery, which is an added advantage over iontophoresis,[9] as peak drug–plasma concentrations may be attained more rapidly.

In order to enhance the extraction of molecules by electroporation, a solution that is hypertonic in relation to the interstitial fluid may be placed on the skin surface to create an osmotic gradient and passively draw water out through pores created by pulsing. As water is flowing to a solution of lower glucose concentration, passive movement of glucose from bodily fluids should also occur. Therefore, a combination of skin electroporation and a hypertonic solution on the skin surface may increase movement of water and its associated solutes through electroporative pathways, leading to enhanced solute and glucose extraction.

The purpose of this study was to evaluate reverse electroporation as a technique to extract glucose through human skin in vitro, using isotonic and hypertonic skin-surface solutions. In order to characterize movement of molecules during reverse electroporation, radiolabelled glucose and tritiated water were used.

Materials and methods

Study design

The study was conducted in two phases (Figure 47.1). First, electrical pulse characteristics (frequency, duration and width of each pulse) were investigated, in order to define the optimal parameters for extracting maximal amounts of glucose through human epidermal membranes, whilst minimizing damage to skin barrier function. These experiments were conducted using the lowest concentrations of glucose likely to be found in the skin (0.03 μmol l^{-1}), in order to provide 'proof of principle' that such low amounts could be extracted. Secondly, the effects of imposing an osmotic gradient (using 10× phosphate-buffered saline or glycerol solution) on the skin surface were evaluated. These experiments were conducted using physiologically more relevant glucose concentrations (4 mmol l^{-1}).

Materials

Tritiated water (^3H_2O, >99% radiochemical purity) and ^{14}C-glucose (^{14}C-GLU, >98% radiochemical purity) were purchased from NEN

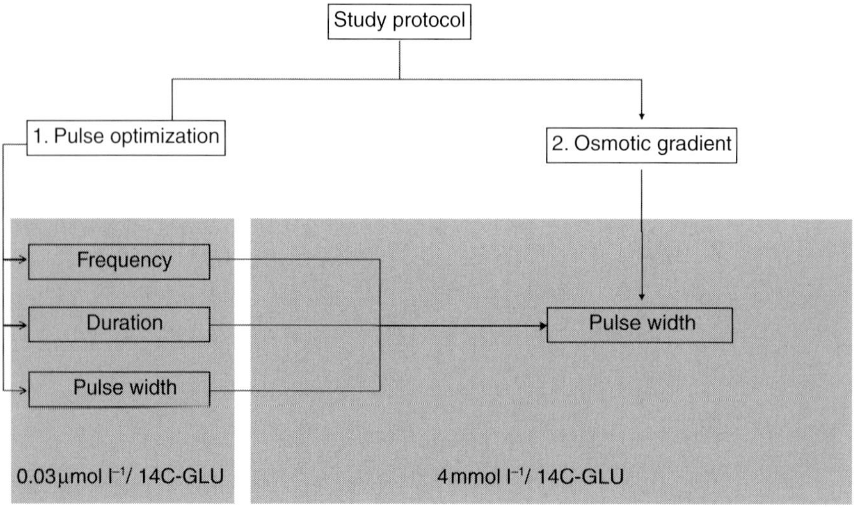

Figure 47.1
Outline study plan for reverse electroporation of glucose through human epidermal membranes.

Biosciences, USA. Sterile Dulbecco's phosphate-buffered saline (sPBS), adjusted to pH 7.4, silver wire (>99.9% purity) and other chemical reagents were purchased from the Sigma Chemical Company, UK. Liquid scintillation-counting (LSC) vials and fluid were purchased from Canberra Packard Life Sciences, UK.

Diffusion cells

Heat-separated human (breast) epidermal membranes[10] were placed into Franz-type glass diffusion cells,[11] consisting of an upper (donor) and lower (receptor) chamber. Receptor chambers were filled with 5 ml sPBS containing 2 µCi 14C-GLU at the appropriate concentration (Figure 47.1). For isotonic conditions (where the osmolarity either side of the membrane was approximately equal), donor chambers were filled with 2 ml sPBS containing 1 µCi ^3H_2O. For hypertonic conditions (where the osmolarity of the donor chamber was approximately 10× that of the receptor), the donor chamber fluid comprised 2 ml 10× concentrated sPBS or 26% glycerol in sPBS (both containing 1 µCi ^3H_2O).

Electroporation

Silver-wire electrodes were placed into both donor and receptor chambers and were connected to a D-330 multi-channel stimulator (Digitimer; Hertfordshire, UK) that controlled the number of 100 V (DC) square wave pulses per second (frequency), duration of each individual pulse (pulse width) and total duration of electroporation (pulse duration). The signal output was verified using a digital cathode ray oscilloscope (CRO; Advanced Digital Storage Oscilloscope; Gould, Essex, UK).

Detection technique

Amounts of ^{14}C-nuclide in the donor chambers and ^3H-nuclide in the receptor chambers were determined by dual label liquid scintillation counting, using a Wallac Model 1409 DSA counter. The amount of radioactivity was converted to the amount of glucose or water, by reference to standard solutions prepared and counted simultaneously.

Results

Pulse optimization

The amounts of ^{14}C-GLU measured in the donor chamber of each diffusion cell were directly proportional to the width (Figure 47.2), duration (Figure 47.3) or frequency (Figure 47.4) of the electroporative signal.

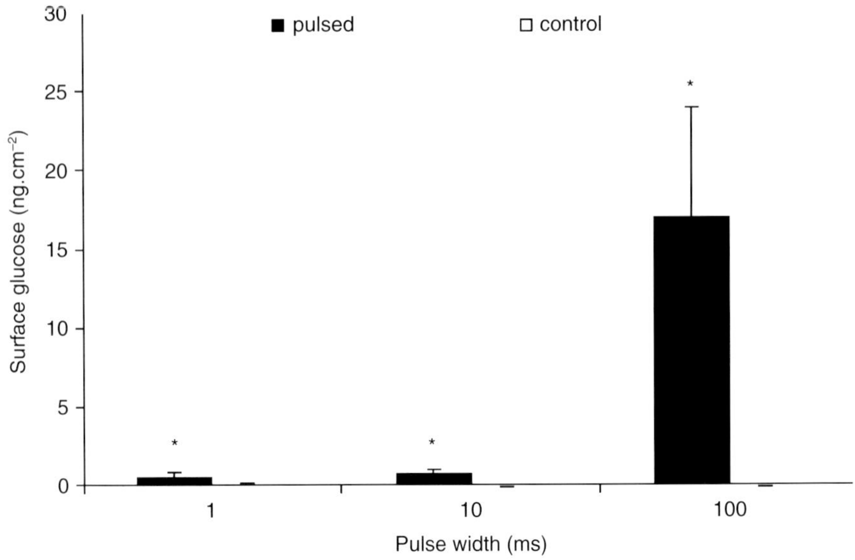

Figure 47.2

Amounts of ^{14}C-GLU measured in buffer (sPBS) bathing the surface of epidermal membranes following electroporation (10 Hz; 60-second duration, variable pulse width) or in controls (non-electroporated) under isotonic conditions (where the osmolarity of receptor and donor chambers were approximately equal). All values are mean ± SD of $n = 6$ membranes (obtained from one individual). Asterisks indicate that result is significantly ($p < 0.05$) different from controls at same time point. Concentration of glucose in the dermal (receptor) fluid was 0.03 μmol l^{-1}. The three different pulse widths were applied in series (with 1 hour between pulses) to the same diffusion cells.

There was a significant increase in the flux of $^{3}H_2O$ from the donor chamber to the receptor chamber under optimal conditions (frequency 10 Hz; pulse width 10 ms; total duration 60 seconds) immediately following electroporation. When applied as a series of three discrete events, $^{3}H_2O$ fluxes decreased back to normal (control) within 1 hour, indicating a reversibility of effect on skin permeability (Figure 47.5).

Effects of an osmotic gradient (hypertonic conditions)

Use of 10× concentrated buffer on the skin surface significantly decreased the extraction of ^{14}C-GLU in comparison with skin, subject to isotonic conditions (Figure 47.6). The cathode ray oscilloscope indicated that the maximum voltage of each pulse through diffusion cells containing the hyperosmotic solution was substantially lower (typically 2–12 V) than under comparable isotonic conditions (100 ± 0.5 V). Thus, 'electroporative' conditions were not attained for epidermal membranes covered with 10× sPBS solution. In contrast to pulse optimization experiments

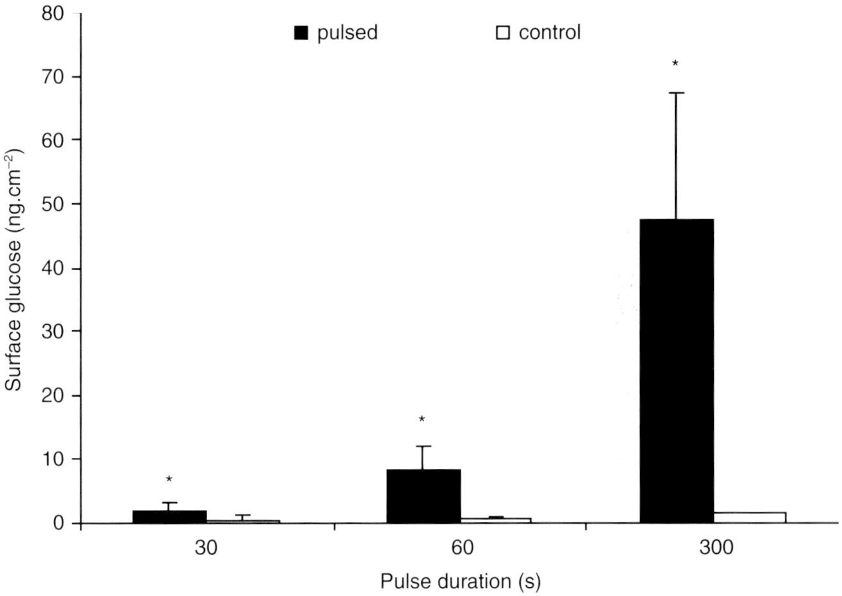

Figure 47.3

Amounts of ^{14}C-GLU measured in buffer (sPBS) bathing the surface of epidermal membranes following electroporation (10 Hz; 10-ms pulse width and variable pulse duration) or in controls (non-electroporated) under isotonic conditions (where the osmolarity of receptor and donor chambers were approximately equal). All values are mean ± SD of $n = 6$ membranes (obtained from one individual). Asterisks indicate that result is significantly ($p < 0.05$) different from controls at same time point. Concentration of glucose in the dermal (receptor) fluid was 0.03 μmol l^{-1}. The three different pulse durations were applied in series (with 1 hour between pulses) to the same diffusion cells.

(using low concentrations of glucose), fluxes of ^3H_2O did not return to control levels after the third in a series of pulse events (Figure 47.7).

Imposition of an osmotic gradient, using glycerol (a non-electrolyte), did not significantly affect glucose extraction 1 hour post electroporation in comparison with isotonic conditions (Figure 47.8). However, after 5 hours, significantly more glucose had been extracted under hypertonic conditions than under isotonic conditions.

Discussion

This study has demonstrated that, following electroporation, there is an enhanced bi-directional flux of material across human epidermal membranes, which permits diffusion of glucose through the membrane from the dermal fluid to the surface. The quantities of glucose extracted were above those required for detection by amperometric biosensors.[12]

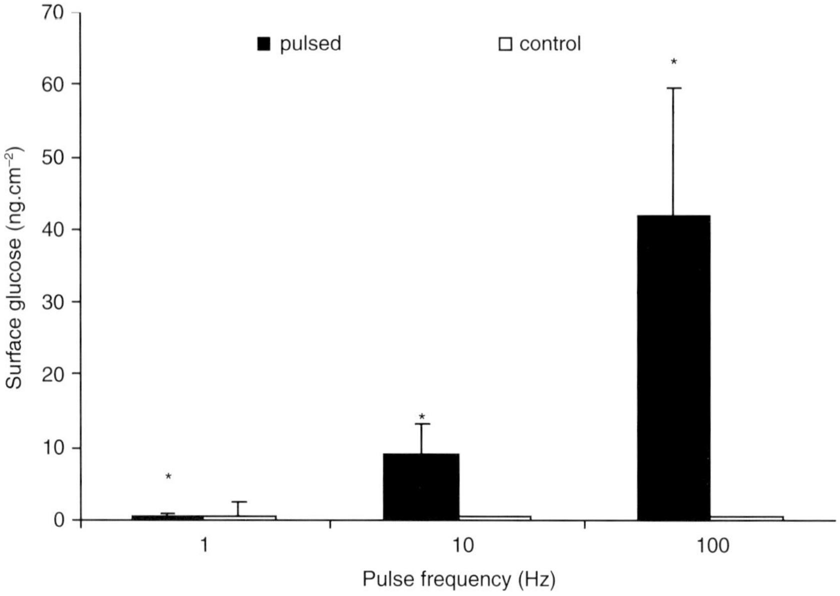

Figure 46.4

Amounts of ^{14}C-GLU measured in buffer (sPBS) bathing the surface of epidermal membranes following electroporation (60-second duration, 10-ms pulse width and variable pulse frequency) or in controls (non-electroporated) under isotonic conditions (where the osmolarities of receptor and donor chambers were approximately equal). All values are mean ± SD of n = 6 membranes (obtained from one individual). Asterisks indicate that result is significantly ($p < 0.05$) different from controls at same time point. Concentration of glucose in the dermal (receptor) fluid was 0.03 μmol l^{-1}. The three different pulse frequencies were applied in series (with 1 hour between pulses) to the same diffusion cells.

Extraction of glucose was accompanied by an enhanced flux of water through the membrane (from the surface to the dermal fluid). The fact that the enhancement in water flux was generally transient indicated that the process was reversible within a 1-hour period.

Surface glucose was detectable within 5 minutes of the onset of electroporation in each experiment. However, there were large variations in the amounts of glucose on the skin surface following shorter (30- and 60-second) pulse durations, indicating that longer (300-second) periods of electroporation may be required to produce reproducible extractions.

The efficiency of electroporative transport may be affected by various factors, including the number and length of pulses, duration of pulsing episodes, and voltage applied during each pulse.[8] In this study, each epidermal membrane was generally exposed to three consecutive pulsing episodes. Thus, the individual effects of each pulse set on skin per-

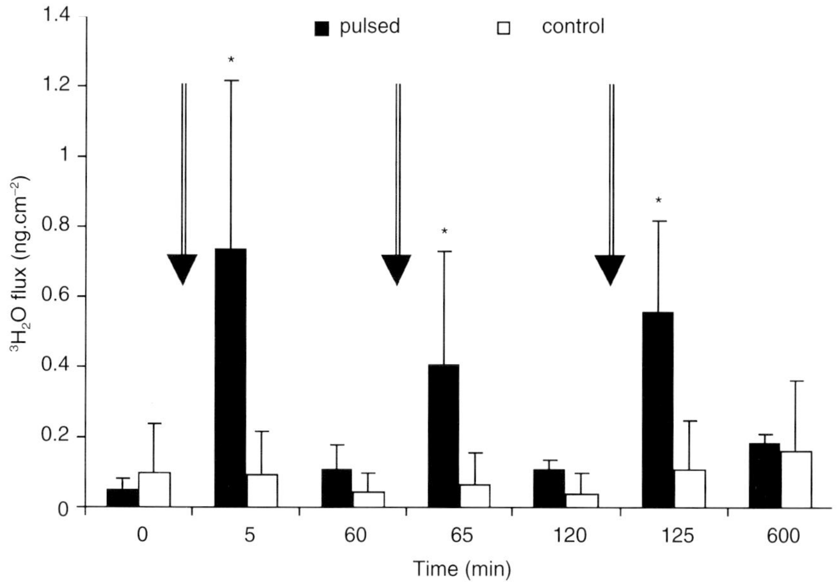

Figure 47.5

Flux of tritiated water (^3H_2O) through human epidermal membranes (from donor to receptor chamber) expressed against time (non-linear axis) in the absence (control) or presence (pulsed) of a series of electroporative pulses (10 Hz, 10-ms pulse width, 60-second duration) administered at 0, 60 and 120 minutes (indicated by arrows). All values are mean ± SD of n = 6 diffusion cells (containing skin from one individual). Asterisks indicate that flux is significantly different ($p < 0.05$) from controls at that time point. Study was conducted using donor and receptor-chamber fluid of equal osmolarity (isotonic conditions). The three different pulse trains were applied in series (with 1 hour between pulses) to the same diffusion cells.

meability should be interpreted with caution, due to the possibility of cumulative interference. Fluxes of ^3H_2O increased immediately after pulsing under all conditions and pulsing regimes, but returned to levels comparable with control cells after 1 hour. This implies that increases in skin permeability were reversible, i.e. no cumulative damage resulted from serial pulsing.

Electroosmosis is thought to be the main mechanism for glucose extraction by reverse iontophoresis.[13,14] However, the effect of electroosmosis on electroporative transport is thought to be negligible, as molecules diffuse through pores in the skin created by pulsing.[9] Application of a hypertonic solution to the skin surface has been found to increase movement of molecules out of the skin in vitro and in vivo.[15,16] By combining this with electroporation, a situation may be created where diffusion of molecules through electroporative pathways is enhanced by an osmotic gradient. The hypertonic buffer and glycerol donor solutions

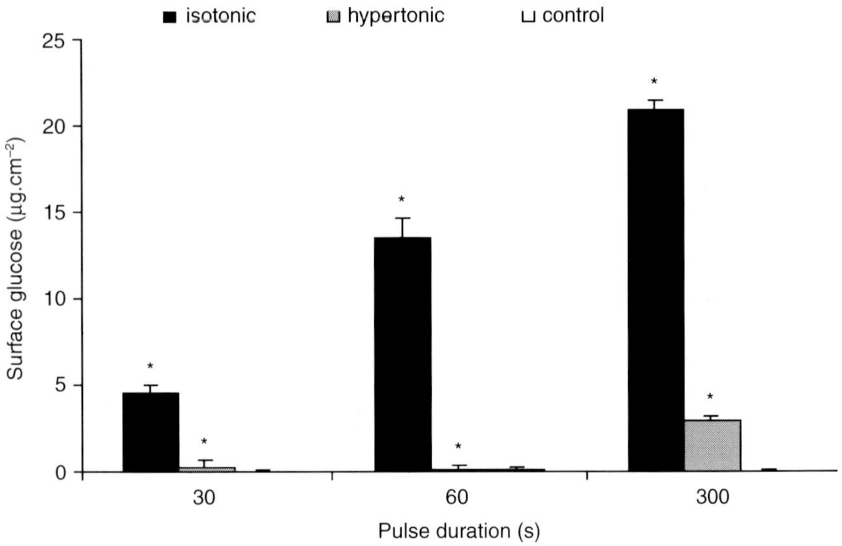

Figure 47.6

Amounts of ^{14}C-GLU measured in buffer (sPBS) bathing the surface of epidermal membranes following electroporation (10-ms pulse width, 10-Hz pulse frequency and variable pulse duration) or in controls (non-electroporated) under isotonic and hypertonic conditions (where the osmolarity of the donor chamber solution was 10× greater than the receptor chamber). All values are mean ± SD of n = 6 membranes (obtained from two individuals). Asterisks indicate that result is significantly ($p < 0.05$) different from controls at same time point. Concentration of glucose in the dermal (receptor) fluid was 4 mmol l^{-1}. The three different pulse durations were applied in series (with 1 hour between pulses) to the same diffusion cells.

used in this study had 10 times the osmotic potential of receptor-chamber fluid. When hypertonic buffer was used, glucose movement was reduced 10-fold in comparison to isotonic conditions. This reduction was most likely due to an increase in the conductivity of donor solutions, caused by the relatively high concentration of sodium and chloride ions.[17] This resulted in a decrease in the applied transdermal voltage, leading to less effective electroporative conditions.[18] When hypertonic solutions of glycerol (a non-electrolyte) were used, the voltages measured across the diffusion cells and the amount of glucose extracted were comparable to those measured under isotonic conditions after 1 hour. However, hypertonic solutions significantly enhanced the amount of glucose extracted after 5 hours, in comparison with isotonic conditions. This effect may be explained either by the presence of a glucose reservoir within the skin[19] or through the stablization of local transport regions induced by electroporation.

This study has shown that glucose may be extracted through epider-

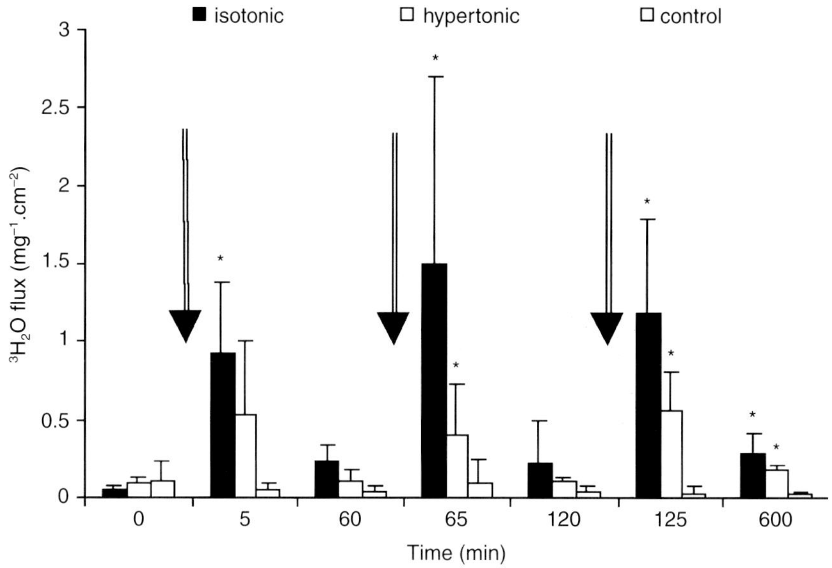

Figure 47.7

Flux of tritiated water (^3H_2O) through human epidermal membranes (from donor to receptor chamber) expressed against time (non-linear axis) in the absence (control) or presence (pulsed) of a series of electroporative pulses (10 Hz, 10-ms pulse width, 60-second duration) administered at 0, 60 and 120 minutes (indicated by arrows). All values are mean $\pm$ SD of $n = 6$ diffusion cells (containing skin from two individuals). Asterisks indicate that flux is significantly different ($p < 0.05$) from controls at that time point. The study was conducted using donor and receptor-chamber fluid of equal osmolarity (isotonic conditions) or using a donor chamber fluid 10× osmolarity of receptor fluid (hypertonic conditions). The three separate pulses were applied in series (with 1 hour between pulses) to the same diffusion cells.

mal membranes using reverse electroporation. The presence of a non-ionic, hypertonic surface solution increased the total amount (but not the rate) of glucose extracted. As electroporation allows larger molecules to penetrate the skin in comparison with iontophoresis,[20] reverse electroporation could potentially widen the scope for non-invasive blood monitoring to encompass other biologically relevant molecules.

Acknowledgements

The authors would like to thank Mr B Stubbs for his technical assistance. This work was funded by the Ministry of Defence (MoD), at facilities operated by the Defence Evaluation and Research Agency (DERA).

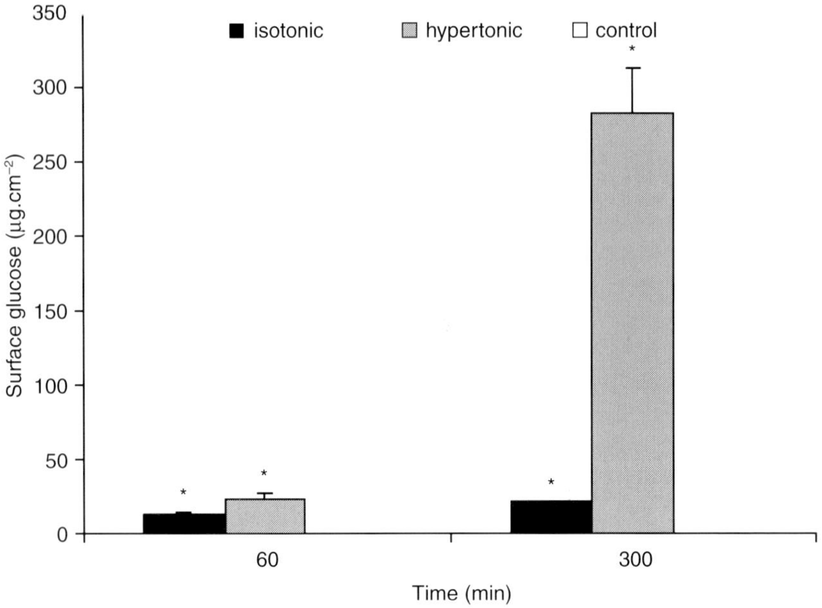

Figure 47.8

Amounts of ^{14}C-GLU measured in buffer (sPBS) bathing the surface of epidermal membranes (expressed against time post-electroporation) following one episode of electroporation (60-second duration, 10-ms pulse width and 10-Hz pulse frequency) or in controls (non-electroporated) under isotonic and hypertonic conditions (where the osmolarity of the donor chamber solution was 10× greater than the receptor chamber). All values are mean ± SD of n = 6 membranes (obtained from two individuals). Asterisks indicate that result is significantly ($p < 0.05$) different from controls at same time point. Concentration of glucose in the dermal (receptor) fluid was 4 mmol l^{-1}.

References

1. Banga AK, Bose S, Ghosh TK. Iontophoresis and electroporation: comparisons and contrasts. Int J Pharmaceut 1999; 179:1–19.
2. Singh P, Maibach HI. Iontophoresis: an alternative to the use of carriers in cutaneous drug delivery. Adv Drug Deliv Reviews 1996; 18: 379–94.
3. Vanbever R, Leroy M, Preat V. Transdermal permeation of neutral molecules by skin electroporation. J Control Release 1998; 54: 243–50.
4. Wang S, Kara M, Krishnan TR. Transdermal delivery of cyclosporin-A using electroporation. J Control Release 1998; 50:61–70.
5. Rao G, Guy RH, Glikfield P et al. Reverse iontophoresis: non-invasive glucose monitoring in vivo in humans. Pharmaceut Res 1993; 12:1869–73.
6. Mize NK, Buttery M, Daddona P et al. Reverse iontophoresis: monitoring prostaglandin E2 associated with cutaneous inflammation in

vivo. Exp Dermatol 1997; 6: 298–302.

7. Bantle JP, Thomas W. Glucose measurement in patients with diabetes mellitus with dermal interstitial fluid. J Lab Clin Med 1997; 130:436–41.
8. Vanbever R, Preat V. In vivo efficacy and safety of skin electroporation. Adv Drug Deliv Reviews 1999; 35:77–88.
9. Prausnitz MR. A practical assessment of transdermal drug delivery by skin electroporation. Adv Drug Deliv Reviews 1999; 35:61–76.
10. Kligman AM, Christophers E. Preparation of isolated sheets of human stratum corneum. Arch Dermatol 1963; 88:70–3.
11. Franz TJ. In vitro vs in vivo percutaneous absorption: on the relevance of in vitro data. J Invest Derm 1975; 64:190–5.
12. Lowry JP. An amperometric glucose-oxidase/poly(o-phenylenediamine) biosensor for monitoring brain extracellular glucose: in vivo characterisation in the striatum of freely-moving rats. J Neurosci Methods 1998; 79:65–74.
13. Glikfield P, Hinz RS, Guy RH. Noninvasive sampling of biological fluids by iontophoresis. Pharmaceut Res 1989; 6:988–90.
14. Rao G, Glikfield P, Guy RH. Reverse iontophoresis: development of a non-invasive approach for glucose monitoring. Pharmaceut Res 1993; 10:1751–5.
15. Hirvonen J, Murtomaki L, Kontturi K. Effect of diffusion potential, osmosis and ion-exchange on transdermal drug delivery: theory and experiments. J Control Release 1998; 56:33–9.
16. Phillips M, Vandervoort RE, Becker CE. Long-term sweat collection using salt-impregnated pads. J Invest Dermatol 1977; 68: 221–4.
17. Asberg A, Holm T, Vassbotn T et al. A non-specific microvascular vasodilation during iontophoresis is attenuated by application of hyperosmolar saline. Microvasc Res 1999; 58:41–8.
18. Jadoul A, Lecouturier N, Mesens J et al. Transdermal alniditan delivery by skin electroporation. J Control Release 1999; 54:265–72.
19. Vanbever R, Leroy M, Preat V. Transdermal permeation of neutral molecules by skin electroporation. J Control Release 1998; 54: 243–50.
20. Banga AK, Prausnitz MR. Assessing the potential of skin electroporation for the delivery of protein- and gene-based drugs. TIBTECH 1998; 16:408–12).

48

Mechanical properties of aging skin – stratum corneum vs dermal changes

W Mok, B Bautista and K Subramanyan

Aims

Skin aging is a complex and multi-factor process, resulting in progressive modifications of the rheological properties of the skin. Despite advances in instrumental development, it remains unclear whether the decrease in skin elasticity with age[1,2] is due to changes in the plasticization of the stratum corneum (SC) or changes in the underlying dermal structure, or both. In this study, we have evaluated the dynamic modulus and the viscoelastic properties of the SC with the Linear Skin Rheometer (LSR; Goodyer Scientific Instruments Ltd, Hathern, UK). The rheological properties of the skin, including and beyond the SC, in the axial direction were studied with the Ballistometer (Dia-Stron Ltd, Andover, UK). The results show that while the Ballistometer measured a decrease in elasticity with age, the LSR does not detect significant differences in the SC rheology between the two age groups. Regional anatomical differences in the mechanical behavior of the SC and dermal layers of skin on the inner and outer forearm were also identified.

Methods

Eighteen young (18–26 years) and twenty-four older (55–65 years) female Caucasian subjects participated in this study. All measurements were taken in a controlled-environment room (20°C and 50 ± 5% relative humidity), where subjects were stabilized for 10 minutes prior to recording measurements. The LSR and the Ballistometer measurements were taken on both the inner and outer forearms with test sites located by a template on the center of the arm, measured 8 cm from the elbow. A two-sample t-test was performed to evaluate the differences between the two age groups for all measurements. A two-tailed matched paired t-test was used to determine differences between test sites (left vs right; inner vs outer forearm) on each subject. A p value less than or equal to 0.05 was considered significant. All procedures involving human subjects received prior approval from the Unilever Research US Institutional Review Board, and all subjects provided written informed consent.

Results

Ballistometer

The alpha parameter of the Ballistometer is a measure of the time-dependent damping of the probe. It is derived by fitting an exponential decay function to the peaks of the bounce profile generated by the probe in response to contact with the skin. A large value indicates an energy-absorbent (inelastic) sample. Older subjects were found to have significantly higher alpha values than the younger subjects ($p < 0.0001$) (Figure 48.1). Additionally, younger subjects displayed higher rebound than the

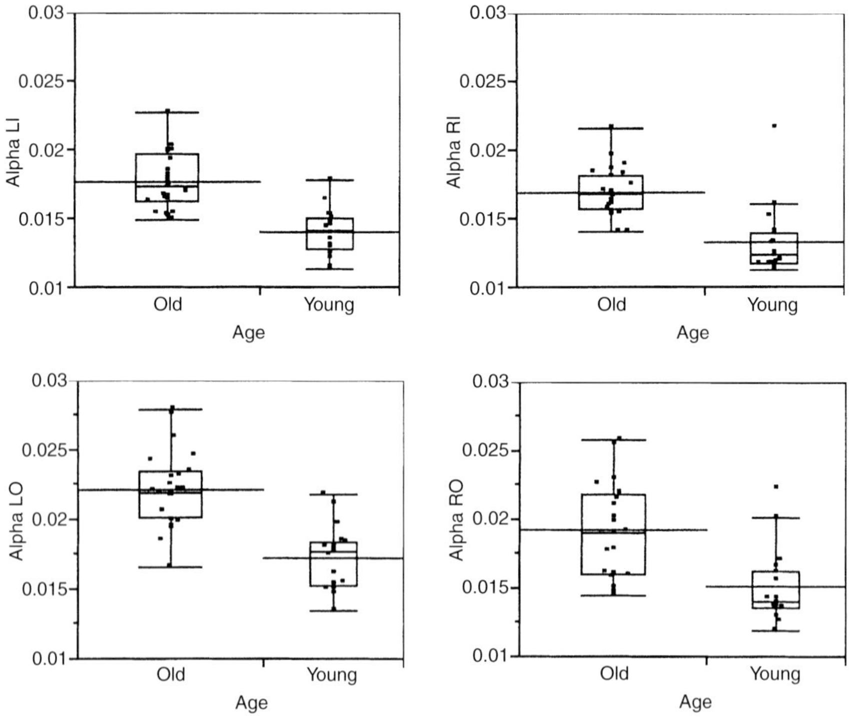

Figure 48.1

Outlier box plots summarize the distribution of the alpha measurements between the two age groups. The dotted line represents the mean, and the uninterrupted line within the box represents the median. The ends of the box are the 25th and 75th quantiles.
LI, left inner; RI, right inner; LO, left outer; RO, right outer.

older subjects ($p < 0.05$) (results not shown), suggesting that younger skin is significantly higher in elasticity compared to older skin. Similar observations have previously been reported with the gravitational Ballistometer, in which older subjects were found to have lower Coefficient of Restitution compared to the younger subjects.[3] Interestingly, a recent study, using the Dia-Stron Ballistometer (energy stored), did not detect any age-related differences.[4] In addition, there were significant differences in elasticity between the inner and outer forearms for all subjects. The outer forearms were significantly lower in elasticity than the inner forearms ($p < 0.05$), perhaps due to a higher susceptibility to environmental damage, and the regional anatomical differences that exist between the outer and inner forearms.[2,5] We did not observe any significant differences in the indentation measurement between the two age groups.

Linear Skin Rheometer

Using the LSR, there were no statistically significant changes in the viscoelasticity or dynamic modulus of the SC upon aging (Table 48.1). The LSR and the Gas Bearing Electrodynamometer (GBE) have been used to measure the viscoelastic properties of the SC, as the technique exerts a negligible normal force and thereby minimizes involvement of the underlying tissue.[6] The LSR is a more sensitive and accurate instrument than the GBE.[7] The LSR measures the dynamic spring rate (DSR) and the energy loss rate (ELR), which correspond to the skin stiffness and softness, respectively. LSR parameters are expressed in g/mm and measures the force required to stretch or compress the skin per unit extension. The LSR has been used to differentiate SC plasticization in response to treatment with moisturizer.[8] Our results show that the inner forearms displayed a significantly higher DSR than the outer forearms

Table 48.1 Comparison between the younger and older age groups by LSR (± SD), with the p-value from the 2-sample t-test.

	Young	Old	p-value
Energy Loss Rate (ELR)			
Left outer	0.61 (± 0.34)	0.78 (± 0.40)	0.28
Left inner	0.33 (± 0.16)	0.49 (± 0.35)	0.13
Right outer	0.69 (± 0.24)	0.94 (± 0.65)	0.16
Right inner	0.35 (± 0.16)	0.34 (± 0.24)	0.51
Dynamic Spring Rate (DSR)			
Left outer	5.71 (± 2.02)	5.20 (± 1.75)	0.91
Left inner	8.13 (± 2.54)	7.95 (± 3.84)	0.92
Right outer	4.99 (± 0.72)	5.05 (± 1.86)	0.65
Right inner	8.04 (± 2.12)	9.30 (± 4.66)	0.14

($p < 0.05$), which can be interpreted as a higher level of firmness. Also, the outer forearms show higher SC viscoelasticity (less elastic), consistent with the observation from the Ballistometer.

Conclusion

The Ballistometer, which measures skin elasticity perpendicular to the skin surface and probes the SC and dermis, clearly shows a decrease in elasticity with age. Similar observations have previously been made with the gravitational Ballistometer.[3] The changes in the dermal elasticity measurement agree with the current findings on the degeneration of elastic tissue in the dermal layer with age.[9,10] The LSR, which has previously been used to differentiate SC plasticization in response to treatment with moisturizer,[5] does not detect significant differences in the SC mechanical responses between the two age groups. This suggests that age-induced changes in the SC mechanical properties are not as significant as changes induced by the SC hydration. Underlying measurement principles in the two methods used imply that the age-related changes in the skin elasticity are predominantly due to changes in the underlying dermal structure. Additionally, significant differences in mechanical properties are observed between the inner and outer forearms of all subjects in both age groups, with the inner forearms showing higher elasticity (SC and below) and increased dynamic modulus (SC) compared to the outer forearms. These differences may reflect the inherent differences in hydration, and other regional anatomical differences between the outer and inner forearms.[5]

References

1. Robert C, Blanc M, Lesty C et al. Study of skin ageing as a function of social and professional conditions: modification of the rehological parameters measured with a noninvasive method-indentometry. Gerontol 1988; 34:284–90.
2. Malm M, Samman M, Serup J. In vivo skin elasticity of 22 anatomical sites – the vertical gradient of skin extensibility and implications in gravitational aging. Skin Res Technol 1995; 1:61–7.
3. Tosti A, Compagno G, Fazzini ML et al. A ballistometer for the study of the plasto-elastic properties of skin. J Invest Dermatol 1977; 69: 315–17.
4. Jemec GBE, Selvaag E, Agren M et al. Measurement of the mechanical properties of skin with ballistometer and suction cup. Skin Res Technol 2001; 7: 122–6.
5. Cua AB, Wilhelm KP, Maibach HI. Frictional properties of human skin: relation to age, sex and anatomical region, stratum corneum hydration and transepidermal water loss. Br J Derm 1990; 123:473–9.
6. Maes D, Short J, Turek BA et al. In vivo measuring of skin softness

using the Gas Bearing Electrodynamometer. Int J Cosmet Sci 1983; 5:189–200.

7. Matt, PJ, Goodyer E. A new instrument to measure the mechanical properties of human stratum corneum in vivo. J Cosmet Sci 1998; 49:321–33.
8. Matts PJ. A new instrument to measure the mechanical properties of human stratum corneum in vivo. Poster presented at the SC II Conference; 1998.
9. Bouissou H, Pieragg MT, Julia M et al. The elastic tissue of the skin. A comparison of spontaneous and actinic (solar) aging. Int J Dermatol 1988; 27:327–35.
10. Herzberg AJ, Dinehart SM. Chronologic aging in black skin. Am J Dermatopathol 1989; 11: 319–28.

49
Improved understanding of skin elasticity by modelling in vivo mechanical tests

PJ Dooling, CW Smith, X Ren, A Burgess, KE Evans, JW Wiechers and N Zahlan

Aims

A wide variety of in vivo mechanical tests are used to prove the efficacy of skincare ingredients by demonstrating improvements in the elasticity of the skin. However, even if we treat the skin as elastic (ignoring time-dependence), the actual deformation produced by any in vivo test is extremely complex. This complexity arises both because of the boundary conditions (the surface is free but the constraints on the lower layers vary with local structure) and the anisotropy of the material properties. By combining numerical modelling and experimental techniques, we aim to extract more meaningful mechanical properties from in vivo tests.

Methods

Because of its wide use in cosmetics ingredients research, we began by using numerical modelling to improve our understanding of the Dermal Torque Meter (DTM) test. A finite element model of the test was developed and applied first to a rubber material with known material properties, and then to human skin. The rubber test results were compared to both finite element model predictions and those from an analytical formula found in the literature.[1] In the case of the skin model, two sets of material properties were used – the first isotropic, and the second with stiffness varying through the thickness, according to the best information obtainable from the literature.

At Exeter University, a technique known as Surface Displacement Analysis (SDA) has been applied to capture the deformation of the skin surface during mechanical testing. As an initial example, data was obtained for an indentation test and compared to finite element model predictions along a nominal axis.

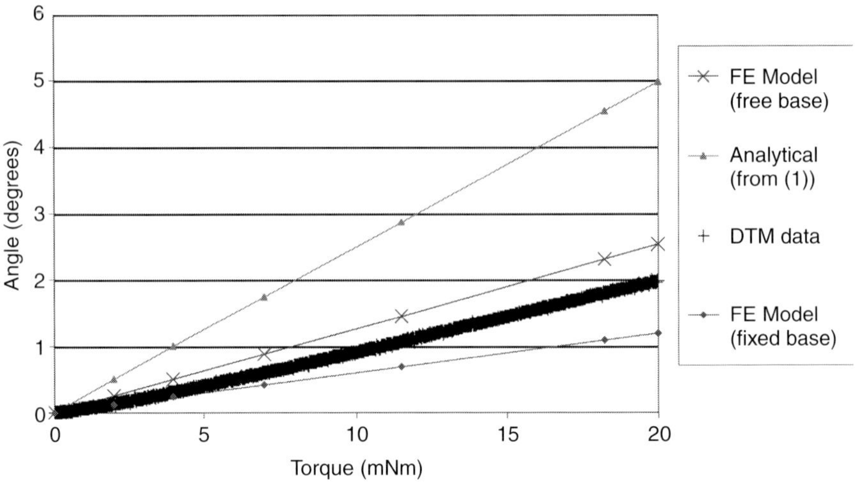

Figure 49.1

Validation using rubber with known mechanical properties. Angle measured by DTM with increasing torque compared with analytical and finite element (FE) model predictions. The data can be seen to lie between the two extreme model boundary conditions (lower surface of material either free to move or fixed).

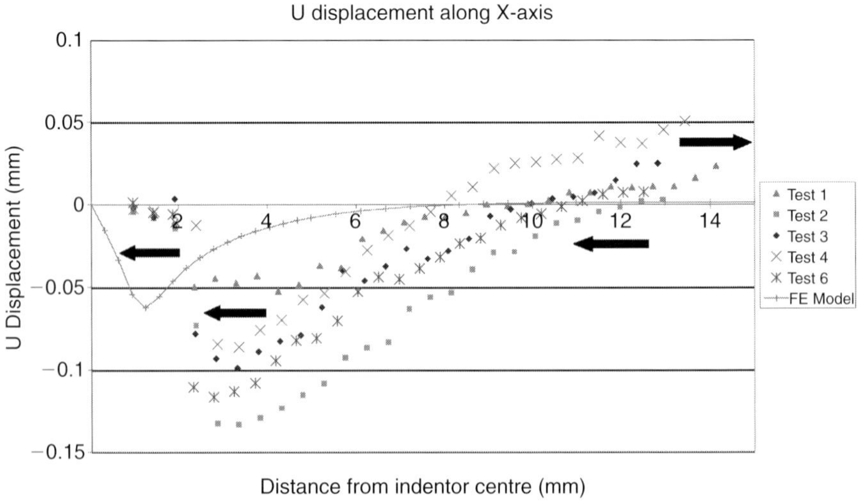

Figure 49.2

Comparison of experimental and predicted surface displacements showing qualitative agreement. The arrows show regions of movement towards and away from the centre of indentation.

Results

The finite element model of the DTM test on the rubber material produced a prediction of angle versus torque that agreed much more closely with the experiment than the analytical formula (Figure 49.1). When modelling skin, we found that the isotropic model based on known whole-skin properties produced a predicted twist in the skin consistent with actual DTM data. However, the layered model was far too stiff.

An isotropic finite element model of the skin was found to reproduce the qualitative behaviour of the indentation test (shape of curve of surface displacement), but not the quantitative behaviour (Figure 49.2).

Conclusions

Because of the complexity of the boundary conditions, analytical solutions are not sufficient to extract mechanical properties from in vivo tests. This may explain the inconsistencies between predictions of modulus for human skin observed when comparing different types of tests.

The results from modelling DTM tests on skin imply that using literature data from in vitro tests on human stratum corneum produces an overestimate of the in vivo stiffness.

The surface displacement technique provides much more information from a given test. Because of this, it is no longer possible to reproduce the results using an isotropic material model. However, by applying these techniques to several different types of tests, it should be possible to obtain a much wider set of mechanical properties.

Reference

1. Agache PG, Monneur C, Leveque JL, de Rigal J. Mechanical properties and Young's modulus of human skin in vivo. Arch Dermatol Res 1980; 269:221–32.

50
Characterization of skin surface: comparison of SIA® and PRIMOS® methods

A Sirvent, M Randeau, C Kurdian, B Closs and F Girard

Introduction

In recent years, intensive work was carried out on the development of optical 3-D surface measurement systems for direct, in vivo skin analysis. In this study, comparative measurements of SIA® and PRIMOS® techniques for skin surface evaluation were done.

Methods

Skin Image Analyser® (SIA®)

Polymer silicone skinprints are studied using the SIA®. Oblique lighting (35°) brings shadows from the replica to the fore, which are then observed with a digital camera linked to a computer. This produces a digitized image, enabling a roughness index to be obtained by analysing the shades of gray (Table 50.1).[1–2]

PRIMOS® (Phaseshift Rapid In vivo Measurement Of Skin)

A parallel-stripe pattern is projected directly on the skin's surface via an optic system, and captured as an image on a digital matrix camera. The parallel-stripe images are rotated to reveal the finest variations in the

Table 50.1 SIA® technical characteristics.

Measured area	1 cm^2
Acquisition time	From 2 to 5 min/replica
z-resolution	$\pm 2\,\mu m$
Minimum surface detection	Furrows $\geqslant 0.03\,mm^2$
Studied parameters	Using Quantiline® + Monaderm software = average roughness

Table 50.2 PRIMOS® technical characteristics.

Projection system	Digital Micromirror Devices (DMD™) with 800 × 600 micromirrors
Area of interest	18 × 13 mm^2
Acquisition time	17 milliseconds, for a single picture ⩾68 milliseconds, for a complete 3-D profile
Calculation of a 3-D picture	5 to 10 seconds
z-resolution	⩾1 µm
x-y distance of the points	17 µm × 17 µm
Use of polarization optics	yes
Studied parameters	Using the PRIMOS® software package: – 2-D or line-roughness parameter – 3-D or star-roughness parameter, depth and volume of wrinkles

skin's surface height, with the degree of rotation providing a qualitative, as well as quantitative, evaluation of each height profile (Table 50.2).[3–5]

Protocol

Population – Fifteen women, aged between 46 and 60 years, with wrinkles in the corners of the eyes.
Product – Polylift® (Silab).
Studied zone – Corner of the eye.
Protocol – At T0: Image acquisition with PRIMOS® followed by polymer silicone skinprints.
Application of 2 µl/cm^2 of cream
– At T2h: Image acquisition with PRIMOS® followed by polymer silicone skinprints.
Skinprints were analysed with SIA®.

Results

SIA® roughness (arbitrary unit)

Two hours after product application, average roughness (Ra) decreased significantly (Table 50.3). A reduction in local difference (Rz) was also observed, although not significant.

These results illustrated the tensing effect of the product.

PRIMOS®

All the studied parameters (Ra, Rt, Rz) decreased significantly 2 hours after application (Table 50.4). The product presented a successful tensing effect (Figure 50.1).

Table 50.3 SIA® results.

	Ra			Rz		
	T0	T2h	Δ (T2h–T0)	T0	T2h	Δ(T2h–T0)
Mean ± sem	36.03 ± 1.62	33.94 ± 1.45	−2.09 ± 0.97	160.05 ± 3.94	157.78 ± 3.88	2.86 ± 2.99
Δ % p*		−5 0.048			−2 0.354	

* Student t-test

Table 50.4 PRIMOS® results.

	Ra			Rt			Rz		
	T0	T2h	Δ (T2h–T0)	T0	T2h	Δ (T2h–T0)	T0	T2h	Δ(T2h–T0)
Mean ±sem	33.50 ±2.72	29.38 ±2.13	−4.12 ±1.87	158.47 ±11.78	138.22 ±11.30	−20.15 ±8.23	241.0 ±19.8	197.5 ±17.6	-43.5 ±17.7
Δ % p*		−5 0.045			−13 0.028			−18 0.027	

* Student t-test

Conclusion

Although both methods present the same tendencies for skin roughness evolution, significant improvements were noted with the PRIMOS® system compared to SIA® analysis. Distorted readings, due to the production of skin replicas, no longer occur with a direct, in vivo system. Image processing techniques developed in parallel allow the precise re-identification of skin areas previously subjected to analysis.

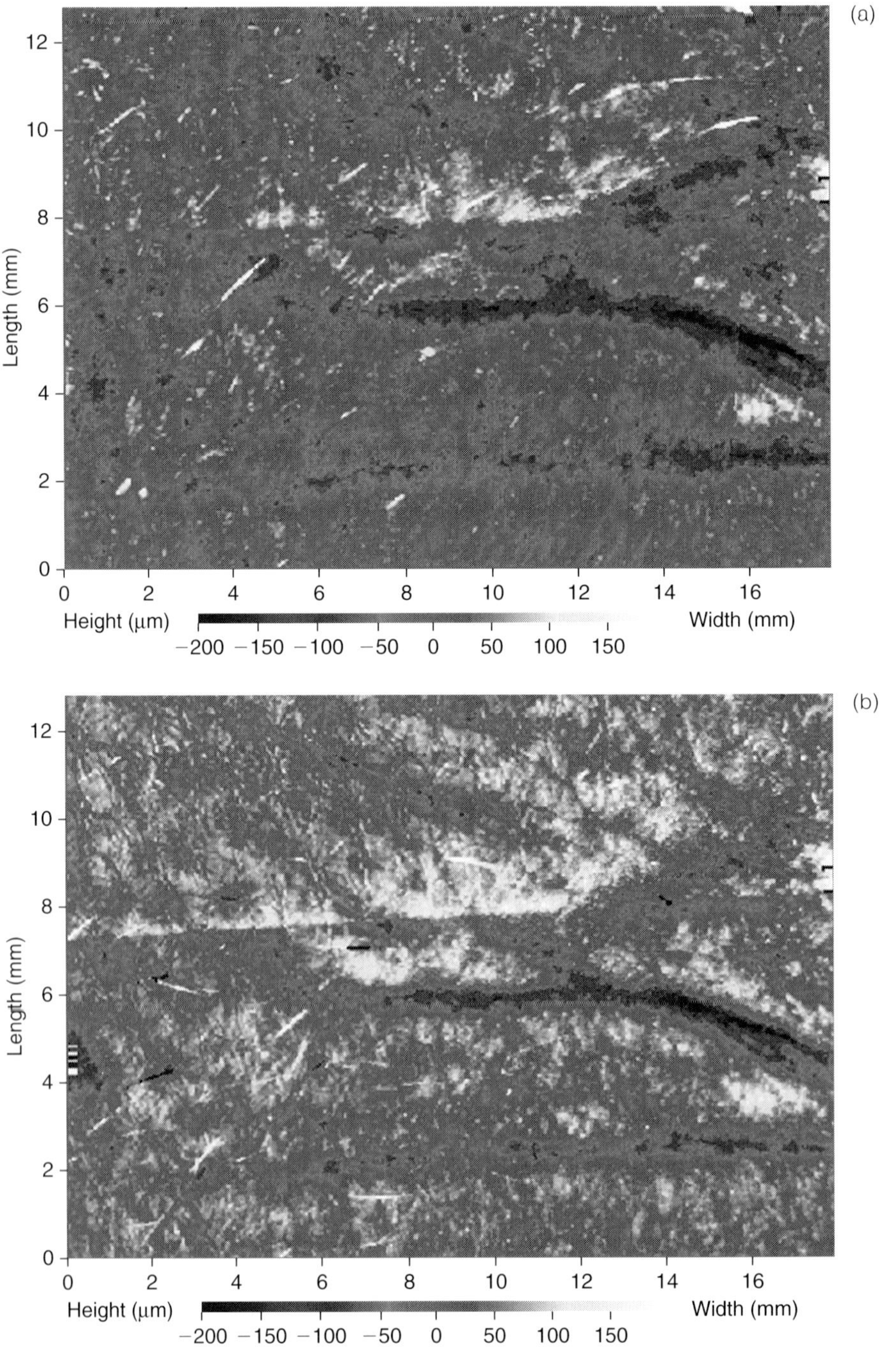

Figure 50.1

Digitized images obtained with PRIMOS®. (a) TO; (b) T2h.

References

1. Makki S, Barbenel JC, Agache P. A quantitative method for the assessment of the microtopography of human skin. Acta Dermatol Venereol 1979; 59:285–91.
2. Corcuff P, Chatenay F, Leveque JL. A fully automated system to study skin surface patterns. Int J Cosm Sci 1984; 6:167–76.
3. Jaspers S, Hopermann H, Sauermann G et al. Rapid in vivo measurement of the topography of human skin by active image triangulation using a digital micromirror device. Skin Res Technol 1999; 5:195–207.
4. Lagarde JM, Rouvrais C, Black D et al. Skin topography measurement by interference fringe projection: a technical validation. Skin Res Technol 2001; 7:112–21.
5. Jaspers S, Bretschneider T, Maerker U et al. Optical topometry with PRIMOS: a powerful tool to prove the efficacy of skin care products in in vivo studies. Proceedings of XXI IFSCC Congress, Berlin 2000:430–4.

51

A new method for contactless in vivo quantitative measurement of stratum corneum gloss attributes: influence of natural active ingredients

V Gillon, G Perie, S Schnebert and G Pauly

Introduction

Background

The gloss appearance of human skin is related to the proportion of the diffuse reflection compared with the specular reflection at the stratum corneum (SC) surface. This specific reflection represents a very slight quantity of light and is mainly influenced by skin roughness and the presence of the hydrolipidic film.

Aim

The aim of our research was to develop a new device for studying complete skin reflection in vivo, in order to evaluate the influence of natural active ingredients on skin complexion.

Principle[1]

According to Fresnel's law about specular-light intensity, the variation of the reflected beam as a function of the angle of incidence is negligible near the normal direction. So, in this condition, it is possible to measure precisely specular reflection.

Because the skin is a very sensitive material, especially concerning its optical properties, it is preferable to evaluate the skin gloss without any contact. A small proportion of the light is reflected at the SC–air interface, due to specular reflectance; this gives a shining skin radiance if well moisturized and tightened.

Materials and methods

Device

As the different apparatus available on the market do not correspond to our needs, we have developed a new device, which is based on an adapted in vivo contactless determination of both specular and diffuse light reflections continuously in numerous directions.

Method[2,3]

An incident polarized light beam is directed at the skin surface to be analysed in one direction, and the reflected beam is simultaneously measured in the same direction.

Specular reflected light, with the same polarization as incident light, is studied, and represents skin shine.

Protocol

Ten healthy female volunteers with dull, rough and dry skin, presenting alteration of cutaneous microrelief on the internal side of the forearms, were recruited and treated twice daily for 3 weeks with two creams: cream containing nacreous components and active ingredients, including VEGESERYL® HGP LS 8572B on one side, and cream containing nacreous components alone on the other side.

Skin optical properties were measured quantitatively by brillanometry after a last standardized application at the end of the 3 weeks of treatment. Skin surface changes have been simultaneously visualized by videomicroscopy.

Results

Brillanometry

After a last standardized application at the end of the 3 weeks of treatment, skin shine was significantly increased with cream containing nacreous components and active ingredients including VEGESERYL® HGP LS 8572B, in comparison with cream containing nacreous components alone (Figure 51.1).

Videomicroscopy

Videomicroscopy results were completely in accordance with those of brillanometry (Figure 51.2).

Tightening and moisturizing active ingredients were in favor of a

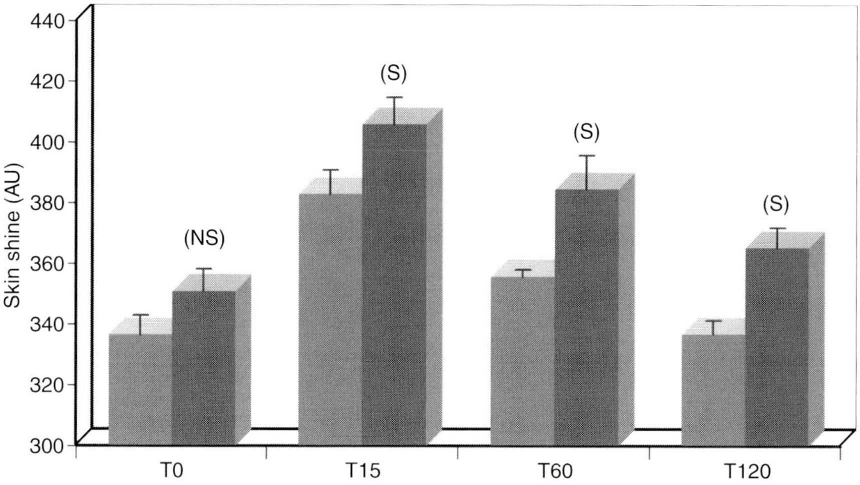

Figure 51.1

In vivo quantification of skin shine by brillanometry. Mean results of 10 volunteers.
■ Cream containing nacreous components alone.
▒ Cream containing nacreous components and active ingredients including VEGESERYL® HGP LS 8572B.
According to Wilcoxon's t-test: (S) significant; (NS) not significant; TSEM 10 volunteers; TO before application; T15, T60, 20: 15, 60, 120 minutes after treatment; AU, arbitrary unit.

microrelief recovery in both directions with more turgescent and larger plates. Under these conditions, efficacy of nacreous components was improved. Skin shine was increased.

Conclusion

A new, contactless device has been built for measuring and studying complete skin reflection in vivo, in order to evaluate the influence of natural active ingredients including vegeseryl® HGP LS 8572B on skin complexion. A combination of active ingredients was added to nacreous components in a cosmetic cream, which was compared with the cream containing nacreous components alone. Quantitative skin shine was significantly increased by the active ingredients, improving skin microrelief with more turgescent and larger plates, and emphasizing the function of nacreous components.

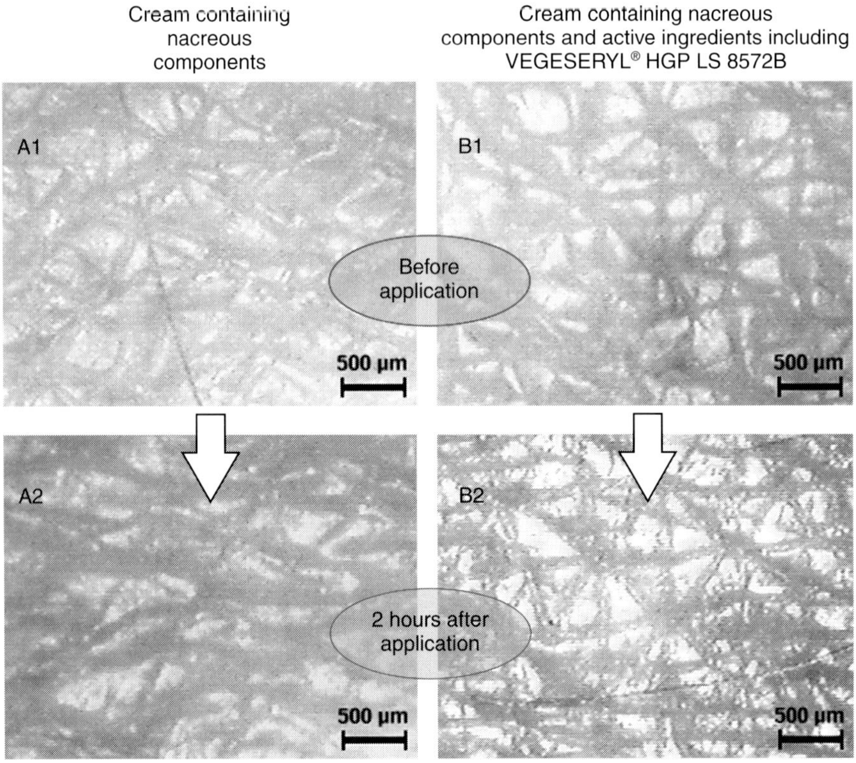

A2/A1: After treatment by cream without tightening and moisturizing active ingredients, destructuring aspect of skin microrelief was observed. Skin remains dull. Efficacy of nacreous components cannot be seen.

B2/B1: After treatment: skin microrelief was well delimited in both directions. Efficacy of nacreous components was largely visible, giving the skin a shining aspect.

Figure 51.2

Visual results by videomicroscopy.

References

1. Smith WJ. *Modern Optical Engineering.* Second edn. New York: McGraw-Hill Inc, 1990.
2. Hundevadt Andersen P. Optical properties of skin. In: Reflectance spectroscopic analysis of selected experimental dermatological models. Skin Res Technol 1997; 3: 8–15.
3. Anderson RR. Polarized light examination and photography of the skin. Arch Dermatol 1991; 127:1000–5.

52
FTIR chemical mapping: a tool for spatially resolved characterization of stratum corneum

P Garidel

Aims

All real-life samples, like tissue samples, are heterogeneous and their chemical composition varies from point to point across the sample. Most methods of analysis either look at one concrete point, or obtain a result that is the average of everything present in the sample. Therefore, the aim of this newly presented technique is the chemical classification and characterization of the distribution of different molecule fractions in the tissue at a spatial resolution of only a few microns. Using this technology, large sample areas can be measured simultaneously, while reducing the acquisition time considerably.

Methods

Fourier transform infrared (FTIR) images were generated from spectra collected on an IRscope II (Bruker) or, alternatively, on a 'Sting-Ray' (BIO-Rad) instrument consisting of a step-scan interferometer coupled to a 64×64 mercury-cadmium-telluride (MCT) focal plane (FP) array detector, which consists of 4096 pixels. The conventional approach for the characterization of a tissue sample would be to acquire sequentially single-point spectra at defined locations from the sample. Focal plane array detector technology performs much like a camera. It uses the multi-channel advantage: instead of one at a time, an array of detectors are working in parallel to produce spectra from different portions of the sample, simultaneously collecting spectra from all the detector pixels. Thus, these IR-microscopes are chemical imaging systems, combining spectroscopy's chemical identification and quantification abilities, with both high spatial resolution (~5 micron) and the power of visualization, in a tool to precisely characterize compositional changes across the sample. This new technique allows us to map a sample area of 400 × 400 micron, generating 4096 spectra, one from each element of the array.

The skin tissue analysed was pig stratum corneum (SC). Using a cryostat, skin sections were frozen and sliced to a thickness of 5 microns. Alternatively, SC was obtained by a biochemical procedure.[1]

Results

We analysed SC and its components by FTIR microscopic imaging.[2] A number of infrared images were generated from these large data sets by measuring and plotting the integrated area of particular spectral components, in each of the 4096 spectra. Figure 52.1 shows a representative FTIR spectrum of SC. The lipid fraction is characterized by the strong asymmetric/symmetric methylene-stretching absorption bands ($\nu(CH_2)$), found between 3000–2800 cm^{-1} and/or carbonyl absorption band (ν (C=O): 1750–1680 cm^{-1}).[3] Characteristic protein bands of the SC are the amide I and amide II bands and $\nu_{as}(CH_3)$ (Figure 52.1).

With this procedure, we can image the distribution of each chemical species through the SC.[2] The spectral intensity is converted in a colour code. Images of SC obtained by using this technique are represented in Figure 52.2. The symmetric and asymmetric methylene-stretching modes

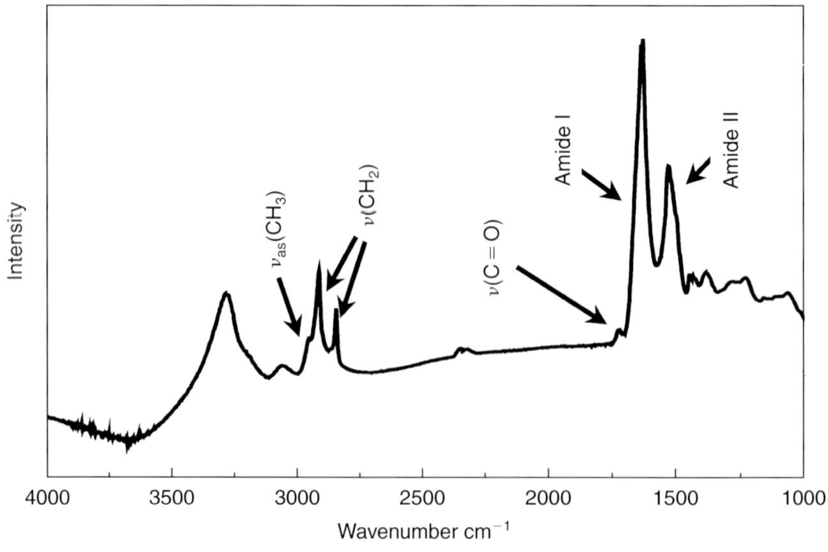

Figure 52.1
FTIR spectrum of stratum corneum (protein and lipid fractions).

are used to map the lipid distribution. The images shown in Figure 52.2b (top) represent the lipid distribution in the tissue. As expected, both images representing the lipid distribution are comparable. Chemical mapping of the proteins is obtained by using the asymmetric methyl and/or amide II mode (Figure 52.2b bottom). The optical micrograph in Figure 52.2a shows a rather homogeneous tissue, whereas FTIR spectrochemical mapping clearly demonstrates that the lipid and protein fractions in the SC are heterogeneously distributed. Large domains of proteins are observed, which are embedded in the surrounding lipid matrix (Figure 52.2b). Comparing the images, mapping the lipid and protein fractions clearly demonstrates that both images representing the lipid and protein distribution are complementary (Figure 52.2b).

Conclusions

FTIR chemical mapping is the generation of a four-dimensional array of data from a sample. Two spatial dimensions (x, y) are obtained and, at every point on the sample, two further dimensions, namely the frequency and the intensity, are obtained.

This method allows us to obtain a realistic molecular difference between protein and lipid areas with an appropriate dimension scale (spatial resolution approaching the IR diffraction limit of ~5 micron). The use of FP-MCT detectors speeds up the data analysis enormously. We look directly at the chemical composition of the molecule fractions, and samples that lack a visible contrast can easily be analysed. It is a non-invasive, non-destructive method. From this study, we can conclude that SC is a rather inhomogeneous tissue, consisting of protein areas embedded in a lamellar lipid matrix.

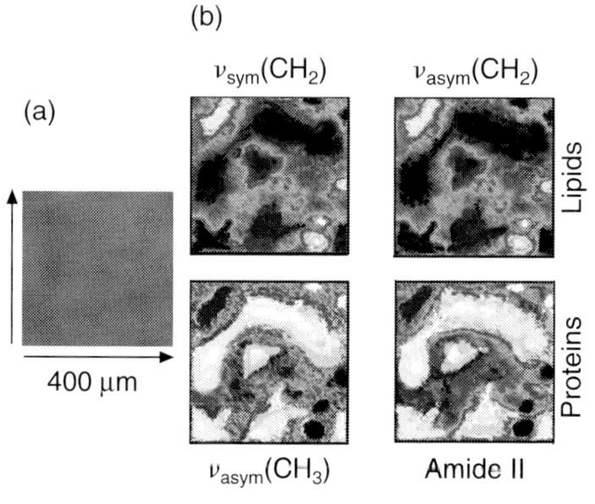

Figure 52.2

(a) Optical micrograph of SC pig skin. (b) IR chemical mapping of the lipid (top) and protein (bottom) fraction. Image size: 400 × 400 μm (white (light): low amount; black (dark): large amount).

Acknowledgements

P Garidel is supported by the Deutsche Forschungsgemeinschaft, which is gratefully acknowledged. R. Mendelsohn and D.J. Moore are acknowledged for introducing me to the field of micro-FTIR technology.

References

1. Goldsmith LA, ed. *Physiology, Biochemistry, and Molecular Biology of the Skin.* 2nd ed. New York and Oxford: Oxford University Press; 1991.
2. Garidel P, Chen HC, Moore DJ et al. Fourier transform infrared microspectroscopic imaging of stratum corneum and its components. Eur Biophys J 2000; 29: 363.
3. Rerek ME, Chen HC, Markovic B et al. Phytosphingosine and sphingosine ceramide headgroup hydrogen bonding: structural insights through thermotropic hydrogen/deuterium exchange. J Phys Chem B 2001; 105:9355–62.

Section IV
Clinical and cosmetic consideration

53
The scale of the problem

R Marks

Introduction

Some 2% of all populations surveyed suffer from psoriasis and even more are affected by an eczematous dermatosis of some sort. These, and several other dermatoses, are marked by scaling of the skin surface, and clearly this physical sign is of major importance in clinical practice. Despite its importance, we know little about its significance, its pathogenesis, its measurement, or its treatment. In what follows, current thinking on these issues will be reviewed.

Pathogenesis

Unlike the scales of fish,[1] in which there is no (or very little) keratinization of any kind, scales in human skin signify abnormal keratinization. Single corneocytes are released imperceptibly from the skin surface in the process of normal desquamation. Any disturbance in the complex process of epidermal differentiation, whether due to an inflammatory process, an inherited metabolic cause or a neoplastic disease process, prevents the final and delicate cleavage of intercorneocyte bonds necessary for desquamation. The net result of this is that corneocytes separate in clumps or lamellae, giving the visual and tactile perception of scaling. The more severe the disease process, thc more pronounced the scaling, although we know very little as to why the appearance of scaling differs in different diseases. In psoriasis, because of the rapid throughput of epidermal cells and the consequent incomplete keratinization, the corneocytes retain in the epidermal nuclei an abnormality known as parakeratosis (Figure 53.1). This differs markedly from the disturbances in the ichthyoses, where the scaling is, for the most part, 'orthokeratotic'. Whether these differences are sufficient to account for all the variations in clinical appearance is not clear. The release of single corneocytes at the skin surface requires the reduction in intercorneocyte-binding forces sufficient to allow the usual, everyday, mechanical stimuli to dislodge the corneocytes from the surface (Figure 53.2). This drop in intercorneocyte

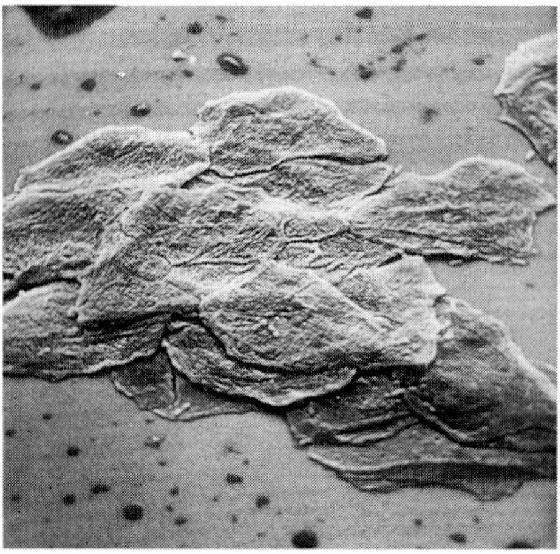

Figure 53.1

Scanning electron micrograph of psoriatic scale showing numerous corneocytes bound together (×500).

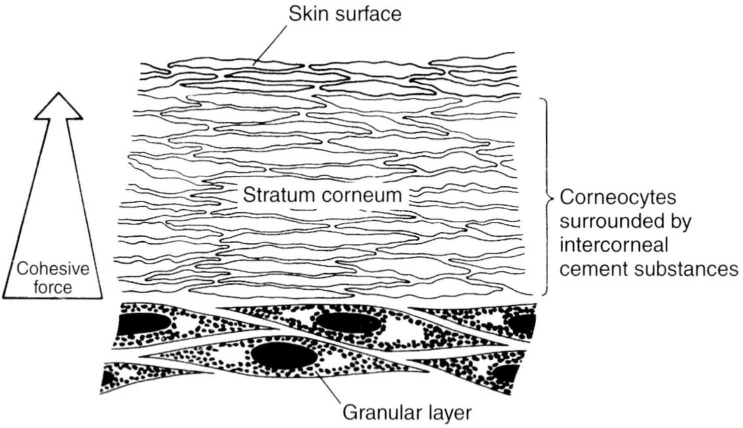

Figure 53.2

Diagram to show reduction of intercorneocyte cohesion towards the surface of the skin.

cohesion (ICC) can be measured using a device termed a cohesograph[2] (Figure 53.3). This instrument has a central piston that possesses a detachable cap, which, in operation, is stuck to the skin surface with a cyanoacrylate adhesive. When the piston is distracted away from the skin, it takes a small segment of stratum corneum (SC) with it – as in the skin-surface biopsy technique.[3] A force transducer measures the force needed to remove the portion of SC. As can be expected, because scaling implies failure in the normal loss of cohesion, all scaling disorders are characterized by an increase in ICC, regardless of the particular pathogenesis. Hydration of the skin surface reduces the tendency of scaling

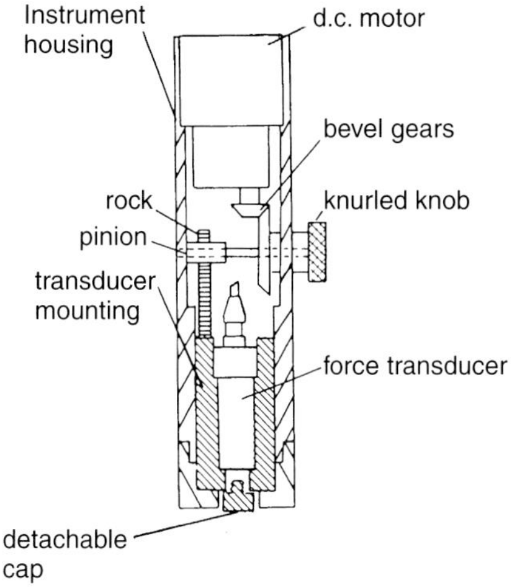

Figure 53.3

Diagram to show main features of cohesograph.

and lowers the ICC. This has enabled us to use the cohesograph as a simple and rapid way to assess the efficacy of moisturizers.

Clinical significance of scaling

The appearance of scaling is inherently unattractive. Somehow, for reasons we do not as yet understand, we are 'hard-wired' to find a scaling skin surface unattractive. Intuitively, we are repulsed by it and avoid contact with affected skin. This societal rejection may be deprecated but it is difficult to do much about. It results in an occupational disadvantage, with eventual economic repercussions. It also causes emotional and interpersonal difficulties, producing social and psychological problems. To add to these little-recognized difficulties experienced by those afflicted by a scaling dermatosis, scaling also results in physical disability. SC affected by scaling doesn't have the excellent extensibility that normal SC possesses and, when an affected part is stretched, painful cracks develop, limiting movement. Involvement of the hands by psoriasis or eczema is the prime example of this problem. Scales also catch on clothes, causing discomfort and annoyance. Scaling and hyperkeratotic areas on the hands prevent fine movement, so that simple manipulations, such as doing up and undoing buttons, become very difficult.

From many points of view, persistent scaling of large areas of skin causes serious disability.

The measurement of scaling

'Why go to the bother of measuring scaling?' is a question sometimes asked. Why go to the bother of using equipment to assess the degree of scaling quantitatively when visual inspection will give 'sufficient information'? The inconvenient truth is that, to assess a patient's progress and to assess the effect of a treatment on a group of patients compared to a similar, untreated (control) group, accurate and reproducible measurement of the degree of scaling is required. In addition, to measure a physical-sign measurement of scaling permits determination of any relationships with other measurable features of a disease, better enabling its characterization. Measurement has become an essential part of modern medicine – unfortunately, as dermatologists, we have been blinded by what we see and have been slow in developing measuring devices.[4] To quote a great dermatological seer "Dermatology won't have arrived till we have a blind dermatologist".

The simplest measuring technique is based on giving numbers to clinical assessments and everyone involved in some way with clinical trials will be familiar with the 0–3 or sometimes 0–4 ordinal scale. The short range of figures to which a scaling skin can be assigned greatly limits the sensitivity of the technique, but, even worse, is the non-equal-interval nature of the scoring system. It is very difficult to rely on such a system or to infer significance from it. Use of a visual analogue scale improves the system somewhat but is still a long way off the ideal.

Adhesive disc methods

The adhesive disc technique in current use is known as the D-Squame disc method. It is simple, convenient, inexpensive, and reliable. Plastic adhesive discs (available commercially as 'D-Squame'®) are applied to the scaling surface to be measured, removed and assessed by comparison with a set of reference diagrams. The latter are a set of discs onto which differing amounts of detachable scale have adhered.[5,6] In order to make the comparison less subjective, the discs may be stained and assessed in a chromameter.

The sticky-disc technique has been used extensively to evaluate dry skin conditions and emollient agents designed for their treatment.[7,8] It is simple and relatively inexpensive. Its disadvantages are that it relies on an arbitrary, short, non-equal internal ordinal scale for the scoring and has a subjective step in the method. Nonetheless, it must be praised as an important step in providing a practical technique for the measurement of scaling.

Profilometric methods for the measurement of scaling

Profilometric methods measure skin surface contour and rely on the fact that a scaling skin surface is more uneven than a normal skin surface and that the degree of unevenness reflects the severity of scaling. The skin surface contour or profile can be measured by taking highly resolved skin-surface replicas and then using a mechanical profilometer, such as the Surfometer® or the Hommeltester®, or by employing an optical technique.

Unfortunately, all methods that depend on taking skin-surface replicas start off with considerable disadvantages. The first of these disadvantages is that applying the silicone elastic material flattens and distorts the scales and, thus, alters what one is trying to measure. One other problem is that the process of making the measurement is cumbersome and time consuming. Yet another potential difficulty is that profilometric scans are linear and in two dimensions, while the skin surface is three-dimensional. However, this latter problem can be surmounted by taking multiple parallel scans. The replicas are taken using a dental-impression material and are, for the most part, too soft for evaluation in a mechanical profilometer. These replicas are 'negative' and hard positive replicas need to be taken from the negatives in order to avoid indentation of the soft negative replica by the diamond stylus of the mechanical profilometer. The profile is measured in units defined by the International Standards Organisation (Table 53.1), but which parameter is chosen for comparison is arbitrary.

Mechanical profilometers have largely been replaced by the laser profilometer, in which the skin surface contour is sensed by a beam of laser light. The contour is tracked by the movement of the unit, holding the laser as the skin surface is kept in focus automatically during scanning over the sample. The excursions of the laser-light housing are an analogue of the skin surface contour; the contour is expressed in the same way as when using the mechanical profilometer, employing the standard roughness parameters.

When a beam of light is shone obliquely on the skin surface, all features and prominences form shadows, the shape and size of which can

Table 53.1 List of symbols and definitions of international surface roughness parameters.

R_a	Arithmetic mean roughness values
R_z (DIN)	Mean peak-to-valley height
R_t	Maximum peak-to-valley height
R_{max}	Maximum individual peak-to-valley height
W_t	Waviness depth
l_{mo}	Measured profile length
N_r	Peak count

be quantified in a number of ways. This principle was used as the basis of a skin-surface assessment technique,[9] in which macrophotographic negatives were scanned by a densitometric device. This scanning macrophotographic and densitometric technique has the advantage of being completely non-invasive but was impractical as a clinical tool because it was a multi-step process and dependent on photographic images. However, television images have also been used instead of photographs and the whole process, including the measurement of the shadowing, can be performed in a one-stage procedure in one 'black box device'.

An image analysis approach to skin-surface assessment has also been adopted by others, but these have also used replicas as the starting point.

In the past few years, a new technology has been developed which relies on analysis of optical fringes. Although such devices are commercially available and have the advantages of being non-invasive and measuring in 'real-time', data on their ability to assess scaling does not appear to be generally available.

Treatment of scaling

Dry, scaly skin is unattractive, itchy and uncomfortable and patients appreciate the simple and effective topical treatments currently available. Emollients are effective in reducing the appearance of scaling within a very short time. These agents flatten out the skin surface contour by hydrating surface horn,[10] but how they reduce scaling is less certain. It may be that the increased water content activates the SC chymotryptic enzyme,[11] which very rapidly cleaves the intercorneocyte desmosomal bonds, so allowing desquamation of single corneocytes. In support of this concept, it is interesting to note that desmosomal connections were retained in mice in dry ambient conditions.[12]

Keratolytics are topical agents that smooth the skin and reduce scaling and hyperkeratosis. They are frequently used for this purpose alone or compounded with other agents. The term 'keratolytic' is curiously inappropriate, as they don't seem to lyse keratin when enhancing desquamation. The traditional and most effective keratolytic available is salicylic acid. Used in a 2–6% concentration in a variety of vehicles, it is regularly successful in reducing scaling and thinning hyperkeratotic patches (Figure 53.4). It also acts as a penetration enhancer, and seems to have a special, and as yet uncharacterized, ability to 'loosen' corneocyte-to-corneocyte bonds. Other agents that have a similar but less predictable effect include the alpha hydroxy acids, such as lactic, glycolic and pyruvic acids. Urea and tretinoin also act as keratolytics. Our understanding of the way these agents work is hopelessly inadequate and, anyway, may

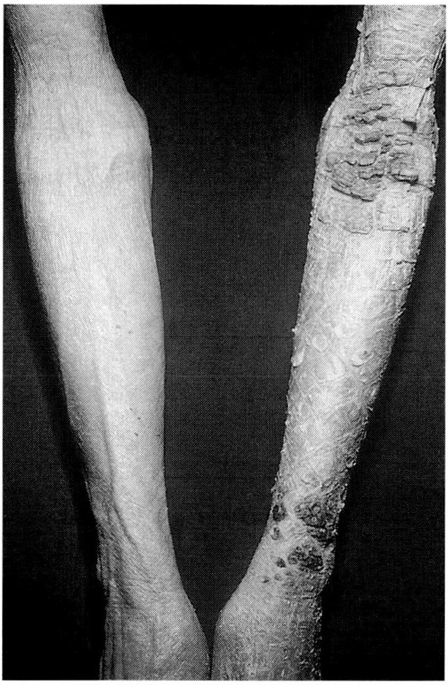

Figure 53.4

This patient has lamellar ichthyosis and has been treated with 6% salicylic acid with white soft paraffin under occlusion on his right arm for one week. The left arm received no treatment during this time.

differ for the different substances. Their actions may also vary with the concentrations employed as, for example, salicylic acid and glycolic acids have a corrosive action at high concentrations.

Conclusion

Scaling is an important clinical sign of disturbed keratinization in many dermatoses. The details of its pathogenesis may vary in the different diseases but the fundamental problem appears to be failure or loss of cohesion between corneocytes at the skin surface so that they separate into clumps. Measurement of the degree of scaling would help in clinical evaluation and in the management of patients. Of the methods available, the simple D-Squame adhesive disc technique is the most practical but newer device-based methods are available. Treatments with emollients and keratolytics are much appreciated and may be effective because they assist in cleavage of intercorneocyte bonds.

References

1. Spearman RIC. The fish integuement. In: *The Integuement: A Textbook of Skin Biology*. Cambridge: Cambridge University Press 1973:59–67.
2. Nicholls S, Marks R. Novel technique for the estimation of intracorneal cohesion in vivo. Br J Dermatol 1977; 96:595–602.
3. Marks R, Dawber RPR. Skin surface biopsy: an improved technique for examination of the horny layer. Br J Dermatol 1971; 84: 117–23.
4. Marks R. Device and rule. Clin and Exp Dermatol 1985; 10: 303–27.
5. Jemec BE, ed. *Non invasive methods and the skin*. CRC Press, 1995:140–51.
6. Schatz H, Kligman A, Mannign S et al. Quantification of dry (xerotic) skin by image analysis of scales removed by adhesive discs (D-squames). J Soc Cos Chem 1993; 44:53–63.
7. El Gammal C, Pagnoni A, Kligman AM et al. A model to assess the efficacy of moisturisers – the quantification of soap induced xerosis by image analysis of adhesive coated discs (D-squames). Clin Exp Dermatol 1996; 21: 338–43.
8. Pierad GE, Pierard-Franchiomon C, Saint-Leger D et al. Squamometry: the assessment of xerosis by colorimetry of D-squame adhesive discs. J Soc Cos Chem 1992; 47: 297–305.
9. Marshall RJ, Marks R. Assessment of skin surface by scanning densitometry of macrophotographs. Clin Exp Dermatol 1983; 8: 121–7.
10. Marks R, ed. *Sophisticated Emollients*. London: Martin Dunitz, 2001.
11. Sondell B, Thornell LE, Egelrud T. Evidence that stratum corneum chymotryptic enzyme is transported to the stratum corneum extracellular space via lamellar bodies. J Invest Dermatol 1995; 104:819–23.
12. Sata J, Denda M, Nakanishi J et al. Cholesterol sulfate inhibits proteases that are involved in desquamation of stratum corneum. J Invest Dermatol 1998; 111:189–93.

54
The interaction of adhesive dressings and stratum corneum

PJ Dykes

Introduction

Removal of adhesive dressings from the skin surface involves two main factors. First, there are the adhesive forces holding the two surfaces together, and, secondly, the cohesive forces within the materials themselves (adhesive or stratum corneum (SC)). A cohesive break in the adhesive will leave adhesive residues on the skin surface. In contrast, a cohesive break in the SC will partially remove SC (skin stripping). The ideal situation is an adhesive break whereby the SC will not be removed and there are no unpleasant adhesive residues left on the skin surface.

One of the dilemmas of wound care is that self-adhesive dressings must stay in place but not damage the surrounding skin on removal. It is well known that, with repeated application and removal of adhesive dressings to the same site, changes in skin barrier function occur.[1] This is followed by a burst of mitosis in the basal epidermal cells (wound-healing response) that is proportional to the extent of the damage.[2–4] Clinically, an inflammatory skin reaction may develop and the management of long-term wound care can be complicated by changes of this nature.

In order to understand the nature of the interaction of adhesive dressings with the skin surface, there is a need for models that simulate clinical usage in a controlled manner. In the studies reported here, we have attempted to (i) measure the amounts of SC removed by different types of adhesive dressings, and (ii) relate the degree of damage caused by adhesive dressings to the forces required for removal.

Methods

Study 1

Study design

The study was an open, within-subject comparison of the effect of

Mepiform® Safetac® soft silicone adhesive dressing (Mölnlycke), Tielle® Hydropolymer Dressing adhesive edge (Johnson & Johnson), and Duoderm® Extra Thin (ConvaTec) on the skin of 12 healthy volunteer subjects (three male and nine female) aged 19–53 years, mean age 35 years. The three adhesive dressings were randomly allocated to three out of four pre-stained test sites (2 × 2 cm) on the flexor aspect of both forearms (four sites per arm), the fourth site on each arm acting as an untreated control. The test materials were removed and discarded after 24 hours. On one arm only, the application and removal were repeated twice more at 24-hour intervals, i.e. three consecutive 24-hour applications.

Staining of the skin surface

The superficial SC in the centre of the test site was stained before application of study materials. A 12-mm aluminium Finn® chamber, containing an 11-mm filter paper disc wetted with 0.03 ml of 1% aqueous methylene blue, was applied to the skin surface for 60 minutes.

Stratum corneum removal and estimation of dye

After application of the test materials, the SC was removed by the skin-surface biopsy procedure.[5] The skin-surface biopsies were extracted with 2 ml dimethyl sulphoxide (DMSO, Analar® grade) and the amount of dye released estimated by measurement of the optical density at a wavelength of 669 nm (peak absorbance).

Statistical analysis

The design of the study was a subject comparison of four treatments and two application schedules. In order to avoid any assumptions about the normality of the data, the analysis used non-parametric procedures. In particular, a multiple comparison procedure, based on the Tukey test, was used. Details of the method can be found in Zar.[6] The data were analysed using UNISTAT® for Windows, version 4.5.

Study 2

Study design

The study was an open, within-subject comparison of the effect of the adhesive edges of Mepilex® Border Safetac® (a self-adherent, soft silicone dressing under development by Mölnlycke), Duoderm® Extra Thin (ConvaTec), Allevyn® Adhesive (Smith & Nephew), Biatain® Adhesive (Coloplast), and Tielle® Hydropolymer Dressing (Johnson & Johnson) on the skin of 20 healthy volunteer subjects (8 male and 12 female) aged 23–64 years, mean age 36 years. The five treatments were randomly allocated to five out of six test sites (3 × 15 cm), previously marked on the back. The sixth site acted as an untreated control site and was covered with non-adherent silicone gauze. All sites were pre-stained with methylene blue. The test materials were removed and discarded after 24 hours. This was repeated twice more at 24-hour intervals, i.e. three consecutive 24-hour applications. The degree of skin-surface damage was assessed by the skin-surface biopsy method.

Peel-force measurement

The test materials were removed under standardized conditions, using a device built by members of the Department of Dermatology, University of Wales College of Medicine, Cardiff (Figure 54.1). The device measures the force required to peel the test materials off the skin surface at an angle of 135° to the skin surface, at a constant speed of 25 mm per second. The steady-state force was measured in mNewtons using a calibrated transducer, the output from which was amplified and recorded using a chart recorder.

Statistical analysis

The mean values for days 2, 3 and 4 were calculated for the steady-state force, and this 3-day mean used for analysis. In order to avoid any assumptions about the normality of the data, subsequent analysis was carried out using the non-parametric multiple comparison procedure, based on the Tukey test.

Results

Study 1

The median absorbance values after one 24-hour application and after three consecutive 24-hour applications are given in Figure 54.2. Sites

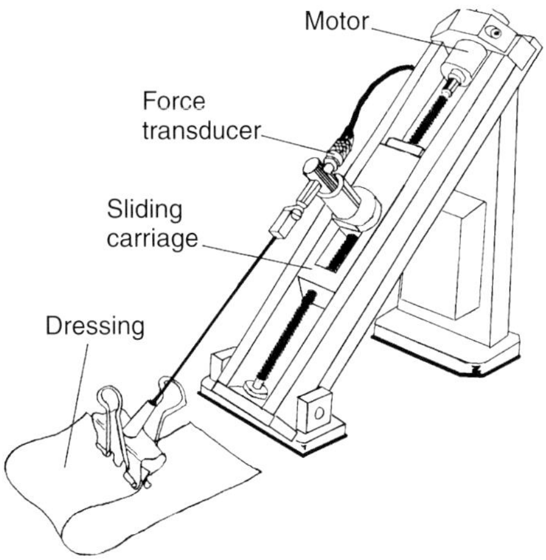

Figure 54.1

Dressing peel-force measurement device.

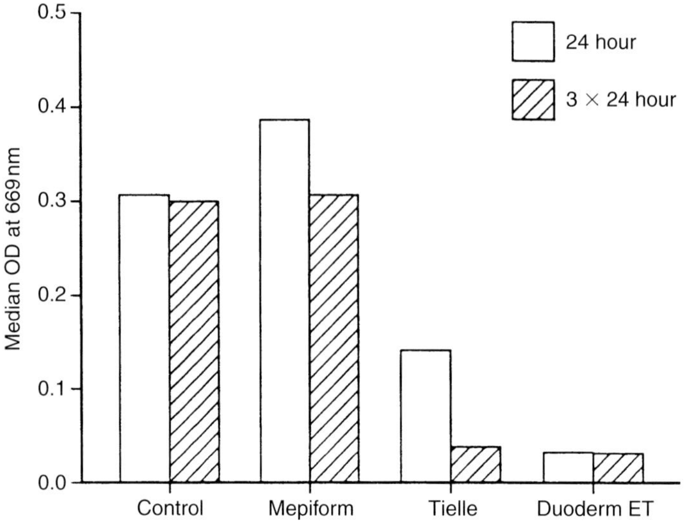

Figure 54.2
Median absorbance values after one 24-hour application and three 24-hour applications.

where Mepiform® Safetac® had been applied showed little SC damage, as indicated by the levels of dye comparable to control values. In contrast, Duoderm®, and, to a lesser extent, Tielle®, showed low levels of dye remaining on the skin surface, indicating removal of greater amounts of superficial SC.

Study 2

The mean steady-state force values (3-day average) are given in Figure 54.3. Statistically significant differences were apparent between some of the products tested, with a rank order from greatest mean force to least mean force as follows: Allevyn Adhesive > Tielle > Duoderm > Mepilex Border Safetac> Biatain Adhesive.

The results of the damage assessment, based on the median absorbance values, indicated that some statistically significant differences were seen with a rank order of most- to least-damaging being: Biatain Adhesive > Duoderm > Allevyn Adhesive > Tielle > Mepilex Border Safetac. When expressed as percentage damage relative to control, a comparison can be made with the steady-state force 3-day mean values (Figure 54.4).

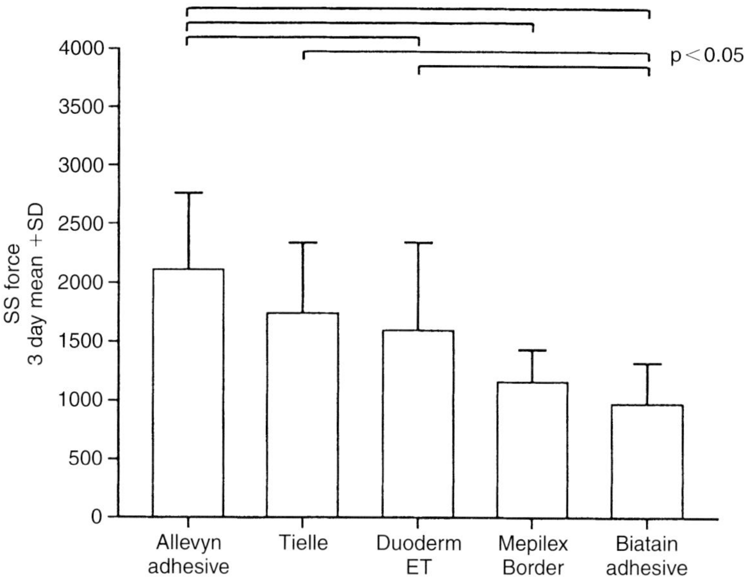

Figure 54.3

Mean steady-state peel force values. Lines indicate statistically significant differences between treatments ($p < 0.05$), according to the multiple comparison procedure (Tukey test).

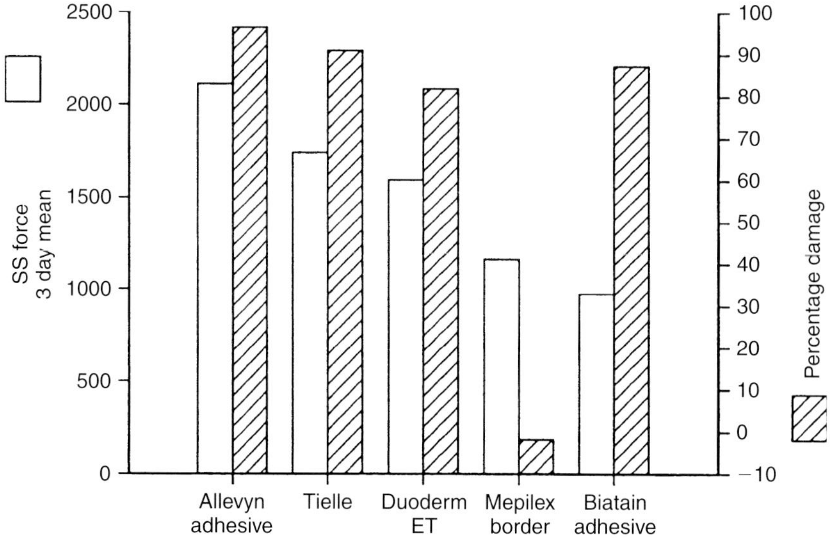

Figure 54.4

Comparison of mean steady-state force with relative damage to control site.

Discussion

The results of Study 1 clearly show statistically significant differences between the adhesive dressings tested, with Mepiform® Safetac® producing less damage to the SC than Tielle® and Duoderm®. These differences may be due to the soft silicone nature of Mepiform® Safetac®. When applied to the skin surface, a more intimate contact with the irregular surface may occur with this product, giving adhesion over a larger surface area. When removed, the peel force is distributed over a larger area, giving reduced damage to the skin surface.

One possible explanation for the differences seen in Study 1 is that the dressings were removed from the skin surface in dissimilar ways. In order to overcome this problem, a device was constructed which removed the dressings in a standardized manner. The results of Study 2 indicate that the device is capable of detecting statistically significant differences between products in terms of steady-state force of removal. Differences in the level of damage to the superficial SC were also detected in this study. However, the relationship between degree of damage and peel force is not clear-cut. For most of the products tested, the percentage damage appears to be related to peel force. Thus, the low peel force of Mepilex® Border Safetac® is associated with a low percentage of damage, and the high peel force of Allevyn® is associated with a high percentage of damage. In contrast, Biatain® Adhesive has a low peel force but a high percentage of damage. Peel force does not, therefore, always correlate with the degree of skin stripping, and other factors must be involved in determining the level of damage to the skin surface.

Choice of wound dressings must take into account many factors, including the patient, the nature of the wound, the frequency of dressing change, and the presence of infection. One problem associated with chronic wound care is the trauma and pain associated with dressing changes that is, in part, due to damage to perilesional skin. This damage is probably linked to the peel force and any skin stripping of the SC which occurs. In the studies reported here, two human models have been developed which quantify the SC removed by different adhesive dressings and measure the peel force of dressing removal. The results presented here are encouraging, and suggest that these models may be useful in helping to develop adhesive dressings that cause minimal trauma to perilesional skin.

Acknowledgements

This study was supported by a grant from Mölnlycke Healthcare AB, Göteborg, Sweden. The data presented in this chapter were published in the Journal of Wound Care, 2001, Volume 10, Number 2.

References

1. Van der Walk PGM, Maibach HI. A functional study of the skin barrier to evaporative water loss by means of repeated cellophane-tape stripping. Clin Exp Dermatol 1990; 15:180–2.
2. Pinkus H. Examination of the epidermis by the strip method. II. Biometric data on regeneration of the human epidermis. J Invest Dermatol 1952; 19:431–46.
3. Hennings H, Elgjo K. Epidermal regeneration after cellophane tape stripping of hairless mouse skin. Cell Tissue Kinetics 1970; 3: 243–7.
4. Komatsu H, Suzuki M. Studies on the regeneration of the skin barrier and the changes in ^{32}P incorporation into the epidermis after stripping. Br J Dermatol 1982; 106: 551–60.
5. Marks R, Dawber RPR. Skin surface biopsy: an improved technique for the examination of the horny layer. Br J Dermatol 1971; 84:117–23.
6. Zar JH. *Biostatistical Analysis*. Second edition. Englewood Cliffs, New Jersey: Prentice-Hall, 1984.

55

Normalization of inflammation and humidity in sodium lauryl sulfate (SLS)-perturbed skin in vivo by gel state phosphatidylcholine

J Gareiss and M Ghyczy

Introduction

Phosphatidylcholine (PC) is the most abundant component of biological membranes. It possesses an intrinsic hydration force, and its metabolites are essential osmoprotectants. PC that is composed of saturated fatty acids (hydrogenated PC), also named gel-state PC or HPC, possesses physical properties that are comparable with those of the components of the skin permeability barrier. When applied to skin, HPC is taken up by the stratum corneum (SC), but it does not cause any irritation. PC, HPC and their metabolites display preventive efficacy in pathological states caused by the redox imbalance and the subsequent formation of free radicals. In the study presented here, HPC increased the humidity of human skin challenged by means of sodium lauryl sulfate (SLS) and ameliorated the inflammatory effects caused by SLS application, but it did not have any effect on transepidermal water loss (TEWL). HPC is an industrially available, easy-to-handle substance, produced according to the GMP standards. These biological effects, together with the above characteristics, suggest the advantages of new topical formulations for the treatment and prevention of frequent skin problems connected with dry skin and the subsequent pathological conditions.

Phosphatidylcholines, bilayers and biological membranes

PC, gel-state PC and ceramides form bilayers functioning as biological barriers which allow the formation of compartments in living organisms. The composition of these bilayers corresponds to the task that the barriers have to perform. The fluid-state membranes of cells and organelles separate aqueous phases and provide means for the generation of chemical and electrical gradients. In the lung, the barrier separates aqueous and gaseous phases, allowing an active gas exchange. In the skin, the bilayers also separate aqueous and gaseous phases, but, in addition, they deal with biological, chemical and mechanical stresses.

These different tasks are reflected in different compositions of the bilayers. The composition changes from fluid-state phospholipids in cell membranes to gel-state PC in the lung, and to the highly crystalline and hydrophobic structure of the skin barrier composed of ceramides, cholesterol and free fatty acids.

Hydrogenated phosphatidylcholine (HPC)

In contrast to fluid-state PC, HPC contains approximately 85% stearic acid and 15% palmitic acid. HPC has a gel-to-liquid transition temperature of 50–55°C, as compared to the 60–63°C of the lipids present in the skin permeability barrier. It possesses thermodynamic properties similar to those of skin ceramides.[1] HPC is well tolerated by skin. In a study on 20 volunteers, the irritation potential of HPC and commercial emulsifiers was compared by quantifying scaling and erythema (Figure 55.1). HPC did not show any irritation potential.[2] A different study on excised skin demonstrated that HPC is taken up by the SC, but does not penetrate to deeper layers.[3] In pharmacy, HPC is used in systemic drug formulations, e.g. to ameliorate the side effects of certain drugs, such as doxorubicin.

Because of these characteristics, HPC is a promising alternative regarding the development of new formulation matrices for topical administration.

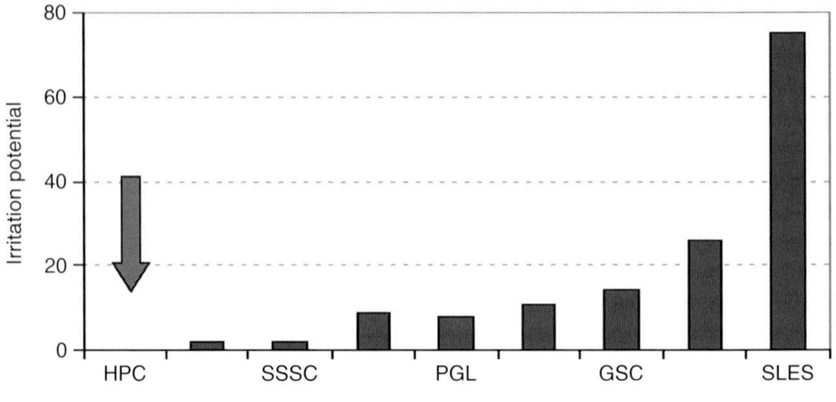

Figure 55.1

Irritation potential of HPC and commercial emulsifiers. SSSC, sorbitan stearate sucrose cocoate; PGL, polyglycerin laurate; GSC, glyceryl stearate citratea; SLES, sodium lauryl ether sulfate.

Aim of the study

The aim of the study was to evaluate the effect of HPC on experimentally caused barrier perturbation and irritation of the skin in vivo. As a means of perturbation, SLS was chosen, as this substance is frequently used and recognized as an experimental model for the identification of protective systems.[4]

Methods

Skin irritation was induced through application of SLS as a 0.01-molar percentage solution on the volar side of the forearm. The volunteers made use of a plastic, foam roller, which was rolled over the skin 50 times, five times per day. The weight of the roller ensured that a specific amount of SLS was applied on the skin surface. 200 μl of a dispersion containing 1% of HPC (Phospholipon® 90 H) were distributed on the skin 30 minutes after the application of SLS. The HPC dispersion was prepared by heating 495 ml of distilled water to 60°C and transferring it to a high-speed mixer. Five grams of HPC were added and the mixture was homogenized at 16000 rpm for 30 minutes. The product was preserved with 0.015% thiomersal and kept at 4°C before use. Skin irritation was measured by Chromameter CR 200, water content in the skin by Corneometer CM 820, and TEWL by Tewameter TM 210. The statistical evaluation was performed by a Wilcoxon pair difference test for combined random samples. The evaluation of the experimental factors took place 12 hours after the last application.[5]

Discussion

HPC formulated in water did not normalize the elevated TEWL (Figure 55.2). This result corresponds to the findings of other laboratories stating that the application of products containing phospholipids[6] or ceramides only[7] would not be sufficient for barrier repair and the ensuing normalization of TEWL in perturbed skin. Somewhat in contrast, the humidity of SC in the challenged skin increased significantly upon the treatment with HPC.

HPC has distinct effects on SLS-perturbed skin with regard to humidity (Figure 55.3) and inflammation (Figure 55.4) in vivo. The first effect can be explained by the intrinsic hydration force of HPC and the osmoprotective properties of its metabolites.[8] The anti-inflammatory effect may be attributed to the preventive efficacy of PC and HPC in redox imbalance conditions in vivo, as reported recently.[9] These findings lead to the conclusion that metabolites of HPC, e.g. betaine, permeate into the part of the dermis where inflammatory processes can be influenced.

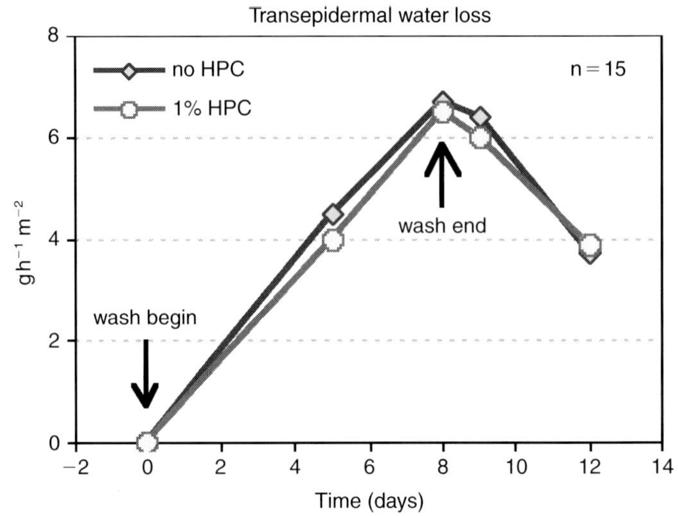

Figure 55.2

Effect of TEWL of human skin in vivo of SLS and SLS plus HPC.

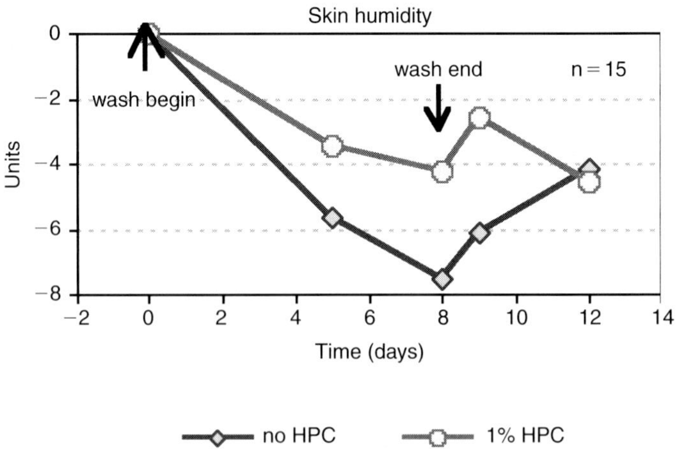

Figure 55.3

Effect of humidity of human skin in vivo of SLS and SLS plus HPC. SKT, - - - .

In earlier studies on human volunteers[10] and animals,[11] it had been reported that the uptake of drugs in the skin was significantly higher if the substances were incorporated in a matrix made of HPC.

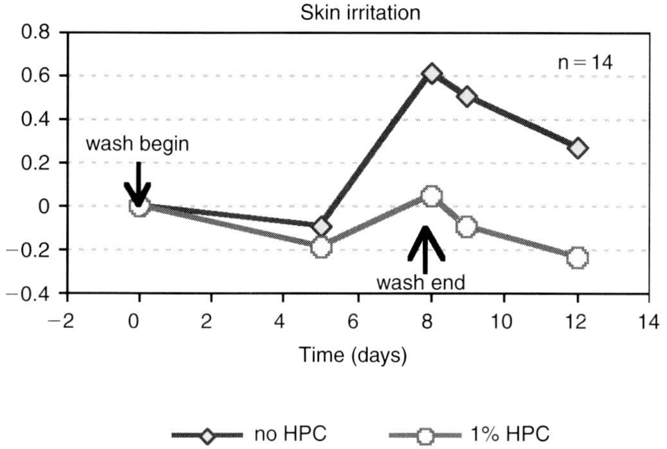

Figure 55.4

Effect on irritation of human skin in vivo of SLS and SLS plus HPC.

Conclusion

Resulting from our own investigations and the findings made by others, we conclude that HPC is an appropriate matrix-forming agent for the topical administration of drugs and cosmetic actives, thereby providing the benefits of:

1. being well tolerated by the skin;
2. normalizing intracellular humidity in the SC;
3. ameliorating inflammatory processes in the skin;
4. forming an adequate permeability barrier matrix in which drugs, lipids and water can be embedded;
5. forming a depot for active substances in the SC followed by an enhanced uptake in deeper layers of the skin.

References

1. Pechtold LA, Abraham W, Potts RO. Characterisation of the stratum corneum lipid matrix using fluorescence spectroscopy. J Invest Dermatol Symp Proc 1998; 3: 105–9.
2. Kutz G, Biehl P, Waldmann-Laue M et al. Zur Auswahl von O/W-Emulgatoren für den Einsatz in Hautpflegeprodukten bei sensibler Haut. SÖFW-Journal 1997; 123: 145–9.
3. Fahr A, Schäfer U, Verma DD et al. Skin penetration enhancement of substances by a novel type of liposome. SÖFW-Journal 2000; 126:49–53.

4. Fartasch M. Ultrastructure of the epidermal barrier after irritation. Microsc Res Tech 1997; 37:193–9.
5. Gehring W, Gloor M, Kleesz P. Predictive washing test for evaluation of individual eczema risk. Contact Dermatitis 1998; 39:8–13.
6. Summers RS, Summers B, Chandar P et al. The effect of lipids, with and without humectant, on skin xerosis. J Soc Cosmet Chem 1996; 47:27–39.
7. Man MQ, Feingold KR, Elias PM. Exogenous lipids influence permeability barrier recovery in acetone-treated murine skin. Arch Dermatol 1993; 129:728–38.
8. Haussinger D. Osmoregulation of liver cell function: signalling, osmolytes and cell heterogeneity. In: Lang F (ed). Cell Volume Regulation. Basel: Karger, 1998: 185–204.
9. Ghyczy M, Boros M. Electrophilic methyl groups present in the diet ameliorate pathological states induced by reductive and oxidative stress: a hypothesis. Br J Nutr 2001; 85:409–14.
10. Foldvari M, Gesztes A, Mezei M et al. Topical liposomal local anesthetics: design, optimization and evaluation of formulations. Drug Dev Indust Pharm 1993; 19: 2499–517.
11. Mezei M, Gulasekharam Y. Liposomes – a selective drug delivery system for the topical route of administration: gel dosage form. J Pharm Pharmacol 1982; 34:473–4.

56

Dandruff is characterized by decreased levels of intercellular lipids in scalp stratum corneum

CR Harding, A Moore, JS Rogers, H Meldrum, A Scott and F McGlone

Introduction

Dandruff, a common scaling disorder of the scalp, is classically associated with the presence of the lipophilic yeast *Malassezia*.[1] However, the observation that this microorganism is also present on healthy scalps suggests that some additional factors are critical for the manifestation of the dandruff lesion. The marked skin scaling observed in this condition indicates that one or more of the processes of stratum corneum (SC) maturation and desquamation is impaired.[2,3] In this study, we have investigated whether an altered level and composition of the intercellular barrier lipids, frequently perturbed in other skin-scaling disorders, e.g. winter xerosis and psoriasis,[4,5] is a characteristic of the dandruff condition.

Methods

Study design

Males and females, aged 20–40 years, were recruited into each study. In the Thai studies, the same subjects were used wherever possible. Scalps were classified as either normal and healthy or as having dandruff, and dandruff severity was scored according to a standard internal protocol. All subjects were placed on a non anti-dandruff shampoo regime for 3 weeks. No hair washing was allowed 48 hours prior to sampling.

Scalp stratum corneum collection and lipid analysis

Exposed scalp sites were swabbed briefly with isopropyl alcohol to remove surface sebum. Sites were sequentially tape-stripped eight times using adhesive tapes, and SC lipids recovered, analysed and quantified.[6]

Assessment of topical response to histamine application

The response to the topical application of a 1% histamine solution was used as an indirect measure of barrier functionality in Thai subjects (n = 220). Subject response was assessed, both qualitatively (using a visual analogue scale assessing the subjective intensity of the itch response), and quantitatively (blood-flow measurement using laser Doppler).

Results

A dramatic decrease in total lipid levels, associated with significant decreases in total ceramides and cholesterol levels, was a characteristic finding in dandruff sufferers in both Caucasian and Thai subjects (Figure 56.1). Triglyceride levels, reflecting sebaceous activity, were also consistently decreased in dandruff. No consistent changes in ceramide subspecies or covalently bound lipid species were observed (data not shown).

Following histamine application, the incidence of hyper-response (i.e. increased blood flow or incidence of reported itch) was highest in individuals with recognizable dandruff (Figure 56.2). The relationship between laser-Doppler measurement and scalp severity score was highly significant ($p < 0.001$, χ^2 (chi-square) = 30.5, Mantel–Haenszel test).

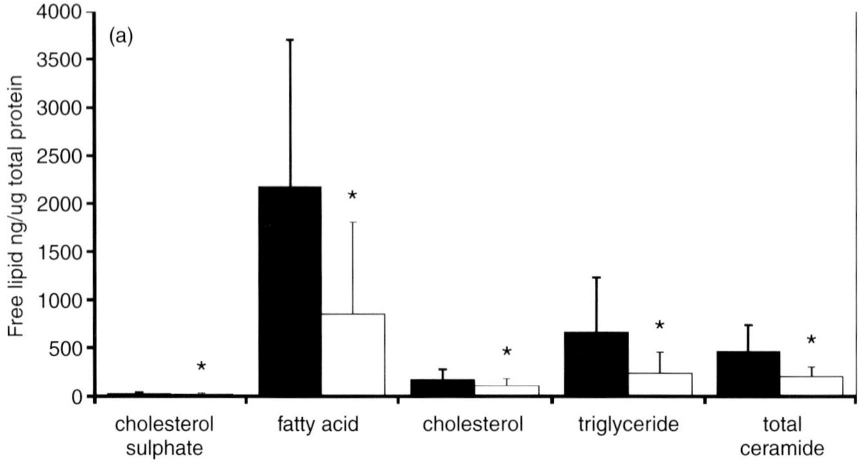

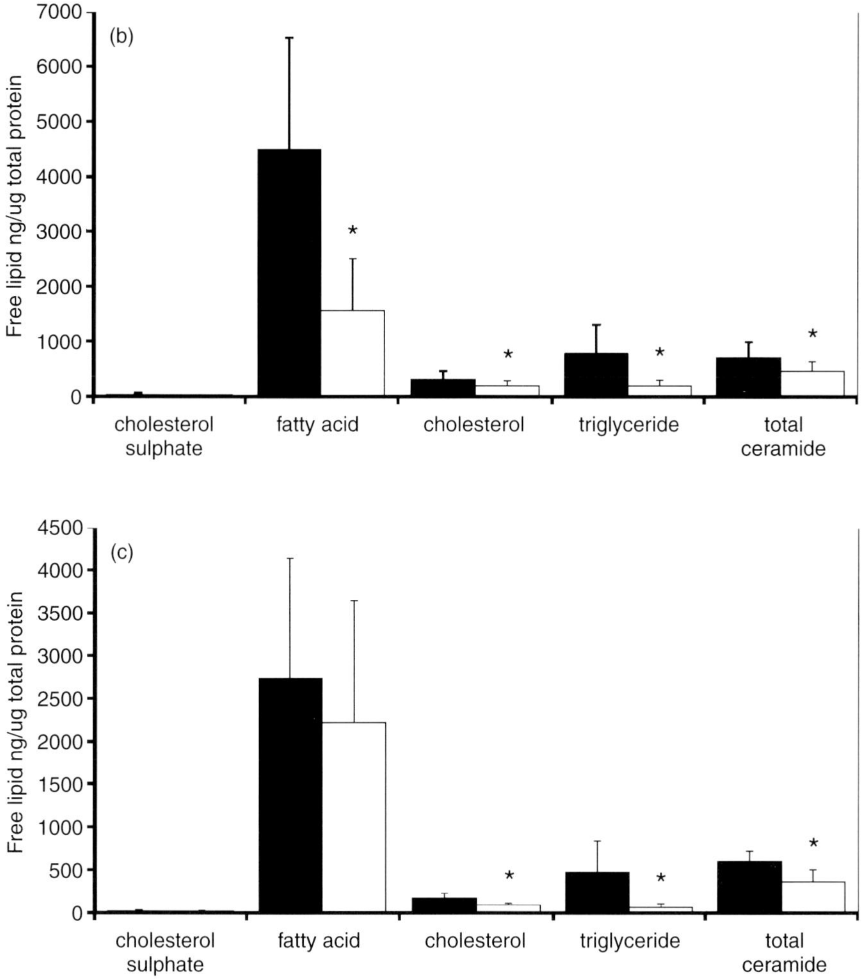

Figure 56.1

Dandruff sufferers have lower levels of free SC lipids. Amounts of cholesterol sulphate, total ceramides, free fatty acids, cholesterol and triglycerides were assayed in tape strips from subjects. Lipids were quantified using a scanning densitometer and were compared to known standards. Asterisk signifies significant difference $p < 0.05$ (Student t-test). (a) Healthy (n = 17, ■) and dandruff (n = 24, □) UK subjects. (b) Healthy (n = 11, ■) and dandruff (n = 20, □) Thai subjects (dry season). (c) Healthy (n = 11, ■) and dandruff (n = 20, □) Thai subjects (humid season).

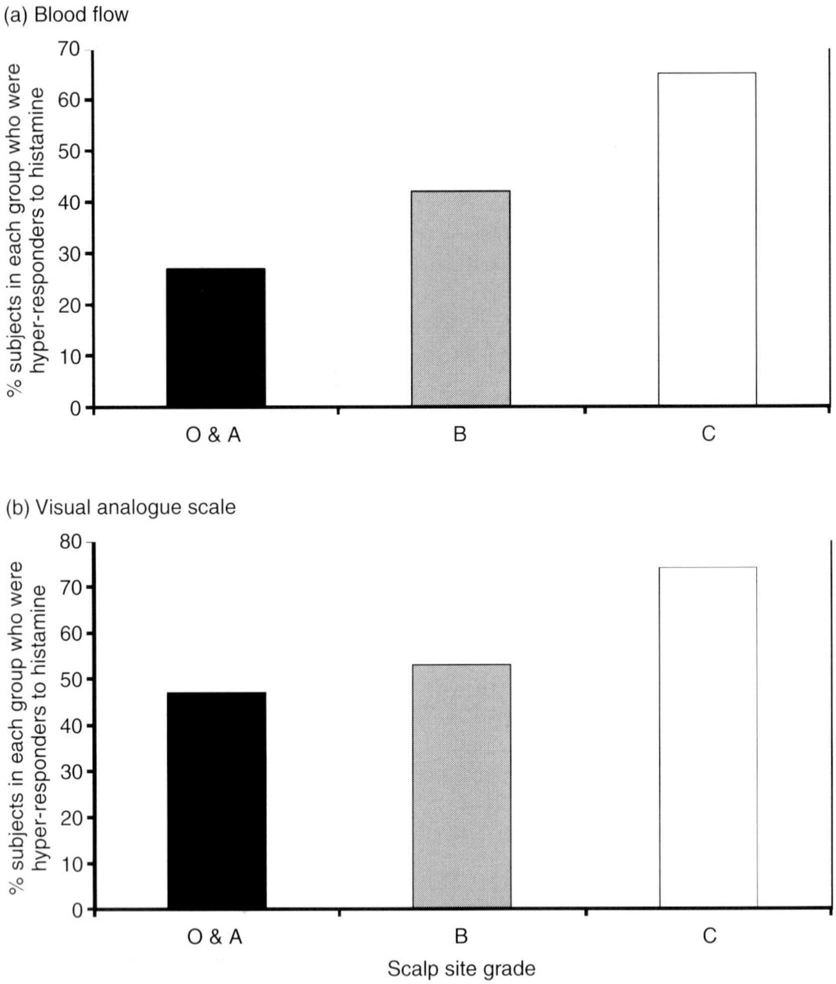

Figure 56.2

Changes in the response to topical histamine application in subjects with dandruff. (a) Objective response (increased blood flow) and (b) subjective response (reported itch) to topically applied histamine measured in subjects with healthy and dandruff scalps. Scalp site grading – O: healthy scalp with no dryness or dandruff; A: fine dryness on scalp surface; B: small powdery flakes partially adhered to scalp; C: moderately flaky scales loosely attached to scalp.

Discussion

The SC, regardless of anatomical site, acts as a primary defence mechanism against environmental stresses. These studies have demonstrated that, in dandruff sufferers, the intercellular lipid content of scalp SC is significantly reduced compared to healthy subjects. This depletion is associated with reduced barrier function, which may leave dandruff sufferers more prone to the adverse, irritant effects of microbial metabolites, surfactants or pollutants present on the scalp surface.

The decreased lipid levels may reflect an impairment of the underlying epidermal differentiation process as a result of irritation induced by *Malassezia*-derived toxins. Alternatively, the reduced levels of SC lipids may reflect a predisposing characteristic of a given individual, i.e. people susceptible to dandruff *inherently* have low SC lipid levels, and a permeability barrier which is readily prone to damage.

We consider it likely that both the intrinsic quality of the SC and the presence of *Malassezia* contribute to the incidence and severity of dandruff. The relative contribution of these two factors towards the manifestation and persistence of this disorder remains to be determined.

References

1. Schuster S. The aetiology of dandruff and the mode of action of therapeutic agents. Br J Dermatol 1984; 111:235–42.
2. Ackerman AB, Kligman AM. Some observations on dandruff. J Soc Cosmet Chem 1964; 20:81–101.
3. Harding CR, Watkinson A, Rawlings AV et al. Dry skin, moisturisation and corneodesmolysis. Int J Cosmet Sci 2000; 22:21–52.
4. Williams ML. Lipids in normal and pathological desquamation. In: Elias PM, ed. *Advances in Lipid Research*. Vol. 24. San Diego: Academic Press, 1991:211–26.
5. Rawlings AV, Hope J, Rogers JS et al. Abnormalities in stratum corneum structure, lipid composition and desmosomal degradation in soap-induced winter xerosis. J Soc Cosmet Chem 1994; 45: 203–20.
6. Rogers JS, Harding CR, Mayo AM et al. Stratum corneum lipids: the effect of ageing and the seasons. Arch Dermatol Res 1996; 288: 765–70.

57

Beneficial corneotherapeutic effects of skin-tolerance-tested moisturizing creams

K De Paepe, J-P Hachem, E Vanpee, D Roseeuw and V Rogiers

Introduction

In the present work, an oil-in-water (o/w) moisturizing cream was applied to experimentally elicited, scaly skin in order to investigate whether the product could promote a more rapid recovery of the disturbed barrier function (as measured by transepidermal water loss (TEWL) measurements) than physiological barrier repair. Experimental models of both irritant (ICD) and allergic (ACD) contact dermatitis were applied. ICD was provoked by sodium lauryl sulfate (SLS), well known for its damaging action on the skin barrier function.[1] The ACD study concerned a nickel-mediated contact allergy patch (CAP) test, carried out in nickel-sensitized volunteers.[2]

Materials and methods

ICD protocol

Baseline measurements (Tewameter TM210®, Courage+Khazaka electronic GmbH) on volar forearm skin ($t_1 = 0$) of twelve female volunteers (mean age 23 ± 3, range 20–29 years) were carried out on three well-defined sites of 2×4 cm. ICD by 24-hour patch test (∅ 20 mm, pore size 200 µm, Sartorius®) with 160 µl of 1.25% (w/v) SLS aqueous solution (Sigma, 99% purity) on two contra-lateral test sites. Application was under occlusion (Dermalock® HDP Medical) and fixed by self-adhesive Fixomull® stretch (Beiersdorf). A test site, covered with a 'blank' patch of 160 µl of water, served as undamaged, control skin. Assessment of SLS irritation was 24 hours after air exposure ($t_2 = 0$).

ACD protocol

ACD on twelve female volunteers (mean age 31 ± 6, range 21–40 years) was provoked by Ni-CAP tests for 48 hours (large Finn Chambers®, ∅20 mm, Epitest) with 0.3 ml of 5% $NiSO_4$ in petrolatum on two contralateral test sites. A third test area contained 150 µl of NaCl (0.9%) and served as undamaged control skin. Assessment of ACD was 24 hours after air exposure (day 1).

Test product

A previously skin-tolerance-tested o/w cream (0.03 ml), which contained 9% glycerin and 4% evening primrose oil (*Oenothera biennis*), was uniformly spread twice daily with an interval of 12 hours for 14 days (ICD protocol) or 4 days (ACD protocol) on one of the damaged skin areas.[3]

Results and discussion

The effect of the cream on ICD in comparison with physiological barrier repair is shown in Figure 57.1. Decreases in TEWL were statistically significant on days 3, 8 and 15. Repeated application of the cream supported the ICD to complete recovery on day 15.

As shown in Figure 57.2, cream application significantly improved the barrier function of ACD on day 5, on which the recorded TEWL values were no longer significantly different from the baseline values. In contrast, values of the untreated ACD skin site remained elevated during the assessment period of 5 days.

In both experimental models, consecutive application of the cream supported barrier recovery before normal physiological barrier repair was

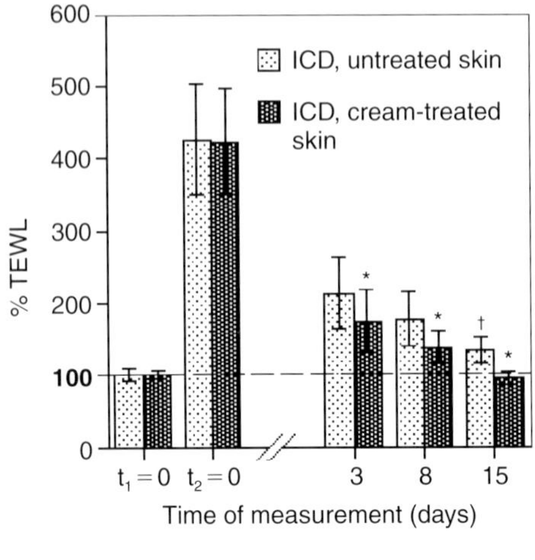

Figure 57.1

Mean values ± SD (n = 12), expressed as a percentage of the TEWL values measured on undamaged, control skin, arbitrarily set at 100% (dashed line). * ($p < 0.01$) significant differences between treated and untreated skin sites; † ($p < 0.01$) significantly different results from values obtained before SLS irritation (Wilcoxon signed-rank test).

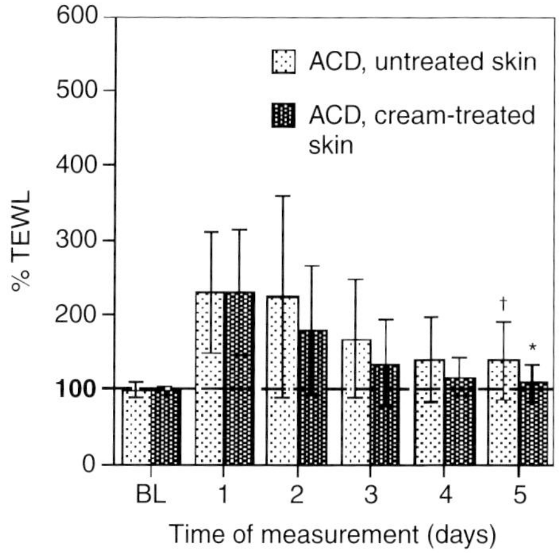

Figure 57.2

Mean values ± SD (n = 12), expressed as a percentage of the TEWL values measured on undamaged, control skin, arbitrarily set at 100% (dashed line). * ($p < 0.05$) statistical difference between treated and untreated skin sites; † ($p < 0.05$) significantly different results from baseline (BL) values (Wilcoxon signed-rank test).0

completed. Due to the hydrating components and the barrier-restoring properties of the lipid phase, well-formulated moisturizing creams can be used to improve subclinical barrier alterations and are substantial adjuvants for corneotherapy.

References

1. Di Nardo A, Sugino K, Wertz PW et al. Sodium lauryl sulfate (SLS) induced irritant contact dermatitis: a correlation study between ceramides and in vivo parameters of irritation. Contact Dermatitis 1996; 35:86–91.
2. Hachem JP, De Paepe K, Vanpee E et al. Combination therapy improves the recovery of the skin barrier function: an experimental model using a contact allergy patch test combined with TEWL measurements. Dermatology 2001; 202:314–19.
3. De Paepe K, Hachem JP, Vanpee E et al. Beneficial effects of a skin tolerance-tested moisturising cream on the barrier function in experimentally-elicited irritant and allergic contact dermatitis. Contact Dermatitis 2001; 44:337–43.

58
How cosmetics interact with the stratum corneum

C Leclerc, F Fouchard, M-P Verdier, C Hadjur, G Madry, G Daty, D Pele, J-C Garson, C Baltenneck, J Leclaire and F Benech-Kieffer

Aims

Skin-care products improve skin condition with an increasing involvement of physiologically active ingredients. Nevertheless, the contribution of other components, globally viewed as the 'vehicle', may be important and has often been observed in clinical studies performed versus 'placebo'.

The aim of this work was to describe the influence of the vehicle on cutaneous physiology and especially on skin barrier function. A selection of cosmetic vehicles corresponding to different physicochemical systems have been chosen: water-in-oil (W/O) and oil-in-water (O/W) emulsions, nanoemulsion, dispersed systems (e.g. nanocapsules and niosomes). They correspond to skin-care products whose clinical and sensorial qualities are highly appreciated.

Methods

The gradual behaviour of the tested vehicles following in vitro application on skin has been evaluated by measuring kinetics of evaporation of volatile phase and by investigating organized structures formed on isolated stratum corneum (SC) surface using X-ray diffraction.

In parallel, using the same method, interaction with intercellular lipids was studied.

The influence of vehicle on cutaneous permeability of a tracer (^{14}C caffeine) was measured.

Finally, its ability to diffuse into the viable epidermis has been indirectly evaluated on human skin ex vivo by following a fluorescent tracer using confocal laser microscopy and optic fluorescent microscopy.

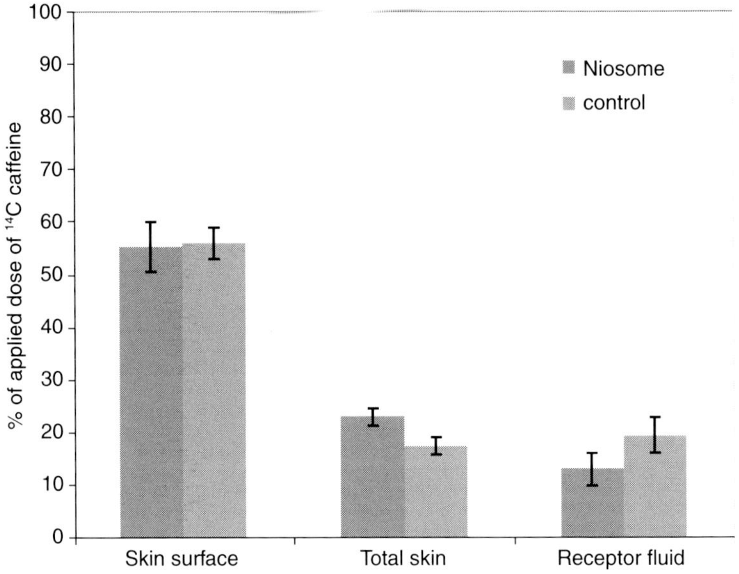

100
90
80
70
60
50
40
30
20
10
0
% of applied dose of ^{14}C caffeine
Niosome
control
Skin surface
Total skin
Receptor fluid

(a)

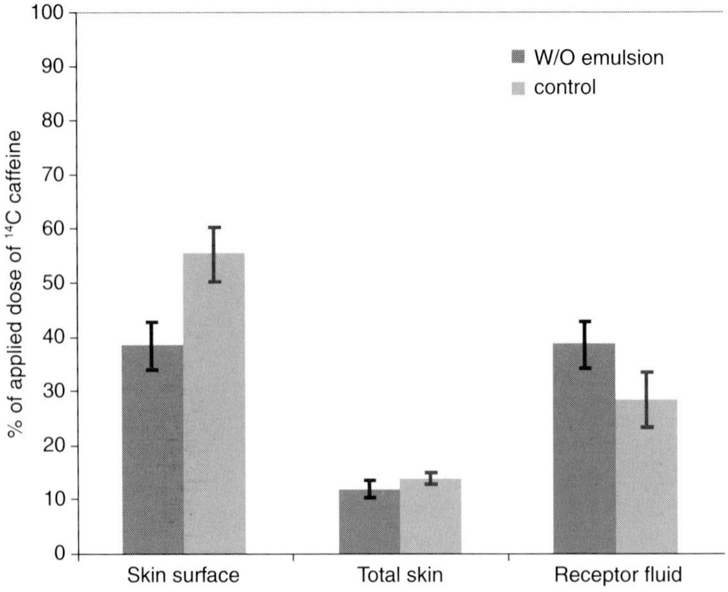

100
90
80
70
60
50
40
30
20
10
0
% of applied dose of ^{14}C caffeine
W/O emulsion
control
Skin surface
Total skin
Receptor fluid

(b)

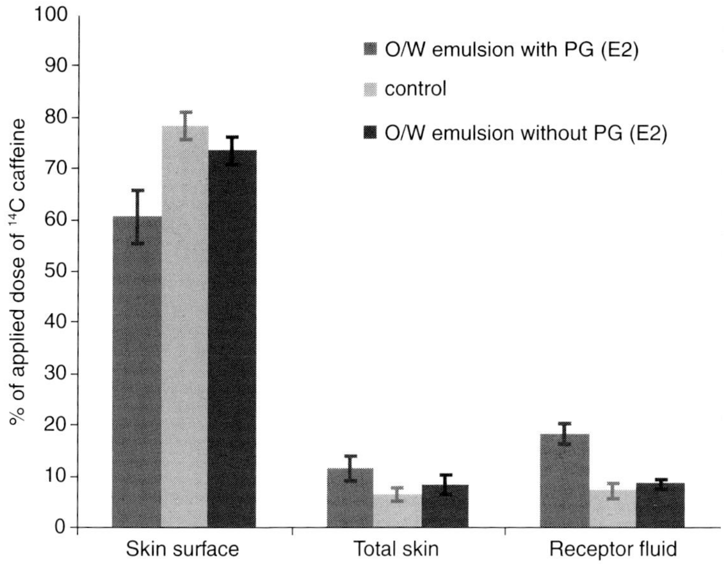

(c)

Figure 58.1

Cutaneous distribution of [^{14}C]caffeine after pre-treatment with (a) niosomes, (b) W/O emulsion, (c) O/W emulsion with and without propylene glycol (PG).

Discussion

Data analysis ranked the vehicles into three groups according to their ability to influence skin barrier function through different mechanisms (Figure 58.1).

No influence on skin barrier function

Niosomes did not influence [^{14}C]caffeine diffusion but improved Nile Red absorption. This vehicle interacted with bilayer lipids with respect to structural characteristics of endogenous lipids. This would confirm the properties of this kind of system to mimic endogenous lipids, maintaining skin barrier function.

Influence by occlusion

W/O emulsion enhanced [^{14}C]caffeine diffusion, probably by the mechanism of occlusion. No interaction with endogenous lipids or diffusion of the fluorescent marker in the SC itself were detected. The kinetic of evaporation of the volatile phase showed no release of water from the vehicle.

Influence by modifying endogenous bilayers lipids

The nanocapsule vehicle enhanced [^{14}C]caffeine diffusion, which could be explained by a swelling of bilayer lipids. Its capacity to deliver Nile Red through the SC confirmed its affinity for SC.

Nanoemulsion interacted with endogenous lipids. Nile Red did not diffuse through SC, whereas [^{14}C]caffeine diffusion was enhanced after the pre-treatment. It seems necessary to measure lipid fluidity to confirm the hypothesis of enhancement of skin diffusion by modifying intercellular lipids.

The O/W emulsion containing propylene glycol interacted with endogenous lipids and also introduced new organized structures into the SC.[1,2] Nevertheless, we confirmed that PG was responsible for the enhancement of [^{14}C]caffeine diffusion by comparison with results obtained with the same emulsion without PG.

Conclusion

We showed that the modifications of skin barrier function may be different according to formulation properties and probably vehicle composition. Further experiments are necessary to understand the mechanism of these modifications and to identify the contribution of some raw materials. Finally, biological responses to these skin modifications should be researched in order to describe better the biological role of these cosmetic vehicles.

Acknowledgements

This work has been performed with cosmetic vehicles supplied by the Research Laboratories at Chevilly Larue. We are particularly grateful to J-T Simonnet, R Lorant and P Delambre.

References

1. Bodde HE, Ponec M, Ijzerman AP et al. In vitro analysis of QSAR in wanted and unwanted effects of azacycloheptanones as transdermal penetration enhancers. Drugs Pharm Sci 1993; 59:99–214.
2. Bouwstra JA, De Vries MA, Goories GS et al. Thermodynamic and structural aspects of the skin barrier. J Control Release 1991; 15:209–20.

59
Strategies to maintain physiological skin moisture

W Baschong

The stratum corneum (SC) forms a water-impermeable barrier between body and environment. It regulates the evaporation of water from the deeper layers (where it amounts to about 70% weight) and impedes the penetration of environmental hazards. Changes in the balance (homeostasis) between supply and loss of water in the SC has an immediate impact on the aspect of the skin. (Figure 59.1).

Water (10–15%) is critical for barrier function. The latter is determined by i) the organization of the lipid bilayers between the corneocytes, ii) the presence of water-retaining factors, i.e. the natural moisturizing factors (NMF), and iii) the flux of water to, and the evaporation from, the SC.

Prevention of evaporation (transepidermal water loss, TEWL) in a dry environment (dry air, cold, wind, etc.) by occlusive formulations

An occlusive layer, such as petrolatum, prevents the skin from losing water when exposed to a dry environment. Prolonged use may downregulate keratinocyte maturation and segregation of NMF and lipids, and eventually deplete barrier constituents and dry out the skin.

Reconstitution of skin moisture in stressed or dry skin

Regular maintenance of skin moisture

Skincare products for daily use (shower gels, body lotions, etc.) usually contain moisturizers. If their use is discontinued and replaced by washing with ordinary soap only, skin moisture may gradually drop and equilibrate at lower, non-physiological levels (Figure 59.2, no moisturizers).

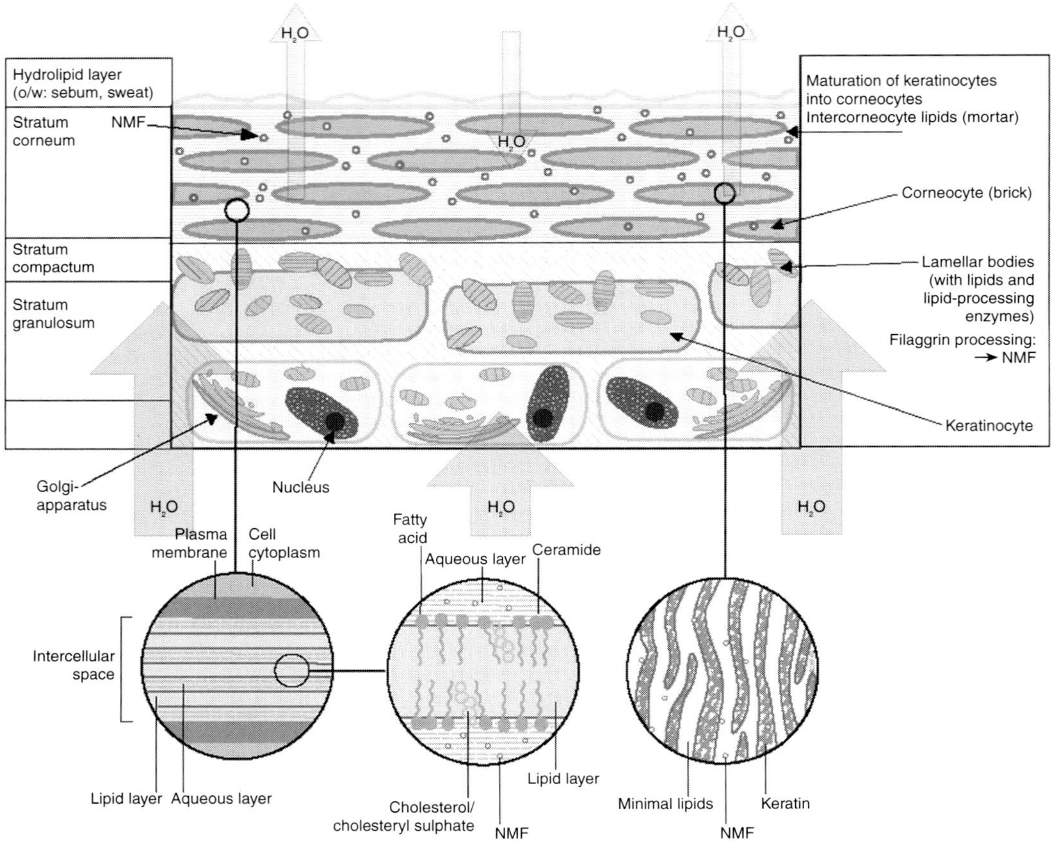

Figure 59.1

Water exchange in the human epidermis (modified brick mortar model).

Reconstitution of skin moisture by formulations containing hygroscopic molecules

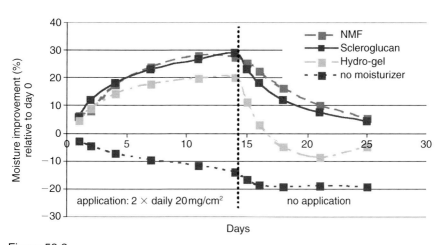

Supplementation of water to the SC by hygroscopic compounds (humectants) such as poly-alcohols (e.g. glycerol, sorbitol, etc.) immediately enhances skin moisture (Figure 59.2, conventional Hydro-gel: water, sodium-carbomer, parabenes, PEG-150, glycerol). Humectants act by stabilizing the water in a formulation during absorption. Eventually, associated water molecules may deposit in the intercorneocyte space and in the corneocytes. Upon discontinuation, hygroscopic molecules still present may desiccate skin, at least temporarily (Figure 59.2, Hydro-Gel), by interfering with intrinsic supplementation of barrier lipids and NMF, and by depleting water from the SC.

Reconstitution of skin moisture by neutral, high-molecular-weight, water-binding polymers

Neutral, high-molecular-weight, water-binding polymers form a layer that decreases water evaporation and enhances SC moisture, and allows for recovery of impaired SC barrier function. Regular application of a natural, triple-helical polysaccharide (0.1% scleroglucan, molecular weight: 5000 KDa: Tinocare™ GL 1% scleroglucan solution from CibaSC) improved skin moisture by about 30%. After discontinuation, skin

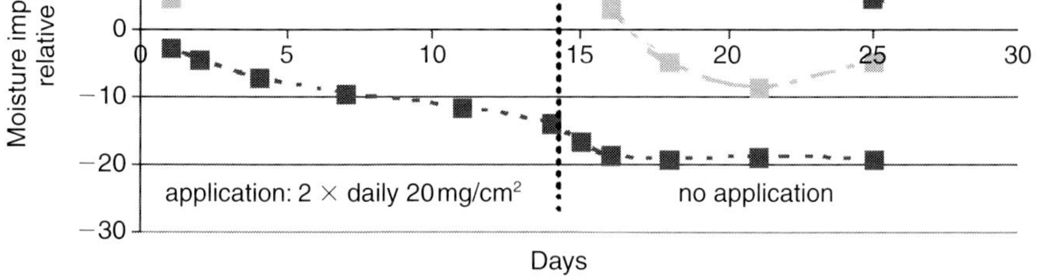

Figure 59.2

Hydro-gel, Scleroglucan and NMF were applied at 20 mg/cm^2 twice daily for 2 weeks (23 applications) to randomly assigned areas (three treated, one non-treated) on the inner forearm of 20 volunteers, who were regular users of skincare products, and had abstained from application for a week prior to treatment. Skin moisture was registered with a Corneometer (Courage & Kazaka; Köln, Germany) on days 0, 1, 2, 4, 7, 11, 14, 15, 16, 18, 21 and 25, and always 12 hours after the last application. Registration was continued after treatment to document the persistence of the moisturizing effect.

moisture decreased only gradually and to a level higher than prior to treatment (Figure 59.2, Scleroglucan).

Reconstitution of skin moisture by supplying natural moisturizing factors (NMF)

The SC contains a mixture of water-storing breakdown products, such as amino-acids (mainly serine, alanine and citrulline), pyrrolidone carboxylic acid (PCA), urea, lactate, glucuronic acid, salts, etc., which are formed and released during keratinocyte maturation and by sweat glands. Consequently, at low NMF, the concentration barrier function is impaired, and supplementing NMF may normalize SC function. 2.5% NMF-liposomes (containing 7% (w/w) encapsulated L-Serine, L-Glycine and L-Alanine: Tinoderm™ NMF from CibaSC) increased skin moisture by up to 30%. After stopping the treatment, moisture remained above the initial level.

Reconstitution of barrier function by supplementing barrier lipids

A complex mixture of phospholipids, cholesterol, neutral lipids and sphingolipids regulates the barrier function. Supplementation of appropriate mixtures, but rarely of single components, may induce functional restoration. Since composition of the barrier lipids varies with skin type, sex, age, and with the skin's pathological condition, choosing the proper mixtures for lipid supplementation is an important task.

60
Seasonal changes in skin biophysical properties in healthy Caucasian women

I Le Fur, F Morizot, S Lopez, C Guinot, J Latreille and E Tschachler

Introduction

The human skin surface has to adapt constantly to changing environmental conditions, such as temperature and relative humidity. Several studies have demonstrated the detrimental effects of winter weather in our countries on the skin[1,2] and seasonal changes in certain biophysical parameters.[3] The work presented here examines seasonal variations of biophysical parameters on facial skin in Caucasian women in France.

Materials and methods

Two similar studies were performed during wintertime and summertime on 123 healthy Caucasian women, aged 20–80 years (mean age ± SD: 49 ± 17).

Registered averaged climatic conditions were mean outside temperature and relative humidity (RH) (data obtained from METEO France, Centre of Paris-Montsouris):

- 6 ± 4°C and 82 ± 8% RH (winter study);
- 21 ± 4°C and 50 ± 13% RH (summer study).

The biophysical properties of the skin, evaluated on the cheeks in a controlled environment (temperature: 21 ± 2°C, RH: 50 ± 5%) after the volunteer had a 30-minute rest period in the laboratory, included:

- capacitance (Corneometer® CM820, Courage and Khazaka Electronic GmbH, Köln, Germany);
- conductance (Skicon®, IBS, Hamamatsu-shi, Japan);
- skin surface temperature (Differential thermometer PT200 from IMPO Electronics);

- skin surface pH (pHmeter®, Courage and Khazaka);
- sebum casual level (Sebumeter® SM810 PC, Courage and Khazaka).

For each biophysical parameter, the study of any 'seasonal' effect was performed using paired Student's t-test.

Results

	Winter Mean ± SD	Summer Mean ± SD	p
Capacitance (μS)	82.0 ± 7.1	81.2 ± 8.2	NS
Conductance (a.u.)	107.6 ± 77.0	115.7 ± 102.8	NS
TEWL ($g/m^2.h$)	11.7 ± 3.5	9.5 ± 2.7	< 0.0001
pH	5.3 ± 0.5	5.0 ± 0.5	< 0.0001
Temperature (°C)	32.9 ± 0.8	32.9 ± 0.7	NS
Sebum casual level (μg/cm^2)	55.2 ± 45.0	57.6 ± 53.8	NS

Discussion/conclusion

These results demonstrate seasonal variations of skin basal values of some biophysical parameters, with an increase of TEWL during wintertime, associated with an increase in skin surface pH. In contrast, these changes were not found to be associated with a decrease in parameters reflecting stratum corneum hydration.

No difference between seasons was observed for sebum, which is in contradiction with previous data demonstrating an increase in sebum related to higher skin temperature found during summertime.[4]

This increase of TEWL during wintertime was associated with low outside mean temperature and high relative humidity, suggesting that inside environmental conditions with high temperature and low humidity (not monitored during our study) may represent important contributing factors in changes of skin barrier function during wintertime.

References

1. Agner T, Serup J. Seasonal variation of skin resistance to irritants. Br J Dermatol 1989; 121:323–8.
2. Uter W, Gefeller O, Schwanitz HJ. An epidemiological study of the influence of season (cold and dry air) on the occurrence of irritant skin changes of the hands. Br J Dermatol 1998; 138:266–72.
3. Black D, Del Pozo A, Lagarde JM et al. Seasonal variability in the biophysical properties of stratum

corneum from different anatomical sites. Skin Res Technol 2000; 6:70–6.

4. Piérard-Franchimont C, Piérard GE, Kligman A. Seasonal modulation of sebum excretion. Dermatologica 1990; 181:21–2.

Index

Note: Page references followed by '**f**' represent a figure and '**t**' represent a table.